Pre-operative Management of the Patient with Chronic Disease

Editors

ANSGAR M. BRAMBRINK
PETER ROCK
JEFFREY R. KIRSCH

MEDICAL CLINICS
OF NORTH AMERICA

www.medical.theclinics.com

Consulting Editors
DOUGLAS S. PAAUW
EDWARD R. BOLLARD

November 2013 • Volume 97 • Number 6

ELSEVIER

1600 John F. Kennedy Boulevard • Suite 1800 • Philadelphia, Pennsylvania, 19103-2899

http://www.theclinics.com

MEDICAL CLINICS OF NORTH AMERICA Volume 97, Number 6
November 2013 ISSN 0025-7125, ISBN-13: 978-0-323-24229-5

Editor: Jessica McCool

Medical Clinics of North America (ISSN 0025-7125) is published bimonthly by Elsevier Inc., 360 Park Avenue South, New York, NY 10010-1710. Months of publication are January, March, May, July, September, and November. Business and editorial offices: 1600 John F. Kennedy Boulevard, Suite 1800, Philadelphia, PA 19103-2899. Periodicals postage paid at New York, NY, and additional mailing offices. Subscription prices are USD $255.00 per year (US individuals), $471.00 per year (US institutions), $125.00 per year (US Students), $320.00 per year (Canadian individuals), $612.00 per year (Canadian institutions), $200.00 per year (Canadian and foreign students), $390.00 per year (foreign individuals), and $612.00 per year (foreign institutions). To receive student/resident rate, orders must be accompanied by name of affiliated institution, date of term, and the signature of program/residency coordinator on institution letterhead. Orders will be billed at individual rate until proof of status is received. Foreign air speed delivery is included in all Clinics' subscription prices. All prices are subject to change without notice. **POSTMASTER:** Send address changes to *Medical Clinics of North America*, Elsevier Health Sciences Division, Subscription Customer Service, 3251 Riverport Lane, Maryland Heights, MO 63043. **Customer Service: Telephone: 1-800-654-2452** (U.S. and Canada); **1-314-447-8871** (outside U.S. and Canada). **Fax: 314-447-8029. E-mail: journalscustomerserviceusa@elsevier.com** (for print support); **journalsonlinesupport-usa@elsevier.com** (for online support).

Reprints. For copies of 100 or more of articles in this publication, please contact the Commercial Reprints Department, Elsevier Inc., 360 Park Avenue South, New York, NY 10010-1710. Tel.: 212-633-3874; Fax: 212-633-3820; E-mail: reprints@elsevier.com.

Medical Clinics of North America is also published in Spanish by McGraw-Hill Interamericana Editores S. A., P.O. Box 5-237, 06500 Mexico, D.F., Mexico.

Medical Clinics of North America is covered in *MEDLINE/PubMed (Index Medicus), Current Contents, ASCA, Excerpta Medica, Science Citation Index,* and *ISI/BIOMED.*

Printed and bound by CPI Group (UK) Ltd, Croydon, CR0 4YY

Transferred to digital print 2012

PROGRAM OBJECTIVE
The goal of the *Medical Clinics of North America* is to keep practicing physicians up to date with current clinical practice by providing timely articles reviewing the state of the art in patient care.

TARGET AUDIENCE
All practicing physicians and other healthcare professionals.

LEARNING OBJECTIVES
Upon completion of this activity, participants will be able to:
1. Review preoperative evaluation and management of patients with neuromuscular disorder, vascular disease, chronic pulmonary disease, endocrine disease, and chronic kidney disease.
2. Discuss perioperative nutritional support.
3. Recognize ischemic heart disease.

ACCREDITATION
The Elsevier Office of Continuing Medical Education (EOCME) is accredited by the Accreditation Council for Continuing Medical Education (ACCME) to provide continuing medical education for physicians.

The EOCME designates this enduring material for a maximum of 15 *AMA PRA Category 1 Credit*(s)™. Physicians should claim only the credit commensurate with the extent of their participation in the activity.

All other health care professionals requesting continuing education credit for this enduring material will be issued a certificate of participation.

DISCLOSURE OF CONFLICTS OF INTEREST
The EOCME assesses conflict of interest with its instructors, faculty, planners, and other individuals who are in a position to control the content of CME activities. All relevant conflicts of interest that are identified are thoroughly vetted by EOCME for fair balance, scientific objectivity, and patient care recommendations. EOCME is committed to providing its learners with CME activities that promote improvements or quality in healthcare and not a specific proprietary business or a commercial interest.

The planning committee, staff, authors and editors listed below have identified no financial relationships or relationships to products or devices they or their spouse/life partner have with commercial interest related to the content of this CME activity:
Brian Barrick, DDS, MD; Jeffrey Berman, MD; Santha Priya Boorasamy; Grace Chen, MD; Thomas G. Deloughery, MD; Samuel M. Galvagno, Jr, DO, PhD; Alina M. Grigore, MD, MHS; Alicia Gruber Kalamas, MD; Michael J. Hannaman, MD; Jessica McCool; Caron M. Hong, MD, MSc; Brynne Hunter; Jeffrey R. Kirsch, MD; Dawn Larson, MD; Sandy Lavery; Marc A. Levitt; Ann-Marie Manley, MD; Robert G. Martindale, MD, PhD; Douglas G. Martz Jr, MD; Jill McNair; Claus U. Niemann, MD; Mary Josephine Njoku, MD; Patrick Odonkor, MB, ChB; Andrea Orfanakis, MD; Lindsay Parnell; William Rayburn; Sarah E. Reck, MD; Peter N. Rock, MD, MBA, FCCM; Marc A. Rozner, PhD, MD; Joseph Salama-Hanna, MBBS; Joshua Sappenfield, MD; Valerie Sera, MD; Palak Turakhia, MD, MPH; David Zvara, MD.

The planning committee, staff, authors and editors listed below have identified financial relationships or relationships to products or devices they or their spouse/life partner have with commercial interest related to the content of this CME activity:
Ansgar M. Brambrink, MD, PhD is a co-investigator on an investigator-initiated multi-center study evaluating videolaryngoscopes in the situation of a difficult airway.
T. Miko Enomoto, MD has a research grant with Actelion Pharmaceuticals, Inc.
Peter Schulman, MD has a research grant from Boston Scientific.
Eric Stecker, MD, MPH has a research grant from Boston Scientific and Biotronik.

UNAPPROVED/OFF-LABEL USE DISCLOSURE
The EOCME requires CME faculty to disclose to the participants:
1. When products or procedures being discussed are off-label, unlabelled, experimental, and/or investigational (not US Food and Drug Administration (FDA) approved); and
2. Any limitations on the information presented, such as data that are preliminary or that represent ongoing research, interim analyses, and/or unsupported opinions. Faculty may discuss information about pharmaceutical agents that is outside of FDA-approved labelling. This information is intended solely for CME and is not intended to promote off-label use of these medications. If you have any questions, contact the medical affairs department of the manufacturer for the most recent prescribing information.

TO ENROLL

To enroll in the *Medical Clinics of North America* Continuing Medical Education program, call customer service at 1-800-654-2452 or sign up online at http://www.theclinics.com/home/cme. The CME program is available to subscribers for an additional annual fee of USD $267.

METHOD OF PARTICIPATION

In order to claim credit, participants must complete the following:

1. Complete enrolment as indicated above.
2. Read the activity.
3. Complete the CME Test and Evaluation. Participants must achieve a score of 70% on the test. All CME Tests and Evaluations must be completed online.

CME INQUIRIES/SPECIAL NEEDS

For all CME inquiries or special needs, please contact elsevierCME@elsevier.com.

MEDICAL CLINICS OF NORTH AMERICA

RELATED INTEREST

Anesthesiology Clinics, Volume 30, Issue 3 (September 2012)
Postanesthesia Care Unit
Scott A. Falk, MD, *Editor*

**DOWNLOAD
Free App!**

Review Articles
THE CLINICS

NOW AVAILABLE FOR YOUR iPhone and iPad

Contributors

CONSULTING EDITORS

DOUGLAS S. PAAUW, MD, MACP
Professor of Medicine, Division of General Internal Medicine, Rathmann Family Foundation Endowed Chair for Patient-Centered Clinical Education; Medicine Student Programs, Professor of Medicine, University of Washington School of Medicine, Seattle, Washington

EDWARD R. BOLLARD, MD, DDS, FACP
Professor of Medicine, Associate Dean of Graduate Medical Education, Designated Institutional Official, Department of Medicine, Penn State-Hershey Medical Center/Penn State University College of Medicine, Hershey, Pennsylvania

EDITORS

ANSGAR M. BRAMBRINK, MD, PhD
Professor, Department of Anesthesiology and Perioperative Medicine, Oregon Health and Science University, Portland, Oregon

PETER ROCK, MD, MBA, FCCM
Martin Helrich Professor and Chair, Department of Anesthesiology, University of Maryland School of Medicine, Baltimore, Maryland

JEFFREY R. KIRSCH, MD
Professor and Chair, Department of Anesthesiology and Perioperative Medicine, Oregon Health and Science University, Portland, Oregon

AUTHORS

BRIAN BARRICK, DDS, MD
Associate Professor, Anesthesiology, UNC Hospitals, University of North Carolina, Chapel Hill, North Carolina

JEFFEY BERMAN, MD
Professor, Anesthesiology, UNC Hospitals, University of North Carolina, Chapel Hill, North Carolina

GRACE CHEN, MD
Assistant Professor, Department of Anesthesiology and Perioperative Medicine, Oregon Health and Science University, Portland, Oregon

THOMAS DELOUGHERY, MD
Department of Medicine, Division of Hematology/Oncology, Oregon Health and Science University, Portland, Oregon

T. MIKO ENOMOTO, MD
Assistant Professor, Department of Anesthesiology and Perioperative Medicine, Oregon Health and Science University, Portland, Oregon

MELISSA J. ERTL, MD
Fellow, Department of Anesthesiology, University of Wisconsin School of Medicine and Public Health, Madison, Wisconsin

SAMUEL M. GALVAGNO Jr, DO, PhD
Assistant Professor, Department of Anesthesiology, Shock Trauma Center, University of Maryland School of Medicine, Baltimore, Maryland

ALINA M. GRIGORE, MD, MHS, FASE
Associate Professor, Department of Anesthesiology, University of Maryland School of Medicine, Baltimore, Maryland

MICHAEL J. HANNAMAN, MD
Assistant Professor, Department of Anesthesiology, University of Wisconsin School of Medicine and Public Health, Madison, Wisconsin

CARON M. HONG, MD, MSc
Assistant Professor, Department of Anesthesiology, University of Maryland School of Medicine, Baltimore, Maryland

ALICIA GRUBER KALAMAS, MD
Department of Anesthesia and Perioperative Care, University of California, San Francisco, San Francisco, California

DAWN LARSON, MD
Assistant Professor, Department of Anesthesiology and Perioperative Medicine, Oregon Health and Science University, Portland, Oregon

ANN-MARIE MANLEY, MD
Assistant Professor, Department of Anesthesiology, Medical College of Wisconsin, Froedtert Memorial Lutheran Hospital, Milwaukee, Wisconsin

ROBERT G. MARTINDALE, MD, PhD
Professor, Department of Surgery, Oregon Health and Science University, Portland, Oregon

DOUGLAS G. MARTZ Jr, MD
Associate Professor of Anesthesiology, University of Maryland School of Medicine, University of Maryland Medical Center, Baltimore, Maryland

CLAUS U. NIEMANN, MD
Department of Anesthesia and Perioperative Care; Department of Surgery, Division of Transplantation, University of California, San Francisco, San Francisco, California

MARY JOSEPHINE NJOKU, MD
Associate Professor, Department of Anesthesiology, University of Maryland School of Medicine, University of Maryland Hospital, Baltimore, Maryland

PATRICK N. ODONKOR, MB, ChB
Assistant Professor, Department of Anesthesiology, University of Maryland School of Medicine, Baltimore, Maryland

ANDREA ORFANAKIS, MD
Assistant Professor, Department of Anesthesiology and Perioperative Medicine, Oregon Health and Science University, Portland, Oregon

SARAH E. RECK, MD
Assistant Professor, Department of Anesthesiology, Medical College of Wisconsin, Froedtert Memorial Lutheran Hospital, Milwaukee, Wisconsin

MARC A. ROZNER, PhD, MD
Professor of Anesthesiology and Perioperative Medicine, Professor of Cardiology, University of Texas MD Anderson Cancer Center, Houston, Texas

JOSEPH SALAMA-HANNA, MBBS
Department of Anesthesiology and Perioperative Medicine, Henry Ford Hospital, Detroit, Michigan

JOSHUA W. SAPPENFIELD, MD
Department of Anesthesiology, University of Maryland School of Medicine, University of Maryland Medical Center, Baltimore, Maryland

PETER M. SCHULMAN, MD
Assistant Professor, Department of Anesthesiology and Perioperative Medicine, Oregon Health and Science University, Portland, Oregon

VALERIE SERA, MD
Clinical Associate Professor, Department of Anesthesiology and Perioperative Medicine, Oregon Health and Science University, Portland, Oregon

ERIC C. STECKER, MD, MPH
Assistant Professor, Knight Cardiovascular Institute, Oregon Health and Science University, Portland, Oregon

PALAK TURAKHIA, MD, MPH
Assistant Professor, Anesthesiology, UNC Hospitals, University of North Carolina, Chapel Hill, North Carolina

Contents

Society. Even clinicians who are not CIED experts should understand the indications for implantation, as well as the basic functions, operations, and limitations of these devices. Before any scheduled procedure, proper CIED function should be verified and a specific CIED prescription obtained. Acquiring the requisite knowledge base and developing the systems to competently manage the CIED patient ensures safe and efficient perioperative care.

When conducting a pre-operative evaluation of a patient with vascular disease, it is crucial to compile a detailed history and perform a thorough physical examination. One must assess for other comorbidities as well as the extent of the disease, as patients with vascular disease often have coexisting ischemic heart disease, hypertension, cerebrovascular disease, or chronic renal insufficiency. The goal of the preoperative evaluation is to identify modifiable risk factors, coordinate a treatment plan with other members of the perioperative care team, and optimize the patient's medical condition to shift the balance of risk/benefit ratio before proceeding with nonemergent surgery.

Chronic pulmonary disease is common among the surgical population and the importance of a thorough and detailed pre-operative assessment is monumental for minimizing morbidity and mortality and reducing the risk of perioperative pulmonary complications. These comorbidities contribute to pulmonary postoperative complications, including atelectasis, pneumonia, and respiratory failure, and can predict long-term mortality. The important aspects of the pre-operative assessment for patients with chronic pulmonary disease, and the value of pre-operative testing and smoking cessation, are discussed. Specifically discussed are pre-operative pulmonary assessment and management of patients with chronic obstructive pulmonary disease, asthma, restrictive lung disease, obstructive sleep apnea, and obesity.

Chronic kidney disease (CKD) is a major public health problem worldwide. Roughly 1 in 10 adult Americans has CKD. These patients are at significant risk for excessive morbidity and mortality during the perioperative period. Given the health and cost burden of end-stage renal disease (ESRD), preventing or avoiding progression of CKD to ESRD is critical. Therefore, identifying risk factors and implementing risk mitigation strategies to prevent further deterioration of renal function during the perioperative period is of paramount importance. This article reviews patient risk stratification, pre-operative evaluation and management, and perioperative interventions for renal protection.

This article summarizes the key features and clinical considerations related to pre-operative management and planning for the care of patients of common endocrine disorders (diabetes mellitus, adrenal insufficiency, thyroid disease), a less common disorder but one that has significant perioperative implications (acromegaly), and two disorders for which pre-operative management is essential to good postoperative outcomes (pheochromocytoma and carcinoid syndrome). There are few evidence-based guidelines for pre-operative management of chronic endocrine disease; hence, this review is based on recent subspecialty society consensus guidelines and professional society clinical practice recommendations.

Patients presenting in an immunocompromised state merit special consideration when being evaluated for fitness to undergo surgery. A variety of immunodeficient conditions and their respective therapies, including human immunodeficiency virus, cancer, and transplantation, exert numerous systemic effects that may lead to multiorgan dysfunction. Understanding the potential impact of these disease manifestations, and their proper evaluation, is essential in achieving optimal perioperative outcomes for these patients.

Surgery, by definition, is a challenge to the hemostatic system. In addition, a surgical procedure may provoke inappropriate venous or arterial thrombosis, such as is suggested historically by Virchow's Triad. For these reasons, proper functioning of the hematologic system is integral in a successful and safe perioperative period. Patients with a disorder of either coagulation or hemostasis, therefore, present an exciting challenge to the pre-operative physician. Diagnosis of a hematologic disorder may be more or less occult. A proper bleeding and clotting history can serve to elucidate such a disorder and is therefore paramount to the pre-operative workup. For those patients with a previously diagnosed disorder of the hematologic system, appropriate laboratory investigation and a concise therapeutic plan for the day of surgery can help to minimize risks in the perioperative period.

One of the most important factors affecting outcome and recovery from surgical trauma is pre-operative nutritional status. Research in perioperative nutritional support has suffered from a lack of consensus as to the definition of malnutrition, no recognition of which nutrients are important to surgical healing, and a paucity of well-designed studies. In the past decade, there has been some activity to address this situation, recognizing the importance of nutrition as a therapy before surgery, after surgery, and possibly even during surgery.

Joseph Salama-Hanna and Grace Chen

Pre-operative evaluation of patients with chronic pain is important because it may lead to multidisciplinary pre-operative treatment of patients' pain and a multimodal analgesia plan for effective pain control. Pre-operative multidisciplinary management of chronic pain and comorbid conditions, such as depression, anxiety, deconditioning, and opioid tolerance, can improve patient satisfaction and surgical recovery. Multimodal analgesia using pharmacologic and nonpharmacologic strategies shifts the burden of analgesia away from simply increasing opioid dosing. In more complicated chronic pain patients, multidisciplinary treatment, including pain psychology, physical therapy, judicious medication management, and minimally invasive interventions by pain specialists, can improve patients' satisfaction and surgical outcome.

Preface

Pre-operative Management of the Patient with Chronic Disease

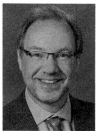 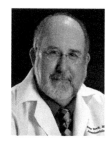 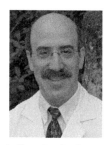

Ansgar M. Brambrink, MD, PhD   Peter Rock, MD, MBA, FCCM   Jeffrey R. Kirsch, MD

Editors

Perioperative medicine is constantly evolving. Today, patients are offered surgical interventions for increasingly difficult medical problems and despite complicated comorbidities or advanced age. Pre-operative options for diagnostic and therapeutic interventions are constantly changing and thereby expanding opportunities for improved patient care. The increased complexity of patients presenting for surgery requires clinicians to remain current with the latest knowledge of and recommendations regarding treatment of specific disease states. This is not only challenging for those treating patients during the perioperative period, but also particularly difficult for the diverse group of clinicians charged with preparing and optimizing patients scheduled for surgery. Moreover, it requires better communication than ever between all clinicians involved in preparing patients for surgery and optimizing their status based on their individual needs.

As active perioperative physicians we were therefore delighted about the opportunity to present an entire issue of articles dedicated to Pre-operative Management of the Patient with Chronic Disease for the *Medical Clinics of North America.* We have invited a number of national experts in anesthesiology and perioperative medicine to summarize current knowledge and advice about optimal pre-operative preparation of patients with pre-existing health problems. While many more chronic health problems exist than can be covered in this issue, we have selected the most prevalent topics that health care workers may encounter during pre-operative preparation of adult patients who are scheduled to undergo surgery. This issue of the *Medical Clinics of North America* compiles outstanding new review articles that will allow all involved clinicians to better identify and address specific pre-operative challenges of their patients.

The presentation of the contributions in this issue follows a system-based approach. Drs Martz and Sappenfield address key challenges in the pre-operative optimization in

Med Clin N Am 97 (2013) xv–xvi
http://dx.doi.org/10.1016/j.mcna.2013.08.002
0025-7125/13/$ – see front matter © 2013 Elsevier Inc. All rights reserved.

patients with diseases of the central nervous system, including cerebrovascular co-morbidities. Dr Turakhia and coauthors in their article on patients with neuromuscular disorders provide systematic information about the different disease entities and important suggestions for optimal preparation of affected patients prior to a planned surgical intervention. Drs Grigore and Odonkor provide advice for the pre-operative preparation of patients with cardiovascular comorbidities in their article addressing the specific challenges in patients with ischemic heart disease, and Dr Schulman and coauthors make recommendations for the care of patients with cardiac rhythm disturbances in their article on considerations in patients with pacemakers or implantable cardioverter defibrillators.

The following articles are dedicated to the pre-operative specifics in patients with vascular disease by Drs Manley and Reck, chronic pulmonary disease by Hong and Galvagno, and chronic kidney disease by Drs Niemann and Kalamas. Systemic diseases and their specific considerations for pre-operative preparation are summarized in articles on patients with chronic endocrine disease by Dr Njoku, patients with immunodeficiency by Dr Hannaman, and patients with disorders of thrombosis and hemostasis by Drs Orfanakis and Deloughery. Specific suggestions for pre-operative preparation of patients requiring nutritional support are provided in an article by Dr Enomoto and coauthors, and for those with chronic pain by Drs Chen and Salama-Hanna.

Our goal as editors of this issue was to provide a systematic overview of the key topics relevant to clinicians charged with preparing patients with chronic diseases for surgery or other interventions that require anesthesia.

Health care workers in all practice environments involved in pre-operative preparation of surgical patients will enjoy reading the different contributions. The information supports specific decision-making, developing a comprehensive care plan and optimization of the patient's medical conditions prior to surgery. It will also support proactive communication between those preparing the patient and the procedural team. By doing so, the result is improved patient care and outcomes for chronically ill patients who require operative interventions.

Ansgar M. Brambrink, MD, PhD
Department of Anesthesiology and Perioperative Medicine
Oregon Health and Science University
Portland, OR 97239, USA

Peter Rock, MD, MBA, FCCM
Department of Anesthesiology
University of Maryland School of Medicine
Baltimore, MD 21201, USA

Jeffrey R. Kirsch, MD
Department of Anesthesiology and Perioperative Medicine
Oregon Health & Science University
Portland, OR 97239, USA

E-mail addresses:
brambrin@ohsu.edu (A.M. Brambrink)
prock@anes.umm.edu (P. Rock)
kirschje@ohsu.edu (J.R. Kirsch)

Dedication

To our families:
Petra, Jan, Phillip, Helen, and Lucas (A.B.)
and
Sue, Katherine, Sarah, and Jim (P.R.)
and
Robin, Jodi, Alan, and Ricki (J.K.)
Thank you for your patience, love, and understanding.

Med Clin N Am 97 (2013) xvii
http://dx.doi.org/10.1016/j.mcna.2013.08.003
0025-7125/13/$ – see front matter © 2013 Published by Elsevier Inc.

Patients with Disease of Brain, Cerebral Vasculature, and Spine

Joshua W. Sappenfield, MD, Douglas G. Martz Jr, MD*

KEYWORDS

- Intracranial disease • Ischemia • Cerebrovascular disease • Neurologic assessment

KEY POINTS

- Patients who present with intracranial masses, vascular lesions, cerebrospinal fluid abnormalities, traumatic injuries, and dementia usually have already sustained a primary insult.
- New onset of a neurologic deficit or acute deterioration of mental status are probable indications for urgent operative intervention.
- All patients should have a focused neurologic assessment of their disability, as well as routine laboratory tests.
- In most cases, a CT or MRI scan is necessary.
- Until definitive treatment of the underlying condition occurs, prevention of secondary injury to the patient's brain is the goal of medical management and important for optimizing final functional outcome.

INTRODUCTION

Several structural abnormalities involving the brain and surrounding structures have perioperative implications. This article reviews the preoperative assessment and preparation of patients with intracranial masses, vascular lesions, cerebrospinal fluid (CSF) abnormalities, traumatic injuries, and dementia.

In general, the assessment of a patient should not delay emergent interventions to prevent morbidity and mortality unless it will directly affect patient outcome. Before urgent interventions, the management of patient care should focus on assessments that optimize the patient's clinical status without unduly delaying necessary procedures. A list of relevant history questions is shown in **Box 1**. With all elective procedures, a full history and indicated tests should be performed before proceeding. A thorough neurologic examination should be performed on the patient, with pertinent findings documented so that other medical providers taking care of the patient will have a reference during the perioperative period. An adequate examination includes the patient's orientation, cognition, Glasgow Coma Scale (GCS), pupil size, sensory

Department of Anesthesiology - S11C, University of Maryland School of Medicine, University of Maryland Medical Center, 22 South Greene Street, Baltimore, MD 21201, USA
* Corresponding author.
E-mail address: DMARTZ@anes.umm.edu

Med Clin N Am 97 (2013) 993–1013
http://dx.doi.org/10.1016/j.mcna.2013.05.007
0025-7125/13/$ – see front matter © 2013 Elsevier Inc. All rights reserved.
medical.theclinics.com

> **Box 1**
> **Pertinent medical history**
>
> Time of onset
>
> Associated symptoms
>
> Neurologic deficits
>
> Baseline functional status
>
> Baseline mental status
>
> Other comorbidities
>
> Current medications
>
> Illicit substance use
>
> Previous cranial/intracranial surgeries

deficits, reflexes, cranial nerve function, and extremity motor strength. A GCS is a composite score of best patient ability to open eyes, speak verbally, and move extremities; the scoring is shown in **Table 1**. When deficits are found, a more detailed examination should focus on the abnormality. Documentation should be clear and legible so that comparisons can be made when suspected changes occur.

GENERAL CONSIDERATIONS

After assessment of the neurologic injury, the goals of treatment are to prevent secondary injury to the brain and manage common sequelae. To prevent further insult, the blood pressure should be maintained or increased to maintain perfusion of tissues where normal autoregulation is absent. Hypocapnea, which causes vasoconstriction, should be avoided to maintain perfusion to the penumbra. Hypoxia worsens the metabolic debt of marginal tissues. The patient should be monitored for metabolic and electrolyte abnormalities, as these are not uncommon. Hypoglycemia and hyperglycemia events are also associated with worsening of neurologic outcomes. All of this information should be taken into consideration when providing care for the primary problem.

SPECIFIC CONSIDERATIONS
Tumors

Supratentorial masses
The overall incidence of new primary central nervous system (CNS) tumors is about 20 per 100,000.[1] The incidence of primary intracranial tumors is about 8 to 10 per

> **Table 1**
> **Glasgow Coma Scale**

Eye Opening	Verbal Response	Motor Response
4: Spontaneously	5: Oriented, speaking clearly	6: Able to follow commands
3: To verbal command	4: Speaks, but disoriented	5: Localizes to pain
2: To pain	3: Speaks incoherently	4: Withdraws to pain
1: No response	2: Incomprehensible words	3: Decorticate posturing
	1: No response	2: Decerebrate posturing
		1: No response

100,000.[2] Primary brain tumors are less common than intracranial tumors secondary to metastasis.[2] Disorders such as Von Hippel–Lindau disease, neurofibromatosis, tuberous sclerosis, Sturge-Weber syndrome, Gorlin syndrome, Turcot syndrome, Gardener syndrome, and Li-Fraumeni syndrome are associated primary brain tumors.[2] Primary CNS lymphoma can also occur in patients who are immunosuppressed (especially in patients with human immunodeficiency virus [HIV] infection or a previous organ transplant).[2] Four-fifths of all intracranial tumors are located in the supratentorial space.[2]

Patients usually present with headache, seizures, or a new neurologic deficit.[2] As the tumor grows, patients may have symptoms related to an increase in intracranial pressure (ICP), cognitive issues, altered mental status, changes in blood pressure, or symptoms from obstructive hydrocephalus.[2] Brain metastases can be asymptomatic and may be found during the workup of the primary cancer.[2]

Resections of brain tumors are elective to semiurgent surgeries, unless a new focal neurologic complaint is present or there is a depressed level of consciousness. A history should be obtained from the patient that includes pertinent information, including how the mass was discovered, any neurologic deficit, or any prior history of seizures. A neurologic examination should be performed and documented. The patient should be assessed using the Karnofsky Performance Scale (**Table 2**) to guide whether surgical intervention is warranted in the patient's care.[2] Routine laboratory tests should be ordered and the patient's comorbidities should be optimized before proceeding with surgery. To evaluate the mass, magnetic resonance imaging (MRI) should be performed to help delineate the etiology of the tumor.[2] If the mass is not in the basal ganglia, posterior fossa, or pineal area, a tissue biopsy should be taken to guide management.[2] For example, if a biopsy shows the mass to be lymphoma, surgical intervention does not improve outcomes in comparison with chemotherapy.[2]

Two medications should be considered when taking care of patients with brain masses, namely steroids and anticonvulsants. Steroids are usually given perioperatively because they decrease brain edema and CSF generation.[2,3] Steroids may improve vasogenic edema by stabilizing endothelial membranes, decreasing the release of toxic substances and electrolyte shifts across capillaries, and increasing cerebral glucose metabolism.

Table 2
Karnofsky Performance Scale

Performance	Patients' Condition
100	Able to work. No signs or symptoms of disease. No assistance required
90	Still has normal function. Minor symptoms
80	Has normal activity with increased effort
70	Symptoms prevent being able to work. Still able to take care of themselves
60	Requires occasional assistance to take care of daily needs
50	Requires frequent assistance and medical care
40	Unable to live by themselves. Requires assistance and special care
30	Severely disabled, possibly requiring hospitalization
20	Hospitalized requiring active supportive interventions
10	Moribund
0	Dead

Data from Schag CC, Heinrich RL, Ganz PA. Karnofsky performance status revisited: reliability, validity, and guidelines. J Clin Oncol 1984;2(3):189.

There is no benefit to administering anticonvulsants to patients with intracranial masses who do not present with seizures. One trial showed no difference in the incidence of seizures of those who received a prophylactic 7-day course of phenytoin, even though the serum drug levels were "therapeutic."[4] The group that received prophylaxis had side effects including rash, elevated liver enzymes, thrombocytopenia, aphasia, altered mental status, ataxia, and photophobia.[4] There is also no benefit to administering phenobarbital or valproic acid prophylactically.[5] However, patients who present initially with a seizure should receive anticonvulsants. The use of levetiracetam (Keppra) for seizures may be indicated because it has a much lower incidence of significant side effects.

Pituitary masses

Pituitary tumors make up about 15% of all new primary CNS tumors.[1] A large number are asymptomatic and are found on computed tomography (CT) or MRI incidentally.[6] Patients may present with visual changes, headache, hypopituitarism, and cranial nerve abnormalities.[6–9] When found incidentally by imaging, other possibilities such as artifact on the image, Rathke cleft cyst, pituitary hypertrophy, hyperfunctioning pituitary secondary primary hormone deficiency, and craniopharyngioma should be considered.[2,6] Four-fifths of these "incidental findings" are actually adenomas while the rest are usually cystic lesions.[6] If found by a CT scan, a follow-up scan with MRI should be performed.

A focused medical history and physical examination should determine whether the patient has any signs and symptoms of a hypofunctioning or hyperfunctioning pituitary, gland and if there are any associated comorbidities (**Table 3**).[6] Besides routine laboratory panels, tests (**Table 4**) can also be ordered to confirm whether the pituitary mass is a functioning adenoma or if the pituitary is hypofunctioning. Pertinent laboratory results may guide recommendations for patient management. For example, prolactin-secreting tumors should be managed with dopamine agonists, whereas growth hormone–secreting tumors require surgery.[2,6,8] Patients who have an adenoma that secretes thyroid-stimulating hormone (TSH) may benefit from receiving somatostatin analogues.[8] Some pituitary tumors may secrete more than one hormone.[8]

Table 3
Associated systemic diseases with pituitary disease

Hypofunctioning Pituitary Gland	Hyperfunctioning Pituitary Gland
Adrenal insufficiency (eg, hypotension)	Hypertension
Infertility	Acromegaly
Amenorrhea	Gynecomastia
Addison disease	Obesity
Impotence	Osteoporosis
Diabetes insipidus	Amenorrhea
Goiter	Hyperthyroidism
Eating disorders	Cardiac disease
	Galactorrhea
	Diabetes mellitus
	Cushing's disease

Data from Refs.[2,6,7]

Table 4
Tests to discriminate functional status of pituitary adenomas status

Pituitary Hormone	Laboratory Tests for Hyperfunction	Laboratory Tests for Hypofunction
Prolactin	Serum prolactin	
Corticotropin	24-h urinary-free cortisol High-dose dexamethasone suppression test Corticotropin stimulation test Adrenocorticotropin hormone level	Corticotropin-releasing hormone stimulation test
Growth hormone	Insulin-like growth factor I Oral glucose tolerance test	Insulin tolerance test Arginine/growth hormone–releasing hormone test
Luteinizing hormone (LH)		LH immunoradiometric assay Gonadotropin-releasing hormone stimulation test Total serum testosterone (in males)
Follicle-stimulating hormone (FSH)		FSH immunoradiometric assay Gonadotropin-releasing hormone stimulation test
Thyroid-stimulating hormone (TSH)	Serum free thyroxine Serum TSH	Serum free thyroxine Serum TSH

Data from Refs.[6–8]

Posterior fossa masses

Posterior fossa masses present in the cerebellum, brainstem, and/or surrounding structures.[2] About one-fifth of all intracranial tumors are located in the posterior fossa.[2] Patients may present with headaches, hydrocephalus, and symptoms caused by compression of the surrounding structures including malaise, anorexia, nausea, vomiting, ataxia, dysarthria, and lower cranial nerve deficits.[2] These patients can decompensate more rapidly because of the limited space in the posterior fossa, and thus may warrant more frequent neurologic assessment.

When assessing patients with tumors of the posterior fossa, a history should be taken with special focus on symptoms arising from the mass. A focused neurologic examination should be performed that includes the cranial nerves and cerebellar function.[2] Besides obtaining an MRI, additional studies that may be beneficial include visual field and vestibular testing, as well as motor and somatosensory evoked potentials.[2] Steroids should be administered in symptomatic patients in whom imaging reveals tumor-associated edema. A transesophageal echocardiogram with bubble study should be performed to elucidate whether the patient has a patent foramen ovale if a surgery in the beach-chair position (eg, sitting upright with head tilted forward) is being planned.[2]

Cerebrovascular Disease

Cerebral aneurysm

The incidence of cerebral aneurysms is 2% to 4%.[2,10] About 6 in 100,000 patients present with subarachnoid hemorrhage (SAH) secondary to cerebral aneurysm rupture annually in the United States.[11] Aneurysms that involve the whole circumference of the cerebral artery are called fusiform aneurysms, whereas ones with involving only part are termed saccular.[12] Aneurysms less than 7 mm in diameter have a 0.1% chance of rupture per year.[13] Increasing size of the aneurysm and location of the aneurysm on the tip of the basilar artery, cavernous artery, and posterior communicating artery places the patient at increased risk of rupture.[13,14] When an unruptured aneurysm is diagnosed, the patient should be adequately assessed and optimized. A list of associated abnormalities is shown in **Box 2**. If a patient has a history of a ruptured intracranial aneurysm, the risk of developing another is between 1% and 2%.[15] Other risk factors for having multiple intracranial aneurysms include female gender and smoking.[16] Grading of the aneurysms is shown in **Table 5**. The Hunt-Hess Scale is the best predictor of mortality in patients with ruptured cerebral aneurysms, and the GCS grading system has the best interrater reliability and correlation with Glasgow Outcome Scale at discharge.[17] Another scale that is commonly used is the World Federation of Neurological Surgeons Scale.

Routine screening for cerebral aneurysms is not warranted,[10,11,15] even if a patient has Ehlers-Danlos syndrome.[10,11] (Type IV Ehlers-Danlos syndrome is caused by a mutation in the type III procollagen gene, leading to defects in the arterial structure.[10,11,20]) Screening in patients with polycystic kidney disease is controversial.[2,10,11,14] If a patient has had a history of SAH or a relative with familial intracranial aneurysm syndrome, screening may be beneficial.[10,11,15] The indications for intervention (endovascular or surgical) in unruptured aneurysms are listed in **Box 3**. However, the clinician should account for rate of aneurysm growth, life expectancy of the patient, and current neurologic function because of the high morbidity and mortality associated with surgical or nonsurgical interventions.[11] If the decision is made not to operate on a patient with an unruptured aneurysm, the patient should be advised to avoid smoking, heavy alcohol use, stimulant drugs, and excessive straining.[10,15] A patient with an unruptured aneurysm and concomitant hypertension should be treated for elevated blood pressure to possibly reduce the likelihood of rupture.[15] Before operating on unruptured aneurysms, not only should a full history and physical of the patient be performed, but studies relevant to identified comorbidities should be ordered so that the patient's treatment can be optimized.

One-tenth to one-quarter of all patients who present to the emergency room with a severe headache of abrupt onset have bleeding into the subarachnoid space.[21] Early intervention (surgery or radiologic endovascular coiling/embolization) reduces the patient's risk of rebleeding and allows institution of therapy to treat vasospasm if it

---

Box 2
Associated diseases with intracranial aneurysms

Arteriovenous malformations

Coarctation of the aorta

Ehlers-Danlos syndrome type IV

Fibromuscular dysplasia

Marfan syndrome

Moyamoya disease

Pituitary gland tumors

Polycystic kidney disease

Pseudoxanthoma elasticum

Data from Refs.[2,10,11,14,15]

Table 5
Cerebral aneurysm grading scale

Classification[a]	Hunt-Hess Scale	WFNSS	GCS Grading System
Grade 0	Unruptured aneurysm	Unruptured aneurysm	Unruptured aneurysm
Grade I	Asymptomatic or minimal headache and slight nuchal rigidity	GCS score of 15	GCS score of 15
Grade II	Moderate to severe headache, nuchal rigidity, no neurologic deficit other than cranial nerve palsy	GCS score of 13 or 14 without focal deficit	GCS score of 12–14
Grade III	Drowsiness, confusion, or mild focal deficit	GCS score of 13–14 with focal deficit	GCS score of 9–11
Grade IV	Stupor, moderate to severe hemiparesis, possibly early decerebrate rigidity and vegetative disturbances	GCS score of 7–12	GCS score of 6–8
Grade V	Deep coma, decerebrate rigidity, moribund appearance	GCS score of 3–6	GCS score of 3–5

GCS is defined in **Table 1**.
Abbreviation: WFNSS, World Federation of Neurological Surgeons Scale.
[a] Serious systemic disease such as hypertension, diabetes, severe arteriosclerosis, chronic pulmonary disease, and severe vasospasm seen on arteriography, result in placement of the patient in the next less favorable category.
Data from Refs.[17–19]

occurs.[15,22] Part of the workup of a suspected aneurysmal rupture should include a CT scan without contrast to diagnose and quantify the injury,[14,15] and either a cerebral angiogram, CT angiogram, or MR angiogram to determine the location of the aneurysm.[11,14] Diagnosis of SAH can also be made with a lumbar puncture if there is a high index of suspicion of SAH and the initial CT is negative.[15] Xanthochromia has sensitivity of 93% and specificity of 95%.[21]

The CT scan can help delineate the risk of cerebral vasospasm, which occurs angiographically in about 70% of all patients with SAH and clinically in about 20% to

Box 3
Indications for intervention on unruptured aneurysms

Large symptomatic intracavernous aneurysms

Symptomatic intradural aneurysms

Coexisting aneurysms to ones who have caused a subarachnoid hemorrhage

Aneurysms larger than 10 mm

Aneurysms that are almost 10 mm in younger patients who have a strong family history, the aneurysm has unique features, or the aneurysm becomes symptomatic

Data from Bederson JB, Awad IA, Wiebers DO, et al. Recommendations for the management of patients with unruptured intracranial aneurysms: a statement for healthcare professionals from the Stroke Council of the American Heart Association. Stroke 2000;31(11):2747–8.

40%.[23,24] The Fisher scale, first described in 1980, is used to grade the hemorrhage after rupture of saccular aneurysms, allowing prediction of the likelihood for subsequent cerebral vasospasm.[25] For the Fisher scale to have the greatest benefit, the CT scan should be performed in the first 24 hours after aneurysm rupture.[26] However, with the improvement in CT scanners and the treatment of aneurysmal bleeds, there is no added predictive value of the Fisher scale over the Hunt-Hess scale when predicting patient outcomes.[23] Routine laboratory panels should be drawn. Many patients may develop electrocardiographic changes (nonspecific ST- and T-wave abnormalities, arrhythmia of various kinds, and so forth), serum elevations in cardiac enzymes, and even left ventricular dysfunction secondary to high levels of circulating catecholamines.[14] These changes usually normalize with improvement in neurologic status of the patient. If the patient is showing signs of cardiovascular instability and/or has a grossly abnormal electrocardiogram, one should consider ordering an echocardiogram, either transesophageal or transthoracic. Correlation of the echocardiogram results with the electrocardiogram and the patient's cardiovascular parameters can help the clinician determine whether the patient is truly undergoing cardiac ischemia or changes from high circulating catecholamines (Takotsubo cardiomyopathy).

The neurologic status of the patient should be monitored. If the patient develops a depressed mental status or is unable to protect the airway, he or she should be intubated.[15] Ventilation mode and parameters should maintain oxygenation and normocarbia.[15] Seizure prophylaxis is usually initiated, as approximately 20% of patients with SAH will develop seizures.[15] However, there is no data to suggest that seizure prophylaxis improves outcomes in these patients.

After the aneurysm has ruptured, measures should be taken to prevent rebleeding until definitive intervention occurs, including bed rest and control of high blood pressure.[15] Antifibrinolytics are sometimes given to decrease the risk of rebleeding after rupture, but have not been widely administered because they increase the risk of cerebral ischemia.[15,27,28] There may be certain subsets of patients who may benefit from antifibrinolytic therapy.[15,28]

After SAH, normotension, euvolemia, and normothermia should be maintained to prevent worsening injury to already damaged brain tissue.[15] Patients should also not be allowed to become hyperthermic.[15] Serial laboratory tests should be conducted to diagnose and treat electrolyte abnormalities, and the patient's blood sugar should be followed to prevent hyperglycemia or hypoglycemia.[15]

Cerebral vasospasm from SAH can occur between 3 and 12 days after the initial hemorrhage.[14] In an effort to prevent the associated delayed neuronal deficit, patients are typically treated prophylactically with calcium-channel blockers,[14,15,29] specifically with nimodipine or nicardipine. Statin therapy has also been shown to be beneficial in 2 small studies.[29] Initiation of hypervolemia, hypertension, and hemodilution ("triple-H" therapy) is indicated in the setting of symptomatic vasospasm.[14,15,24] However, induced hypertension should only be used after the aneurysm is secured. It is also possible to use balloon angioplasty or to selectively administer vasodilators.[15] Intra-arterial application of vasodilators such as papaverine, verapamil, and nicardipine has been shown to effectively treat vasospasm.[24] Balloon angioplasty is effective at treating vasospasm, but can cause structural damage to the arteries (including rupture) and may make them less responsive to vasodilators.[24] The use of endothelin antagonists, intracisternal fibrinolysis, and low molecular weight heparin has not been proven to be beneficial.[29]

There are factors that may further delineate the risk of poor outcome after intervention in patients, and these should be considered before proceeding with open or endovascular repair. Risk factors for worsening of neurologic status after surgery include previous episode of ischemic stroke, an aneurysm greater than 9 mm in size, calcification of the aneurysm on CT, increasing age of the patient, location of the aneurysm on the tip of the basilar artery, and symptoms related to the aneurysm besides rupture.[10,30] Specifically, an age greater than 50 years is associated with worse outcomes, and risk continues to worsen as the patient gets older.[13] However, the relationship between age and outcomes may be less significant when the aneurysm is managed endovascularly.[10,13] Patients who receive endovascular treatment of their intracranial aneurysms seem to have better perioperative and postoperative mortality and morbidity in comparison with open surgical management.[10,14,22,31] The disadvantage of endovascular coiling is that about one-third to half of aneurysms may be incompletely embolized on the first attempt,[11,31] whereas clipping may incompletely occlude a little less than one-fifth.[31] Another disadvantage of coiling is that the aneurysm may recanalized, which occurs in one-fifth to one-third of all coiled aneurysms.[14] Carotid disease and concomitant arteriovenous malformations (AVMs) are important when considering repair of intracranial aneurysms. Aneurysms associated with AVMs are more likely to rupture, and before surgical correction of the AVM the aneurysm should be fixed.[10] Aneurysmal rupture has also been associated with carotid endarterectomies, which should be taken into consideration before operating.[10]

Cerebral arteriovenous malformations

AVMs are usually present at birth but usually do not become symptomatic until later in life. Patients with AVMs present with headaches, intracranial hemorrhaging, seizures, neurologic deficits, or loss of consciousness.[2,32,33] The most common presentation is after hemorrhage.[2] As more imaging is being performed, some are also being found incidentally. The incidence in the United States is estimated to be about 0.1%.[2] Patients who present with hemorrhage should quickly be evaluated for herniation, midline shift, and the presence of venous pouches or aneurysms inside the AVM.[33] All of these findings would be indications for more emergent intervention because they are signs of impending neurologic sequelae or early recurrent hemorrhage.[33] There are 3 options for intervention: surgery, endovascular embolization, and radiosurgery.[2,32,33] The greatest limitation of radiosurgery is the time it takes to reduce the size of the AVM.[33]

AVMs should be distinguished from cavernous hemangiomas, capillary telangiectasias, developmental venous anomalies, Moyamoya disease, cerebral proliferative angiopathy, and cerebrofacial arteriovenous metameric syndrome (CAMS).[33] CT angiography, MR angiography, and arterial angiography are all useful in evaluating these vascular lesions.[32,33] Delineation of the specific vascular lesion is important because treatment is different for each of the abnormalities. For example, developmental venous anomalies require no treatment.[33] If they are discovered after intracranial hemorrhage, a concomitant pathologic condition should be sought.[33]

Patients with CAMS will most likely have multiple AVMs; however, they usually do not hemorrhage.[33] Cerebral proliferative angiopathy is also slightly different from classic AVMs and usually presents with focal neurologic findings, transient ischemic attacks, seizures, and headaches.[33] Presentation with intracranial hemorrhage is rare.[33]

It is important to identify on imaging whether dural arteriovenous fistulas have cortical venous reflux, as this finding is associated with a more malignant course.[33] If imaging reveals signs of venous congestion or parenchymal ischemia, there is a higher risk of hemorrhage.[33] Besides previous hemorrhage, other risk factors for AVM hemorrhage include aneurysms, venous stenosis, single or deep venous drainage, and location in the posterior fossa or deep structures of the brain.[2,33] There are multiple risk factors for neurologic deficit, including arterial steal, high-flow shunting, venous congestion, venous obstruction, and adjacent gliosis.[33]

Patients who present for surgery should have a focused neurologic assessment of their deficits. Frequent neurologic assessments are necessary to monitor for changes. Besides routine laboratory tests, the patient undergoing open repair should have blood type and cross-match performed for potential use in the operating room. Severe electrolyte and metabolic abnormalities should be corrected before proceeding with any planned procedures.

Hydrocephalus

Hydrocephalus is defined as an abnormal collection of CSF.[2] CSF production in a healthy adult varies from 360 to 500 mL of CSF per day.[2] The majority of CSF production occurs in the choroid plexus, flows through the ventricular system and out of the fourth ventricle, then is reabsorbed into systemic circulation through the arachnoid villi.[2]

Patients with hydrocephalus present with the signs and symptoms listed in **Table 6**. However, in the setting of chronic hydrocephalus the onset may be insidious. The assessment of hydrocephalus should begin with a focused history looking for symptoms such as headaches, problems with vision, and urinary incontinence. A neurologic examination should focus on possible abnormalities of cranial nerves, cerebellar function, and gait. Imaging of the head is necessary with either CT or MRI. A workup of the etiology of the hydrocephalus should take place, as this will define not only prognosis but also treatment options.[2] Frequently these patients require an extraventricular drain if the symptoms are severe. As a temporizing intervention, acetazolamide and furosemide can be given to decrease CSF production,[2] or a lumbar puncture for CSF drainage after structural lesions have been ruled out.

Nonobstructing hydrocephalus usually occurs in adults secondary to subarachnoid hemorrhage, meningitis, or traumatic head injury.[2] Another variant is normal-pressure hydrocephalus. Such patients present with hydrocephalus but, as the name implies, do not have increased ICP.

Another similar disease process is pseudotumor cerebri, which is increased ICP not caused by hydrocephalus, tumor, or trauma. In most cases the cause is unknown. However, there is an association with obese females, although it can less often be caused by medications, infections, or venous flow issues.[2,34] A proposed mechanism is a decrease in CSF reabsorption, leading to an increase in "brain water accumulation," decreasing cerebral compliance.[2] Patients present with headaches, visual changes, dizziness, and nausea.[2] The physical examination findings are papilledema,

Table 6	
Signs and symptoms of hydrocephalus	
Symptoms	**Signs**
Vomiting	Papilledema
Visual disturbance	Loss of upward gaze
Incontinence	Abducens nerve palsy
Unsteady gait	Brisk deep tendon reflexes
Headaches	Unsteady gait
Neck pain	Altered mental status
Drowsiness	
Cognitive decline	

Data from Lumenta CB, Di Rocco C, Haase J, et al, editors. Neurosurgery. Berlin, Heidelberg (Germany): Springer; 2010. http://dx.doi.org/10.1007/978-3-540-79565-0.

enlarged blind spots, and sometimes abducens nerve palsy.[2] Imaging should be obtained, either CT or MRI, and a lumbar puncture performed.[2] Patients who have been diagnosed with pseudotumor cerebri should have regular follow-ups with an ophthalmologist.[2] Medications that may be beneficial are acetazolamide, furosemide, and topiramate, as these agents reduce CSF production.[2] Lastly, a CSF shunt can be placed to decrease ICP and alleviate symptoms.

Head injury

Severe brain injury is defined as a GCS of 8 or less, or an abbreviated injury score 3 or greater.[35] The percentage of severe brain injury caused by motor vehicle crashes is about 56%, and about 31% is caused by falls.[35] Roughly half to two-thirds of patients with moderate to severe brain injuries have isolated brain injuries while the rest have multiple traumatic injuries.[35,36] About two-thirds of the patients with a GCS of 8 or less will die, whereas the mortality drops to about 1 in 10 for a GCS of 9 to 12.[35] Sixty percent of all deaths will occur before the patient reaches the hospital, while another quarter will pass in the first 2 days after admission.[35] Older age and higher Injury Severity Scores are associated with an increase in mortality in traumatic brain injury (TBI).[36,37] Patients taking warfarin and who have intracranial bleeding or a loss of consciousness are also at an increased risk of dying.[38] Taking antiplatelet medications such as aspirin and clopidogrel increases the risk of mortality in TBI, but taking more than 1 antiplatelet medication does not create an additive risk.[37,39] Studies on trauma and anticoagulants have been retrospective, and the subjects had concomitant comorbidities for which they were taking anticoagulants so it is difficult to confer how much of the increased risk is from the medication. Hypothermia at admission of the trauma patient is associated with an increase in mortality, even in the setting of isolated TBI.[40] Management and treatment of the traumatically injured brain revolves around preventing secondary injury to the injured brain and the surrounding uninjured brain.[41,42]

The standard of care is to prevent patients from developing hypotension (systolic blood pressure <90 mm Hg) and hypoxia (arterial partial pressure of oxygen [$Paco_2$] <60 mm Hg or O_2 saturation <90%).[41–43] A single systolic blood pressure less than or equal to 90 mm Hg is a strong predictor of worse outcome before the patient reaches the hospital, doubling the patient's risk of mortality.[43] After the patient reaches the hospital, having 1 episode of hypotension and each additional episode increases the risk in mortality even further.[36,43] Duration of oxygen saturation less than 90% is an independent predictor of mortality.[43] The decrease in blood pressure or oxygen saturation is detrimental to the patient who has isolated TBI or multiple injuries.[36]

The $Paco_2$ is just as important. Prophylactic hyperventilation is not recommended.[41,44] Aggressive hyperventilation could cause cerebral ischemia.[44] Temporary hyperventilation may be appropriate to lower ICP; however, it should be avoided in the first 24 hours when patients are at risk for hypoperfusion.[41,44] Although the minute ventilation is important for managing cerebral blood flow and ICP, the tidal volumes should be limited. Patients who have a TBI and have tidal volumes greater than 10 mL/kg of predicted body weight are more likely to develop acute respiratory distress syndrome.[45]

In the acute resuscitation phase of the traumatically injured patient, every effort should be made to prevent hypotension and hypoxia. The blood pressure should be supported with volume (with a goal to maintain normovolemia) and vasopressors to prevent secondary injury to the brain. Albumin should not be used in the resuscitation of this subset of patients.[46] The airway should be secured early to, not only prevent hypoxia and hypercapnea, but also prevent aspiration and further decompensation of the patient's respiratory status. If possible, the provider should obtain relevant history about the patient including the mechanism of injury, current comorbidities, and current medications (especially anticoagulants). The patient should be examined systematically for other possible injuries that require treatment, such as hemorrhage from a femur fracture, neurogenic shock from a spinal cord injury, or myocardial dysfunction from a myocardial contusion.

CT can be useful to determine the extent of the brain injury and to plan surgical management. Repeat CT scans are useful during the patient's hospital stay, especially if there are any neurologic changes. Patients with evidence of intracranial bleeding and concomitant use of warfarin should have their anticoagulation reversed with fresh frozen plasma.[38] The use of tranexamic acid in traumatic brain injury is controversial. It does not have approval from the Food and Drug Administration for use in trauma, and has not been shown to decrease mortality from TBI when given after trauma.[27,28,47–49] Tranexamic acid has also not been studied in isolated TBI. However, in an underpowered, randomized controlled trial, it showed an almost significant reduction in mortality and no increase in the incidence of focal cerebral ischemic lesions.[49]

Monitoring the ICP in trauma patients is the standard of care, and is used to help guide management.[50] The indications for ICP monitoring are shown in **Table 7**. Elevated ICPs should be correlated and compared with neurologic examination.[41,51] No absolute value for ICP has been established for the treatment of intracranial hypertension, although treatment is recommended for ICP of 20 mm Hg or greater.[41,51] Treatment of increased ICP consists of elevating the head of the bed, drainage of CSF, administration of hypertonic saline or mannitol, and barbiturate coma in extreme cases.[41] The clinician should also consider surgical consultation for decompression.[41] A nonrandomized prospective study showed a relative risk reduction in mortality of 41% in patients treated with an ICP monitor.[52] The concept of using ICP monitors to guide treatment has recently been challenged by a randomized controlled trial that demonstrated no difference in mortality in patients with ICP monitors and those without after TBI.[53] The group without ICP monitors, however, received a longer duration of brain-specific treatment, more hypertonic saline/mannitol, and more hyperventilation.[53] The ICP-monitor group was more likely to receive high-dose barbiturates and develop decubitus ulcers.[53] A systematic review has also highlighted that all the previous studies were observational, with the potential for significant selection bias.[54] Because of the previous studies' designs, it has been very difficult to compare results between studies.[54]

Table 7
Indications for ICP monitoring in patients with a GCS ≤8

One of the Following CT Findings	Normal CT Scan, and Two of the Following
Hematoma	Age >40 years
Contusion	Motor posturing
Swelling	Systolic blood pressure <90 mmHg
Herniation	
Compressed basal cistern	

Data from Haddad SH, Arabi YM. Critical care management of severe traumatic brain injury in adults. Scand J Trauma Resusc Emerg Med 2012;20:12. http://dx.doi.org/10.1186/1757-7241-20-12; and Brain Trauma Foundation, American Association of Neurological Surgeons, Congress of Neurological Surgeons, et al. Guidelines for the management of severe traumatic brain injury. VI. Indications for intracranial pressure monitoring. J Neurotrauma 2007;24(Suppl 1):S37. http://dx.doi.org/10.1089/neu.2007.9990.

Implanting an ICP monitor allows for calculation of the cerebral perfusion pressure (CPP). CPP is equal to the mean arterial blood pressure minus the ICP or the central venous pressure, depending on which is greater. Continuous monitoring of the CPP has been linked to an improvement in outcomes.[55,56] Patients who have longer periods of time with CPP less than 60 mm Hg are more likely to have a worse condition (eg, severe disability or vegetative state) at time of discharge, and a higher mortality.[55–57] However, raising the CPP in a patient who does not have intact autoregulation may increase the ICP and increases the patient's risk of developing acute respiratory distress syndrome.[56] Therefore, it is not recommended to artificially raise the CPP to a level above 60 mm Hg.[41,56]

After TBI, patients are at risk for abnormalities in their electrolytes, and should be monitored regularly in the posttraumatic period. Patients are also at risk for coagulopathy early after trauma, and this has been reported up to 5 days after the initial TBI.[58] Hyperglycemic and hypoglycemic periods can worsen outcomes in patients with TBI, and should be monitored and treated.[41,42] Urine output should be monitored, as diabetes insipidus is a common cause of patients becoming hypovolemic.[41] Patients with a GCS of 10 or less, intracranial hematoma, depressed skull fracture, contusion, penetrating trauma, or a seizure within 24 hours of head injury are at a higher risk of having posttraumatic seizures.[41,59,60] These patients should be monitored and prophylactic medications administered. Phenytoin, levetiracetam, and valproate have been shown to reduce seizures in the first 7 days after injury.[59–62] However, valproate should not be used routinely because of the possible increase in associated mortality.[59] Patients who sustain a TBI are at risk of developing deep venous thrombosis and pulmonary embolism; therefore, mechanical prophylaxis (ie, graduated compression stockings or intermittent pneumatic compression stockings) is indicated.[41,63] Pharmacologic strategies for prevention of thrombi are more effective than mechanical means; however, they also increase the risk of enlarging hematomas and intracranial bleeding.[41,63] Sedatives can be given to the patient with increased ICP, but clinicians should avoid causing hypotension secondary to their administration.[41,64]

Because patients who have a TBI become hypermetabolic, they have a reduction in mortality if full caloric replacement is obtained within 7 days.[65] Patients should be fed enterally if possible,[41] and there may be some benefit from zinc supplementation.[65] Each patient should also be put on gastric stress ulcer prophylaxis with H2 antagonists or proton-pump inhibitors.[41] Infusion of intravenous magnesium has not been shown to improve outcomes.[66] Routine exchange of ventricular catheters or prophylactic antibiotic administration with ventricular catheters does not improve outcomes.[41,67] However, the CSF can be monitored daily for infection by measuring glucose, protein, cell count, and Gram stain.[41] Steroids should not be given to patients with TBI, as this medication been shown to increase mortality.[3,68]

Patients who present for surgery unrelated to their TBI should have documentation of their neurologic examination. If ICP is being monitored, part of the preoperative assessment is to make sure ICP is not unacceptably high when the patient is laid flat. Besides routine laboratory tests, if the patient has sustained multiple traumatic injuries a type and cross-match of blood products may be prudent to maintain oxygen-carrying capacity to the injured brain. Any electrolyte or metabolic abnormalities should be corrected before the patient proceeds to the operating room.

Spinal cord injury

A significant percentage of all patients with multiple severe traumatic injuries have concomitant spinal cord injuries.[69] Patients who have a GCS of 8 or less are at much higher risk for spinal injury.[69] The incidence of severe neck injury is the highest in rollovers and the lowest in rear-end collisions.[70] Patients who are ejected from their vehicle are likely to have a more severe neck injury.[70] It is rare for patients who were wearing their seat belt to have a severe neck injury.[70] Damage to the cervical spinal cord usually results from hyperextension of the neck secondary to the head impacting another structure such as the windshield.[70]

The initial assessment of a patient with suspected spinal trauma should thus be the same as for all other traumatically injured patients. The patient's airway, breathing, and circulation should be assessed rapidly. A quick neurologic examination should be performed, which should include purposeful movement of the extremities and pupil size. The patient should then be exposed to identify all other life-threatening injuries, followed by a systematic examination of the patient. Spine precautions should be adhered to, such as c-collars and log rolling for patient transfers.[69] Relevant history should be ascertained, such as time of injury, mechanism of injury, location of any pains, presence of any paresthesias/dysesthesias, weakness in any extremities, and baseline musculoskeletal function. A thorough neurologic examination should then be performed on the patient to identify the level of the injury and whether it is a complete or partial injury. A good examination should include motor strength, sensory perception, and the presence of reflexes. The back of the patient should also be examined for bruising, tenderness to palpation, and any widening of the spaces between spinous processes.[69] If the patient is unconscious, the clinician may have to rely on reflexes and rectal tone.[69]

Just as after TBI, hypotension and hypoxia should be avoided.[71] The patient should be resuscitated with intravenous fluids to a euvolemic state using best clinical judgment and vasopressors given to support a mean arterial blood pressure greater than 85 mm Hg.[71] Part of the workup for suspected spine injury should include a chest radiograph and pelvic radiograph, followed by a CT scan.[69] Assessment of the patient with isolated spinal cord injury should be rapid, to minimize the time to initiation of treatment. Compression of the spinal cord for longer than 6 hours has been shown to cause irreversible neurologic damage in dogs.[72] There does not appear to be a role for steroids in the treatment of spinal cord injury. In fact, it may increase morbidity related to infectious complications.[69,71]

Neurogenic shock occurs as a complication of cervical spine injuries in about one-fourth of all cervical spine traumas and in about 9% of all spinal cord injuries.[73] Neurogenic shock is caused by a loss of the "descending supraspinal fibers that activate the preganglionic sympathetic neurons," which results in the patient becoming hypotensive and bradycardic.[74] The patient can also have unopposed parasympathetic activity.[74] This effect can be seen on the day of injury and up to 2 weeks after spinal cord injury.[74] It is also associated with the possible development of cardiac-rhythm abnormalities and significant hypotension.[74] Treatment consists of the maintenance of normovolemia and inotropes to support the patient's hemodynamics.

If a patient presents for surgery after remote injury to the spinal cord, a focused neurologic examination of the patient's disability should be performed. The clinician should also seek out any history from the patient of a previous episode of autonomic hyperreflexia. Autonomic hyperreflexia is usually evident after stimulation to the bowel or bladder, and causes vasoconstriction below the level of the spinal cord injury and vasodilation above the spinal cord injury. Symptoms include headache, flushing, sweating, visual changes, anxiety, nasal congestion, palpitations, angina, or dyspnea. For patients who have had a cervical fusion, preoperative assessment should include a history of any intubation or anesthesia complications arising from decreased range of motion of the neck.

Dementia

Dementia is common in the elderly population, with a prevalence of about 7% in persons older than 65 years.[75] With increasing age, the patient is more likely to have comorbidities that should be evaluated before undergoing elective surgery. Age by itself is a risk factor for developing postoperative pulmonary complications.[76] As dementia progresses it becomes more difficult to obtain a complete or reliable history from the patient. It is logical to elicit medical history from family members, caregivers, and patient records from previous medical care providers.[77]

Along with comorbidities, the type of the proposed surgery should be taken into consideration. The preoperative physician should not misled into considering laparoscopic surgery as having less cardiac risk than open procedures.[78] For larger surgeries that may require hospitalization, it may be important to assess the patient's instrumental activities of daily living, as well as perform a Mini-Mental State Examination (MMSE) and shortened Geriatric Depression Scale (GDS). Having a single deficit in the instrumental activities of daily living, a MMSE score of less than 20, or a shortened GDS score of greater than 6 are all associated with an increase in mortality at 2 years.[79] Another important assessment is of functional capacity. A functional capacity of less than 4 metabolic equivalents (METs) is linked with an increase in perioperative cardiac risk.[76] Although functional status and capacity may not be modifiable, known deficits should indicate the need for preoperative counseling to the patient and family of possible outcomes and aggressive interventions in the early postoperative period. Patients should also be evaluated for dysphagia, which would put the patient at increased risk of aspiration.

Specifically for dementia, the etiology should be elucidated because it could have perioperative implications. For example, a patient with vascular dementia should be treated differently to a patient with Alzheimer disease. The patient with vascular dementia should probably undergo evaluation of their carotids by vascular duplex to identify if there is any significant occlusive disease.

Alzheimer disease is by far the most common cause of dementia[77]; other causes include Creutzfeldt-Jakob disease, Pick disease, Huntington disease, Parkinson disease, HIV, and high-flow shunts from intracranial AVMs.[33,77] Cognitive dysfunction can also occur after exposure to toxic substances such as lead and ecstasy.[77] Certain diseases are also associated with dementia. For example, diabetes is a risk factor for both Alzheimer disease and vascular dementia.[76]

Advanced age and dementia are both risk factors for developing cognitive dysfunction after surgery.[76,80,81] Other risk factors for postoperative cognitive dysfunction include duration of anesthesia, respiratory complications, and postoperative infections.[81] Higher levels of education and benzodiazepine administration before surgery seem to be protective against postoperative cognitive dysfunction.[81] Postoperative cognitive disorders are important because they are associated with increased length of hospital stay and decreased quality of life.[76] There are several modifiable risk factors such as visual impairment, hearing deficits, malnutrition, dehydration, and medications (ie, benzodiazepines and anticholinergics).[76] These factors should be addressed in the preoperative setting for elective cases, and minimized in urgent cases to improve perioperative outcomes.

It is unclear whether postoperative cognitive dysfunction is related to inflammation from surgery, toxicity from anesthetic medications, or patient-specific factors.[80] It does not seem to matter whether the patient receives a general or regional anesthetic.[82] There is some evidence to suggest that postoperative cognitive dysfunction merely unmasks already existing cognitive decline in patients. A large retrospective study showed no difference in cognitive decline in patients with an average age from 77 to 82 years, regardless of whether they had surgery or illness in comparison with controls.[83] The topic of postoperative cognitive dysfunction remains controversial and has not been fully elucidated.[80]

SUMMARY

Patients who present with intracranial masses, vascular lesions, CSF abnormalities, traumatic injuries, and dementia usually have already sustained a primary insult. New onset of a neurologic deficit or acute deterioration of mental status is a probable indication for urgent operative intervention. All patients should have a focused neurologic assessment of their disability, along with routine laboratory panels. In most cases, imaging is necessary as well. Until definitive treatment of the underlying condition occurs, prevention of secondary injury to the patient's brain is the goal of medical management and is important to optimize final functional outcome.

REFERENCES

1. Dolecek TA, Propp JM, Stroup NE, et al. CBTRUS statistical report: primary brain and central nervous system tumors diagnosed in the united states in 2005-2009. Neuro Oncol 2012;14(Suppl 5):v1–49. http://dx.doi.org/10.1093/neuonc/nos218.
2. Lumenta CB, Di Rocco C, Haase J, et al, editors. Neurosurgery. Berlin, Heidelberg (Germany): Springer; 2010. http://dx.doi.org/10.1007/978-3-540-79565-0.
3. Brain Trauma Foundation, American Association of Neurological Surgeons, Congress of Neurological Surgeons, et al. Guidelines for the management of severe traumatic brain injury. XV. Steroids. J Neurotrauma 2007;24(Suppl 1): S91–5. http://dx.doi.org/10.1089/neu.2007.9981.
4. Wu AS, Trinh VT, Suki D, et al. A prospective randomized trial of perioperative seizure prophylaxis in patients with intraparenchymal brain tumors. J Neurosurg 2013. http://dx.doi.org/10.3171/2012.12.JNS111970.
5. Sirven JI, Wingerchuk DM, Drazkowski JF, et al. Seizure prophylaxis in patients with brain tumors: a meta-analysis. Mayo Clin Proc 2004;79(12):1489–94. http://dx.doi.org/10.4065/79.12.1489.
6. Lania A, Beck-Peccoz P. Pituitary incidentalomas. Best Pract Res Clin Endocrinol Metab 2012;26(4):395–403. http://dx.doi.org/10.1016/j.beem.2011.10.009.
7. Cooper O, Melmed S. Subclinical hyperfunctioning pituitary adenomas: the silent tumors. Best Pract Res Clin Endocrinol Metab 2012;26(4):447–60. http://dx.doi.org/10.1016/j.beem.2012.01.002.
8. Melmed S, Conn PM, editors. Endocrinology: basic and clinical principles. 2nd edition. Totowa (NJ): Humana Press; 2005. http://dx.doi.org/10.1007/978-1-59259-829-8.
9. Fernandez-Balsells MM, Murad MH, Barwise A, et al. Natural history of nonfunctioning pituitary adenomas and incidentalomas: a systematic review and metaanalysis. J Clin Endocrinol Metab 2011;96(4):905–12. http://dx.doi.org/10.1210/jc.2010-1054.
10. Wiebers DO, Piepgras DG, Meyer FB, et al. Pathogenesis, natural history, and treatment of unruptured intracranial aneurysms. Mayo Clin Proc 2004;79(12): 1572–83. http://dx.doi.org/10.4065/79.12.1572.
11. Bederson JB, Awad IA, Wiebers DO, et al. Recommendations for the management of patients with unruptured intracranial aneurysms: a statement for healthcare professionals from the Stroke Council of the American Heart Association. Stroke 2000;31(11):2742–50.

12. Health Quality Ontario. Coil embolization for intracranial aneurysms: an evidence-based analysis. Ont Health Technol Assess Ser 2006;6(1):1–114.
13. Wiebers DO. Unruptured intracranial aneurysms: natural history, clinical outcome, and risks of surgical and endovascular treatment. Lancet 2003; 362(9378):103–10. http://dx.doi.org/10.1016/S0140-6736(03)13860-3.
14. Brisman JL, Song JK, Newell DW. Cerebral aneurysms. N Engl J Med 2006; 355(9):928–39. http://dx.doi.org/10.1056/NEJMra052760.
15. Bederson JB, Connolly ES Jr, Batjer HH, et al. Guidelines for the management of aneurysmal subarachnoid hemorrhage: a statement for healthcare professionals from a special writing group of the Stroke Council, American Heart Association. Stroke 2009;40(3):994–1025. http://dx.doi.org/10.1161/STROKEAHA.108.191395.
16. Qureshi AI, Suarez JI, Parekh PD, et al. Risk factors for multiple intracranial aneurysms. Neurosurgery 1998;43(1):22–6 [discussion: 26–7].
17. Oshiro EM, Walter KA, Piantadosi S, et al. A new subarachnoid hemorrhage grading system based on the Glasgow coma scale: a comparison with the Hunt and Hess and World Federation of Neurological Surgeons scales in a clinical series. Neurosurgery 1997;41(1):140–7 [discussion: 147–8].
18. Hunt WE, Hess RM. Surgical risk as related to time of intervention in the repair of intracranial aneurysms. J Neurosurg 1968;28(1):14–20. http://dx.doi.org/10.3171/jns.1968.28.1.0014.
19. Ogungbo B. The World Federation of Neurological Surgeons Scale for subarachnoid haemorrhage. Surg Neurol 2003;59(3):236–7 [discussion: 237–8].
20. Pepin M, Schwarze U, Superti-Furga A, et al. Clinical and genetic features of Ehlers-Danlos syndrome type IV, the vascular type. N Engl J Med 2000; 342(10):673–80. http://dx.doi.org/10.1056/NEJM200003093421001.
21. Dupont SA, Wijdicks EF, Manno EM, et al. Thunderclap headache and normal computed tomographic results: value of cerebrospinal fluid analysis. Mayo Clin Proc 2008;83(12):1326–31. http://dx.doi.org/10.1016/S0025-6196(11)60780-5.
22. Phillips TJ, Dowling RJ, Yan B, et al. Does treatment of ruptured intracranial aneurysms within 24 hours improve clinical outcome? Stroke 2011;42(7): 1936–45. http://dx.doi.org/10.1161/STROKEAHA.110.602888.
23. Lindvall P, Runnerstam M, Birgander R, et al. The Fisher grading correlated to outcome in patients with subarachnoid haemorrhage. Br J Neurosurg 2009; 23(2):188–92. http://dx.doi.org/10.1080/02688690802710668.
24. Eddleman CS, Hurley MC, Naidech AM, et al. Endovascular options in the treatment of delayed ischemic neurological deficits due to cerebral vasospasm. Neurosurg Focus 2009;26(3):E6. http://dx.doi.org/10.3171/2008.11.FOCUS08278.
25. Fisher CM, Kistler JP, Davis JM. Relation of cerebral vasospasm to subarachnoid hemorrhage visualized by computerized tomographic scanning. Neurosurgery 1980;6(1):1–9.
26. Dupont SA, Wijdicks EF, Manno EM, et al. Timing of computed tomography and prediction of vasospasm after aneurysmal subarachnoid hemorrhage. Neurocrit Care 2009;11(1):71–5. http://dx.doi.org/10.1007/s12028-009-9227-7.
27. Roos Y, Rinkel G, Vermeulen M, et al. Antifibrinolytic therapy for aneurysmal subarachnoid hemorrhage: a major update of a Cochrane review. Stroke 2003; 34(9):2308–9. http://dx.doi.org/10.1161/01.STR.0000089030.04120.0E.
28. Gaberel T, Magheru C, Emery E, et al. Antifibrinolytic therapy in the management of aneurysmal subarachnoid hemorrhage revisited. A meta-analysis. Acta Neurochir (Wien) 2012;154(1):1–9. http://dx.doi.org/10.1007/s00701-011-1179-y [discussion: 9].

29. Weyer GW, Nolan CP, Macdonald RL. Evidence-based cerebral vasospasm management. Neurosurg Focus 2006;21(3):E8.

30. Eftekhar B, Morgan MK. Preoperative factors affecting the outcome of unruptured posterior circulation aneurysm surgery. J Clin Neurosci 2011;18(1):85–9. http://dx.doi.org/10.1016/j.jocn.2010.07.121.

31. Molyneux AJ, Kerr RS, Yu LM, et al. International subarachnoid aneurysm trial (ISAT) of neurosurgical clipping versus endovascular coiling in 2143 patients with ruptured intracranial aneurysms: a randomised comparison of effects on survival, dependency, seizures, rebleeding, subgroups, and aneurysm occlusion. Lancet 2005;366(9488):809–17. http://dx.doi.org/10.1016/S0140-6736(05) 67214-5.

32. Al-Shahi R, Warlow C. A systematic review of the frequency and prognosis of arteriovenous malformations of the brain in adults. Brain 2001;124(Pt 10): 1900–26.

33. Geibprasert S, Pongpech S, Jiarakongmun P, et al. Radiologic assessment of brain arteriovenous malformations: what clinicians need to know. Radiographics 2010;30(2):483–501. http://dx.doi.org/10.1148/rg.302095728.

34. Wall M. Idiopathic intracranial hypertension. Neurol Clin 1991;9(1):73–95.

35. Bouillon B, Raum M, Fach H, et al. The incidence and outcome of severe brain trauma—design and first results of an epidemiological study in an urban area. Restor Neurol Neurosci 1999;14(2):85–92.

36. Manley G, Knudson MM, Morabito D, et al. Hypotension, hypoxia, and head injury: frequency, duration, and consequences. Arch Surg 2001;136(10): 1118–23.

37. Ohm C, Mina A, Howells G, et al. Effects of antiplatelet agents on outcomes for elderly patients with traumatic intracranial hemorrhage. J Trauma 2005;58(3): 518–22.

38. Mina AA, Bair HA, Howells GA, et al. Complications of preinjury warfarin use in the trauma patient. J Trauma 2003;54(5):842–7. http://dx.doi.org/ 10.1097/01.TA.0000063271.05829.15.

39. Mina AA, Knipfer JF, Park DY, et al. Intracranial complications of preinjury anticoagulation in trauma patients with head injury. J Trauma 2002;53(4):668–72. http://dx.doi.org/10.1097/01.TA.0000025291.29067.E9.

40. Sappenfield JW, Hong CM, Galvagno SM. Perioperative temperature measurement and management: moving beyond the surgical care improvement project. J Anesthesiol Clin Sci 2013;2(1):8. http://dx.doi.org/10.7243/2049-9752-2-8.

41. Haddad SH, Arabi YM. Critical care management of severe traumatic brain injury in adults. Scand J Trauma Resusc Emerg Med 2012;20:12. http://dx.doi.org/10.1186/1757-7241-20-12.

42. Curry P, Viernes D, Sharma D. Perioperative management of traumatic brain injury. Int J Crit Illn Inj Sci 2011;1(1):27–35. http://dx.doi.org/10.4103/2229-5151.79279.

43. Brain Trauma Foundation, American Association of Neurological Surgeons, Congress of Neurological Surgeons, et al. Guidelines for the management of severe traumatic brain injury. I. Blood pressure and oxygenation. J Neurotrauma 2007;24(Suppl 1):S7–13. http://dx.doi.org/10.1089/neu.2007.9995.

44. Brain Trauma Foundation, American Association of Neurological Surgeons, Congress of Neurological Surgeons, et al. Guidelines for the management of severe traumatic brain injury. XIV. Hyperventilation. J Neurotrauma 2007; 24(Suppl 1):S87–90. http://dx.doi.org/10.1089/neu.2007.9982.

45. Mascia L, Zavala E, Bosma K, et al. High tidal volume is associated with the development of acute lung injury after severe brain injury: an international observational

study. Crit Care Med 2007;35(8):1815–20. http://dx.doi.org/10.1097/01.CCM. 0000275269.77467.DF.

46. Finfer S, Bellomo R, Boyce N, et al. A comparison of albumin and saline for fluid resuscitation in the intensive care unit. N Engl J Med 2004;350(22):2247–56. http://dx.doi.org/10.1056/NEJMoa040232.

47. Cyklokapron—ShowLabeling.aspx. 2013. Available at: http://labeling.pfizer. com/ShowLabeling.aspx?id=556. Accessed March 17, 2013.

48. CRASH-2 Trial Collaborators, Shakur H, Roberts I, et al. Effects of tranexamic acid on death, vascular occlusive events, and blood transfusion in trauma patients with significant haemorrhage (CRASH-2): a randomised, placebo-controlled trial. Lancet 2010;376(9734):23–32. http://dx.doi.org/10.1016/S0140-6736(10)60835-5.

49. CRASH-2 Collaborators, Intracranial Bleeding Study. Effect of tranexamic acid in traumatic brain injury: a nested randomised, placebo controlled trial (CRASH-2 intracranial bleeding study). BMJ 2011;343:d3795. http: //dx.doi.org/10.1136/bmj.d3795.

50. Brain Trauma Foundation, American Association of Neurological Surgeons, Congress of Neurological Surgeons, et al. Guidelines for the management of severe traumatic brain injury. VI. Indications for intracranial pressure monitoring. J Neurotrauma 2007;24(Suppl 1):S37–44. http://dx.doi.org/10.1089/ neu.2007.9990.

51. Brain Trauma Foundation, American Association of Neurological Surgeons, Congress of Neurological Surgeons, et al. Guidelines for the management of severe traumatic brain injury. VIII. Intracranial pressure thresholds. J Neurotrauma 2007;24(Suppl 1):S55–8. http://dx.doi.org/10.1089/neu.2007.9988.

52. Farahvar A, Gerber LM, Chiu YL, et al. Increased mortality in patients with severe traumatic brain injury treated without intracranial pressure monitoring. J Neurosurg 2012;117(4):729–34. http://dx.doi.org/10.3171/2012.7.JNS111816.

53. Chesnut RM, Temkin N, Carney N, et al. A trial of intracranial-pressure monitoring in traumatic brain injury. N Engl J Med 2012;367(26):2471–81. http: //dx.doi.org/10.1056/NEJMoa1207363.

54. Mendelson AA, Gillis C, Henderson WR, et al. Intracranial pressure monitors in traumatic brain injury: a systematic review. Can J Neurol Sci 2012;39(5):571–6.

55. Kirkness CJ, Burr RL, Cain KC, et al. Effect of continuous display of cerebral perfusion pressure on outcomes in patients with traumatic brain injury. Am J Crit Care 2006;15(6):600–9 [quiz: 610].

56. Brain Trauma Foundation, American Association of Neurological Surgeons, Congress of Neurological Surgeons, et al. Guidelines for the management of severe traumatic brain injury. IX. Cerebral perfusion thresholds. J Neurotrauma 2007;24(Suppl 1):S59–64. http://dx.doi.org/10.1089/neu.2007.9987.

57. Clifton GL, Miller ER, Choi SC, et al. Fluid thresholds and outcome from severe brain injury. Crit Care Med 2002;30(4):739–45.

58. Lustenberger T, Talving P, Kobayashi L, et al. Time course of coagulopathy in isolated severe traumatic brain injury. Injury 2010;41(9):924–8. http: //dx.doi.org/10.1016/j.injury.2010.04.019.

59. Temkin NR, Dikmen SS, Anderson GD, et al. Valproate therapy for prevention of posttraumatic seizures: a randomized trial. J Neurosurg 1999;91(4):593–600. http://dx.doi.org/10.3171/jns.1999.91.4.0593.

60. Brain Trauma Foundation, American Association of Neurological Surgeons, Congress of Neurological Surgeons, et al. Guidelines for the management of severe traumatic brain injury. XIII. Antiseizure prophylaxis. J Neurotrauma 2007;24(Suppl 1):S83–6. http://dx.doi.org/10.1089/neu.2007.9983.

61. Temkin NR, Dikmen SS, Wilensky AJ, et al. A randomized, double-blind study of phenytoin for the prevention of post-traumatic seizures. N Engl J Med 1990; 323(8):497–502. http://dx.doi.org/10.1056/NEJM199008233230801.
62. Inaba K, Menaker J, Branco BC, et al. A prospective multicenter comparison of levetiracetam versus phenytoin for early posttraumatic seizure prophylaxis. J Trauma Acute Care Surg 2013;74(3):766–73. http://dx.doi.org/10.1097/TA.0b013e3182826e84.
63. Brain Trauma Foundation, American Association of Neurological Surgeons, Congress of Neurological Surgeons, et al. Guidelines for the management of severe traumatic brain injury. V. Deep vein thrombosis prophylaxis. J Neurotrauma 2007;24(Suppl 1):S32–6. http://dx.doi.org/10.1089/neu.2007.9991.
64. Brain Trauma Foundation, American Association of Neurological Surgeons, Congress of Neurological Surgeons, et al. Guidelines for the management of severe traumatic brain injury. XI. Anesthetics, analgesics, and sedatives. J Neurotrauma 2007;24(Suppl 1):S71–6. http://dx.doi.org/10.1089/neu.2007.9985.
65. Brain Trauma Foundation, American Association of Neurological Surgeons, Congress of Neurological Surgeons, et al. Guidelines for the management of severe traumatic brain injury. XII. Nutrition. J Neurotrauma 2007;24(Suppl 1): S77–82. http://dx.doi.org/10.1089/neu.2006.9984.
66. Temkin NR, Anderson GD, Winn HR, et al. Magnesium sulfate for neuroprotection after traumatic brain injury: a randomised controlled trial. Lancet Neurol 2007;6(1):29–38. http://dx.doi.org/10.1016/S1474-4422(06)70630-5.
67. Brain Trauma Foundation, American Association of Neurological Surgeons, Congress of Neurological Surgeons, et al. Guidelines for the management of severe traumatic brain injury. IV. Infection prophylaxis. J Neurotrauma 2007; 24(Suppl 1):S26–31. http://dx.doi.org/10.1089/neu.2007.9992.
68. Roberts I, Yates D, Sandercock P, et al. Effect of intravenous corticosteroids on death within 14 days in 10008 adults with clinically significant head injury (MRC CRASH trial): randomised placebo-controlled trial. Lancet 2004;364(9442): 1321–8. http://dx.doi.org/10.1016/S0140-6736(04)17188-2.
69. Schmidt OI, Gahr RH, Gosse A, et al. ATLS(R) and damage control in spine trauma. World J Emerg Surg 2009;4:9. http://dx.doi.org/10.1186/1749-7922-4-9.
70. Huelke DF, O'Day J, Mendelsohn RA. Cervical injuries suffered in automobile crashes. J Neurosurg 1981;54(3):316–22. http://dx.doi.org/10.3171/jns.1981.54.3.0316.
71. Hurlbert RJ. Strategies of medical intervention in the management of acute spinal cord injury. Spine (Phila Pa 1976) 2006;31(Suppl 11):S16–21. http://dx.doi.org/10.1097/01.brs.0000218264.37914.2c [discussion: S36].
72. Delamarter RB, Sherman J, Carr JB. Pathophysiology of spinal cord injury. Recovery after immediate and delayed decompression. J Bone Joint Surg Am 1995;77(7):1042–9.
73. Mallek JT, Inaba K, Branco BC, et al. The incidence of neurogenic shock after spinal cord injury in patients admitted to a high-volume level I trauma center. Am Surg 2012;78(5):623–6.
74. Piepmeier JM, Lehmann KB, Lane JG. Cardiovascular instability following acute cervical spinal cord trauma. Cent Nerv Syst Trauma 1985;2(3):153–60.
75. Norton S, Matthews FE, Brayne C. A commentary on studies presenting projections of the future prevalence of dementia. BMC Public Health 2013;13:1. http://dx.doi.org/10.1186/1471-2458-13-1.
76. Bettelli G. Preoperative evaluation in geriatric surgery: comorbidity, functional status and pharmacological history. Minerva Anestesiol 2011;77(6):637–46.

77. Verborgh C. Anaesthesia in patients with dementia. Curr Opin Anaesthesiol 2004;17(3):277–83.
78. Gurusamy KS, Koti R, Samraj K, et al. Abdominal lift for laparoscopic cholecystectomy. Cochrane Database Syst Rev 2012;(5):CD006574. http://dx.doi.org/10.1002/14651858.CD006574.pub3.
79. Inouye SK, Peduzzi PN, Robison JT, et al. Importance of functional measures in predicting mortality among older hospitalized patients. JAMA 1998;279(15):1187–93.
80. Brambrink AM, Orfanakis A, Kirsch JR. Anesthetic neurotoxicity. Anesthesiol Clin 2012;30(2):207–28. http://dx.doi.org/10.1016/j.anclin.2012.06.002.
81. Moller JT, Cluitmans P, Rasmussen LS, et al. Long-term postoperative cognitive dysfunction in the elderly ISPOCD1 study. ISPOCD investigators. International study of post-operative cognitive dysfunction. Lancet 1998;351(9106):857–61.
82. Williams-Russo P, Sharrock NE, Mattis S, et al. Cognitive effects after epidural vs general anesthesia in older adults. A randomized trial. JAMA 1995;274(1):44–50.
83. Avidan MS, Searleman AC, Storandt M, et al. Long-term cognitive decline in older subjects was not attributable to noncardiac surgery or major illness. Anesthesiology 2009;111(5):964–70. http://dx.doi.org/10.1097/ALN.0b013e3181bc9719.

Patients with Neuromuscular Disorder

Palak Turakhia, MD, MPH*, Brian Barrick, DDS, MD,
Jeffey Berman, MD

KEYWORDS

- Neuromuscular disorders • Preoperative management • Multiple sclerosis
- Myasthenia gravis • Peripheral neuropathy

KEY POINTS

- Neuromuscular disorders are a rare and varied group of diseases.
- These disorders can affect anterior horn cells, nerve roots, plexi, peripheral nerves, neuro-muscular junction, and muscles.
- Patients may have multisystem involvement, including the respiratory and cardiac systems.
- Patients may be at risk for intraoperative complications such as malignant hyperthermia, rhabdomyolysis, and idiopathic reactions to muscle relaxants.
- These various comorbidities must be optimized before surgery, involving a multidisciplinary approach.

Neuromuscular disorders are a heterogeneous group of disorders that affect various elements of the nervous system, including the anterior horn cells, nerve roots, plexi, peripheral nerves, neuromuscular junction, and muscles. These disorders can be genetic or acquired defects, and can present at any age.[1] Because these entities often affect multiple organ systems, optimal perioperative management is best achieved using a multidisciplinary approach, whereby there is expert management of each of the associated comorbidities. Careful attention to current medication regimens is very important to maintain patients' homeostasis and avoid adverse drug interactions (**Table 1**).

Many neuromuscular disorders have unique anesthetic implications. Those potential problems and attendant risks ought to be addressed by the entire perioperative team to assure that patients are in optimal physiologic condition preoperatively. When patients are in tenuous condition or have end-stage disease, a comprehensive

Anesthesiology, UNC Hospitals, University of North Carolina, N2198, CB# 7010, Chapel Hill, NC 27599-7010, USA
* Corresponding author.
E-mail address: pturakha@webmail.mfa.gwu.edu

Med Clin N Am 97 (2013) 1015–1032
http://dx.doi.org/10.1016/j.mcna.2013.05.005
0025-7125/13/$ – see front matter © 2013 Elsevier Inc. All rights reserved.

Table 1
Commonly affected organ systems

Organ System	Type of Dysfunction
Central nervous system	Developmental delay, mood disorders, spasticity, chronic pain, progressive loss of function, demyelination, atrophy
Respiratory	Respiratory muscle weakness, bulbar muscle weakness, impaired cough reflex
Cardiac	Arrhythmias, autonomic dysfunction, myopathy
Endocrine	Glucose intolerance secondary to chronic steroid use
Gastrointestinal	Impaired swallowing, delayed gastric emptying, dysfunctional gastrointestinal motility, impaired nutritional status

discussion with the patient and family should delineate a plan of care regarding resuscitation measures and/or postoperative ventilation (**Table 2**).

The purpose of this article is to give general guidelines for preoperative optimization of patients with more commonly seen disorders. The disorders are grouped according to the anatomic location of the lesion (**Fig. 1**).

LESIONS OF THE CENTRAL NERVOUS SYSTEM
Amyotrophic Lateral Sclerosis

Amyotrophic lateral sclerosis (ALS) is a progressive disorder involving upper and lower motor neurons, located in the motor cortex and the anterior horn of the spinal cord, respectively. Patients can present with both upper and lower motor neuron findings, including weakness of both upper and lower extremities and slurred speech (primary lateral sclerosis). Those with pseudobulbar palsy, in which conduction from upper motor neurons to corticobulbar pathways is disrupted, may demonstrate cranial nerve findings. Juvenile forms of ALS exist, but generally present early in life and are rare. The pathogenesis of adult ALS is debated but has been attributed to genetic, environmental, autoimmune, and viral etiology.

Treatment of ALS is palliative, aimed toward symptom control and improvement of quality of life.[2] Riluzole has been shown to result in a modest increase in survival in patients with ALS.[3] Although it preferentially blocks sodium channels, riluzole is thought to increase glutamate uptake and slow the progression of cellular destruction. Patients taking riluzole need close follow-up, including liver function tests.

Table 2
Anesthetic implications of neuromuscular disease

Agent	Implication
Nondepolarizing neuromuscular blocking drugs	Prolonged paralysis and need for postoperative ventilation
Succinylcholine (a depolarizing neuromuscular blocking drug)	Hyperkalemia (many disorders associated with synthesis of extrajunctional acetylcholine receptors)
Any sedative agent (intravenous or inhaled volatile agent)	Risk of postoperative weakness, delirium, cognitive dysfunction
Spinal or epidural techniques	Risk of symptom exacerbation (multiple sclerosis)
Inhaled anesthetic agents	Risk of rhabdomyolysis and/or malignant hyperthermia-like reaction (muscular dystrophies)

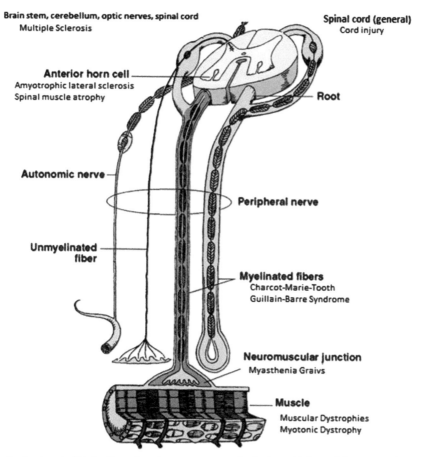

Fig. 1. Anatomic distribution of various neuromuscular lesions. (*Adapted from* Bertorini TE. Overview and classification of neuromuscular disorders. In: Bertorini TE, ed. Clinical Evaluation and Diagnostic Tests for Neuromuscular Disorders. Woburn (MA): 2002, Butterworth-Heinemann; 2002; with permission.)

Surgery for ALS is generally palliative and is directed toward better management of dysphagia, malnutrition, drooling, and aspiration. Such procedures may include tracheotomy and gastrostomy-tube placement.[4]

Preoperative considerations

Bulbar dysfunction Up to 25% of patients with ALS have onset of symptoms beginning with the bulbar muscles.[5] These patients are at high risk for perioperative complications associated with general anesthesia. Signs of bulbar dysfunction include weight loss, dysarthria, and difficulty whistling or using a straw. Nutritional and fluid status should be optimized preoperatively. If a review of systems and cardiopulmonary examination suggest a recent pneumonia, chest radiographs should be taken. Alternatives to general anesthesia in patients with advanced bulbar dysfunctional ought to be considered.

Respiratory insufficiency Respiratory failure is the principal cause of death in patients with ALS. A decline in respiratory muscle strength correlates closely with death. Patients have impaired cough and decreased ability to clear airway secretions. Measures used to detect pulmonary dysfunction include forced vital capacity (FVC) and nocturnal oximetry.[6] Noninvasive positive pressure ventilation (NPPV)[7] and mechanically assisted cough techniques[8] should be considered to compensate for respiratory muscle dysfunction. Frank discussions regarding the potential need for postoperative ventilation, prolonged intubation, and inability to wean from mechanical ventilation should occur with these patients and their family before surgery.

Mood disorders Depression is often seen in patients with ALS. Up to 50% of patients also have pseudobulbar affect, one of the manifestations of which is emotional lability.[9] Tricyclic antidepressants (TCAs) are commonly used to treat these disorders.[10] TCAs can prolong the QT interval. Recommendations exist to taper TCAs, although the risks and benefits of this must carefully be assessed. If the decision is made to taper, it should be done at least 2 weeks before surgery to avoid withdrawal. If the decision is made to continue, a preoperative electrocardiogram (ECG) should be obtained. If the QT interval is indeed prolonged, intraoperative drugs that increase the QT interval (such as ondansetron and droperidol) should be avoided. Excessive prolongation of the QT interval puts patients at risk for developing polymorphic ventricular tachycardia (torsades de pointes). Selective serotonin reuptake inhibitors have also been used successfully to treat depression associated with ALS,[11] and these should be continued with preoperatively.[12]

Spinal Muscle Atrophy

Spinal muscle atrophy (SMA), or Werdnig-Hoffmann disease, is a genetic neurodegenerative disorder of infants and children. Disruption of the SMN1 gene, which encodes a protein necessary for motor neuron survival, leads to degeneration and death of the motor neurons of the spinal cord. The overall result is hypotonia and muscle weakness. SMA is divided into several clinical types. Type I is the most severe and often results in death in early childhood. Type II is of intermediate severity, with respiratory dysfunction being a common cause of death during adolescence. Patients with Types III and IV have significant heterogeneity, and patients may live normal adult lives.[13] Patients who survive into adulthood have a high incidence of scoliosis, and often require corrective surgery to prevent further respiratory compromise.[14]

Preoperative concerns

Respiratory Patients with SMA often have respiratory compromise. In a prospective study, it has been shown that 100% of patients lose height-adjusted FVC, predisposing them to aspiration, pulmonary infections, and pneumonia.[15] Patients may also have a restrictive respiratory defect secondary to scoliosis. Patients undergoing scoliosis surgery may continue to deteriorate with regard to respiratory function, as pulmonary impairment is multifactorial in these patients.[16]

Cardiac Cardiac involvement in the form of cardiomyopathy and severe bradyarrhythmias has recently been demonstrated in a mouse model of SMA.[17] The cardiomyopathy manifests as a small-for-body-size heart with impaired inotropy. The reduction of pumping efficacy related to bradycardia is debatable. There is increasing evidence suggesting that cardiomyopathy may exist in humans with SMA Types I and III. There are also several case reports of cardiac arrhythmias and congenital septal defects in patients with SMA Type I and in patients with adult-onset SMA (Kugelberg-Welander syndrome).[18,19] However, a smaller retrospective study showed no increase in cardiac involvement in patients with SMA Types II and III.[20] Preoperative ECG is not recommended for every patient, but should be considered for patients who report dyspnea on exertion, palpitations, or other symptoms of possible cardiac dysfunction.

Multiple Sclerosis

Multiple sclerosis (MS) affects between 250,000 and 300,000 people in the United States and 1 million people worldwide. Most patients present between the ages of 20 and 40 years, although there are reports of patients who presented when younger than 10 years and older than 60. Women are affected twice as often as men. The progression of MS can be split into 3 main categories: primary progressive, secondary progressive, and relapsing-remitting. Most patients (85%–90%) are in the relapsing-remitting category.[21]

MS is thought to be an immune-mediated disorder occurring in genetically susceptible people. Environmental factors are also thought to have a role. Demyelinated plaques, often visible on magnetic resonance imaging (MRI), are pathognomonic for MS. These plaques are frequently observed in the optic nerves, brainstem, cerebellum, and spinal cord. Patients often present with optic neuritis, sensory disturbances, diplopia, limb weakness, ataxia, and neurogenic bowel and bladder. As the disease progresses, patients may develop cognitive impairment, depression, dysarthria, dysphagia, progressive quadriparesis, sensory loss, and pain.

Corticosteroids are the mainstay of the treatment of acute flares in relapsing disease. Interferon-β is also used, and glatiramer acetate is an alternative. Azathioprine and intravenous immunoglobulin have been shown to reduce the rate of relapse. Immunosuppressants, such as methotrexate, cyclophosphamide, and cyclosporine,[22] have demonstrated moderate benefit in patients with progressive MS. However, these drugs have significant adverse side effects (**Table 3**).

Preoperative considerations

Preoperative counseling Patients should undergo a thorough neurologic examination before surgery. Anesthesia and perioperative stress have been implicated in relapses, and patients should be counseled regarding such risk.[23] Controversy exists regarding the best type of anesthesia for patients with MS. There are no substantive data supporting any anesthetic approach as being the best. There are multiple case reports, but no well-designed studies, that describe idiopathic reactions with both regional[24] and neuraxial (ie, epidural or spinal) anesthesia.[25] Therefore, regardless of which anesthesia technique is used, candid conversation and education regarding the risks, benefits, and alternatives of anesthetic approaches must be held with patients, who must be active participants in the decision-making process.

Autonomic dysfunction Patients with MS can have autonomic dysfunction, which generally is due to brainstem lesions.[26] This disorder can lead to hemodynamic instability under anesthesia, including hypotension and arrhythmias. Patients should therefore be assessed for signs of autonomic instability such as orthostatic hypotension, sexual dysfunction, and gastroparesis.

Table 3
Immunosuppressants used for the treatment of multiple sclerosis

Medication	Side Effects
Methotrexate	Hepatotoxicity, nephrotoxicity, myelosuppression, pulmonary damage
Interferon-β	Hepatotoxicity, leukopenia
Azathioprine	Anemia, thrombocytopenia, leukopenia
Cyclophosphamide	Neutropenia, cystitis, prolongation of neuromuscular blockage with succinylcholine
Cyclosporine	Nephrotoxicity, electrolyte disturbances

Respiratory dysfunction Respiratory dysfunction is common in MS. Aspiration and pneumonia are common causes of mortality in patients with end-stage disease, but respiratory involvement is also seen earlier in the disease course, especially with relapses. Patients may have bulbar dysfunction, muscle weakness, and impaired voluntary muscle control.[27] Patients with worsening neurologic dysfunction (wheelchair confinement, involvement of the upper limbs) tend to have more severe pulmonary dysfunction.[28] Before surgery, patients should be assessed for the presence of pulmonary infections. If such is the case, proper treatment and postponement of elective procedures until optimal condition is achieved should be the course of action.

Medications Literature is sparse, but most of the reviews involving immunosuppressant use in the perioperative period are from patients with rheumatoid arthritis[29] and renal transplantation. The literature also tends to evaluate infectious risk and wound healing in the postoperative period. It is difficult to make recommendations on the continuation of these medications in the perioperative period but, at minimum, patients should be assessed for the various toxicities before surgery (see **Table 3**).

Spinal Cord Injury

In the United States there are approximately 12,000 new cases of spinal cord injury per year. In 2005 the average age at injury was 40.2 years, with 8:1 male predominance. Motor vehicle crashes account for 42.1% of reported cases of spinal cord injury, followed by falls (26.7%) and acts of violence (15.1%).[30]

Spinal cord injury is divided into 3 phases. At the time of the initial injury, acute compression or transection of the spinal cord can lead to a variety of arrhythmias and hypertension secondary to increased sympathetic and parasympathetic activity. The second phase consists of neurogenic shock, and lasts anywhere from a few days to a few weeks. Patients are areflexic, hypotensive, and bradycardic secondary to vasodilation and decreased preload. The third phase is characterized by a gradual return of reflexes and muscle tone, and is known as the "reflex" phase.[31]

Goals in perioperative management of patients with acute spinal cord injury are differ somewhat from those for patients with chronic injury. In acute injury, the goal is to limit or stop secondary injury. Surgical decompression, steroids, methylprednisolone, and other agents are used to prevent further cord injury.[32] Data supporting early intervention, particularly high-dose methylprednisolone therapy, is still inconclusive, although it remains a common practice (**Figs. 2** and **3**).[33]

With chronic spinal cord injury, return of sympathetic output below the level of the injury can result in exaggerated autonomic reflexes. The term for this is autonomic hyperreflexia, the pathophysiology of which is shown in **Fig. 2**.[34] The likelihood of development and intensity of the hyperreflexia increase as the level of the spinal cord lesion becomes more cephalad. Patients often develop secondary medical issues that both interfere with quality of life and lead to early morbidity and mortality. Such issues include pressure ulcers, atelectasis, recurrent pneumonia, deep vein thrombosis/pulmonary embolism, and recurrent urinary tract infections.[35]

Acute spinal cord injury

Respiratory Atelectasis, pneumonia, pulmonary edema, pulmonary embolism, and aspiration pneumonitis are seen in two-thirds of patients with cervical and upper thoracic spinal cord injury. The degree of respiratory dysfunction generally correlates with the level of the cord injury. Initiation of mechanical ventilation usually improves hypoxemia and hypercapnia. Patients who do not require mechanical ventilation should undergo aggressive pulmonary hygiene in the perioperative period.

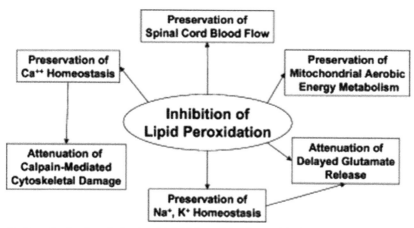

Fig. 2. Hypothesized central role of inhibition of lipid peroxidation in the neuroprotective effects of high-dose methylprednisolone in acute spinal cord injury. (*From* Hall ED, Springer JE. Neuroprotection and acute spinal cord injury: a reappraisal. NeuroRX 2004;1(1):82.)

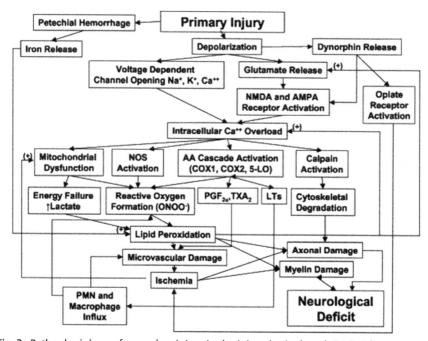

Fig. 3. Pathophysiology of secondary injury in the injured spinal cord. 5-LO, 5-lipoxygenase; AA, arachidonic acid; AMPA, 2-amino-3-(3-hydroxy-5-methyl-isoxazol-4-yl)propanoic acid; COX, cyclooxygenase; LTs, leukotrienes; NMDA, N-methyl-D-aspartate; ONOO$^-$, peroxynitrite anion; PGF$_{2\alpha}$, platelet-derived growth factor 2α; PMN, polymorphonuclear leukocyte; TXA$_2$, thromboxane A$_2$. (*From* Hall ED, Springer JE. Neuroprotection and acute spinal cord injury: a reappraisal. NeuroRX 2004;1(1):81.)

Neurogenic shock Neurogenic shock presents with bradycardia and hypotension, and is thought to be secondary to decreased peripheral resistance and cardiac output.[36] Patients should be given aggressive fluid resuscitation, and invasive monitoring should be undertaken to guide pressor therapy.[37] Drugs that are useful in this setting include phenylephrine (a pure α1-agonist) and norepinephrine. Norepinephrine should be considered especially if the patient is bradycardic, because a vagally mediated reflex bradycardia may result from phenylephrine use.

Chronic spinal cord injury
Autonomic dysfunction Autonomic hyperreflexia occurs in 85% of patients with injuries above the T7 level.[38] A variety of stimuli can trigger autonomic hyperreflexia, including phlebotomy, rectal examination, bladder catheterization, and pressure ulcers. However, the most common precipitating events are bowel or bladder distention. Autonomic hyperreflexia can be a medical emergency. Manifestations are severe hypertension, diaphoresis, flushing, and headache. Patients should be counseled to maintain meticulous bowel and bladder hygiene and to treat pressure ulcers aggressively. For patients who have frequent episodes, consideration should be made toward treatment with a calcium-channel blocker or guanethidine.[39] General or spinal anesthesia should be strongly considered for procedures below the level of the lesion, even if the patient is insensate in the area in question. Both have been shown to decrease sympathetic output and decrease the incidence of this reflex.[40]

Respiratory dysfunction Respiratory illness is one of the most common causes of death in patients with spinal cord injury. Respiratory mechanics need to be optimized pending surgery. Useful techniques include assisted cough, respiratory muscle training, mechanical insufflations, and (if needed) respiratory muscle pacing.[41] Lung infection, of course, should be treated before elective surgery.

Gastrointestinal Patients with spinal cord injury have varying degrees of gastroparesis.[42] These patients should strictly adhere to standard NPO (nothing by mouth) guidelines. Additionally the use of metoclopramide has been shown to reduce gastric emptying times in these patients.[43] If used, metoclopramide therapy should be instituted well before surgery, and the patient should be monitored for extrapyramidal side effects.

Spasticity Spasticity is seen in more than 70% of patients 1 year after injury.[44] Baclofen is often the treatment of choice for spasticity. For patients who do not respond to oral baclofen, intrathecal baclofen has been used successfully.[45] While baclofen causes downregulation of central γ-aminobutyric acid receptors, the drug itself is responsible for increased inhibitory tone in the central nervous system. Acute discontinuation of oral baclofen can induce acute withdrawal, manifested as seizures, hallucinations, worsening spasticity, or hyperthermia. Withdrawing intrathecal baclofen abruptly can be life-threatening and may result in death.[46] Thus, patients who present with intrathecal drug-delivery systems should have their infusion continued and undergo device interrogation in both the preoperative and postoperative period.[47]

LESIONS OF THE PERIPHERAL NERVOUS SYSTEM
Charcot-Marie-Tooth Disease

Charcot-Marie-Tooth disease (CMT) is one of the most commonly inherited neuromuscular disorders, affecting approximately 1 in 2500 people. It is actually a heterogeneous group of disorders, with 80% of cases being the demyelinating form. It is usually inherited as an autosomal dominant disorder, but X-linked inheritance is not uncommon.[48]

Defects in genes that encode proteins within myelin, Schwann cells and axons, result in demyelination and axonal degeneration. Many patients develop symptoms early in life. Weakness and muscle wasting start in the lower extremities, then gradually affect the upper extremities. Sensory loss is also present, and also develops from distal to proximal. Patients may develop tremors, muscle cramps, and bony deformities. High-arched feet and hammer-toe deformity are common orthopedic manifestations.

Treatment of CMT remains mostly supportive, involving rehabilitation. Patients often undergo surgical correction of the various bony deformities. Overall, general anesthesia is well tolerated in patients with CMT, and reported complications have been rare.[49]

Preoperative considerations

Respiratory The incidence of respiratory dysfunction is lower than for other neuromuscular disorders, reported as anywhere from 0% to 30% in the literature. When present, CMT is usually a restrictive defect secondary to respiratory muscle weakness. Patients may have a higher than average risk of obstructive sleep apnea, making them more sensitive to sedative medication. Diaphragm dysfunction may increase the risk of prolonged neuromuscular blockade. Patients in certain subtypes may also have paralysis of the vocal cords, placing them at higher risk for aspiration.[50] Respiratory care needs to be tailored to the individual patient.

Cardiovascular There have been several case reports of arrhythmias associated with CMT, including patients undergoing anesthesia.[51] An increased incidence of mitral prolapse is seen. However, prospective studies have not shown an increase in frequency of cardiac dysfunction in comparison with the general population.[52] A preoperative electrocardiogram may not be necessary in every patient with CMT, but patients who have a review of systems suggestive of cardiac involvement (palpitations, episodes of dizziness) should be further evaluated. Patients with mitral prolapse need not be premedicated for routine procedures unless concomitant mitral regurgitation exists.

Guillain-Barré Syndrome

Guillain-Barré syndrome (GBS) is actually a heterogeneous group of disorders. An acute inflammatory demyelinating polyradiculoneuropathy accounts for 85% to 90% of cases. It has become the leading cause of acute flaccid paralysis in Western countries since the eradication of polio. Patients report a preceding infection in 60% to 65% of cases, with the most common being upper respiratory tract infections (20%–47%), influenza (13%–25%), and gastrointestinal infections (11%–21%). *Campylobacter jejuni* infections have been identified as a trigger in various case-control studies in 13% to 72%.[21]

Patients with GBS present with progressive bilateral and symmetric weakness of the limbs, and may also have numbness, weakness, and paresthesias.[53] Related comorbidities include respiratory insufficiency requiring prolonged mechanical ventilation, autonomic dysfunction, venous thromboembolisms from prolonged immobility, and pain. Treatment of GBS includes plasma exchange and intravenous immunoglobulin, which have both been shown to hasten recovery.[54]

Preoperative considerations

Respiratory Seventeen percent to 30% of patients with GBS may develop respiratory compromise, often requiring intubation.[55] Risk factors include rapid disease progression; inability to cough, stand, lift the elbows, or lift the head; and an increase in liver function tests. Bulbar muscle dysfunction predisposes to aspiration pneumonitis.

Diaphragm and intercostal muscle weakness can affect the patient's ability to cough and clear secretions, resulting in atelectasis and shunt. Tongue and retropharyngeal muscle weakness and can lead to obstruction.[56] In patients who are not mechanically ventilated, incentive spirometry and aggressive pulmonary toilet are crucial. These patients will not present for any surgeries other than emergent procedures.

Autonomic dysfunction Evidence of autonomic dysfunction is seen in up to 20% of patients with GBS. Severe bradycardia provoked by endotracheal suctioning or positive pressure ventilation is not unusual. In extreme cases, temporary transvenous pacing may be required to avoid progression to asystole.[57]

Fatal outcomes have been linked to paroxysmal dysfunction, severe hypertension, and blood-pressure lability. Patients should be assessed for warning signs of autonomic dysfunction, including postural hypotension, facial flushing, and electrocardiographic changes. Patients with autonomic dysfunction should be treated with short-acting medications, intravenous fluids, and pacing, if necessary.[58]

Pain Pain is an early symptom in 33% to 71% of patients with GBS, and can precede weakness.[59] Gabapentin[60] and carbamazepine[61] have both been shown to improve pain in patients with GBS. Opioids have also been used, but patients should be in a monitored setting. In addition to decreasing the respiratory drive, opioids such as morphine are associated with histamine release, which may exacerbate autonomic dysfunction.

Corticosteroids Steroids alone have not been shown to affect recovery time or long-term outcome. There is moderate evidence, however, that steroids as part of combination therapy may hasten recovery. Diabetes requiring insulin is one of the complications in patients with GBS treated with steroids.[62] For patients on chronic steroids, glucose levels should be monitored and, if elevated, treated appropriately.

DISORDERS OF THE NEUROMUSCULAR JUNCTION
Myasthenia Gravis

Myasthenia gravis (MG) is an autoimmune disease thought to be the result of an antibody-mediated attack on the acetylcholine receptors at the neuromuscular junction. Patients present with weakness that improves with rest and worsens with repeated activity. More than 50% of patients initially present with ocular features, including diplopia and ptosis. The generalized weakness affects limb muscles and can also affect bulbar muscles. There has been an increase in prevalence in the last several decades, which has been attributed to improved diagnosis, an aging population, and prolonged survival with the disease.[63]

Physostigmine, also known as Mestinon, is the mainstay of MG therapy. This drug increases the availability of acetylcholine at the neuromuscular junction. Moreover it does not cross the blood-brain barrier, so patients are not prone to central cholinergic symptoms. Corticosteroids modulate the immune response, and are often a second-line drug in therapy. Immunosuppressants such as azathioprine, cyclosporine, tacrolimus, and mycophenolate mofetil may be needed in some patients.[64] In patients with acute exacerbation, plasma exchange and intravenous immunoglobulins are used. Thymectomy is commonly used to treat patients with generalized MG, and has resulted in remission rates of greater than 50%.[65]

Preoperative considerations
Weakness Patients with increased weakness should be evaluated and treated before surgery. Therapies range from increased dosing of medication to hospital admission

for plasma exchange. Although plasma exchange is the standard of care,[66] intravenous immunoglobulin therapy has also been used with comparable results.[67] Another study showed plasma exchange to be superior to intravenous immunoglobulin, but both studies showed more side effects with plasma exchange. Complications are associated with vascular access and fluid shifts, and include venous thrombosis, infection, pneumothorax, hypotension, bradycardia, and congestive heart failure.[68] Plasma exchange may result in a prolonged duration of action of succinylcholine, as this drug requires plasma cholinesterase for metabolism. Perioperative drugs that rely on nonspecific plasma and tissue esterases, such as esmolol and remifentanil, should not have their duration affected to as great a degree.

Medication Pyridostigmine should be continued in the perioperative period. Intravenous supplementation may be necessary if a patient is due for a dose of pyridostigmine intraoperatively. The dose conversion from intravenous to oral, according to the pharmacy references at the authors' institution, is 1:30, owing to high first-pass metabolism. Some sources report a conversion rate of up to 1:90. It should be noted that if an overdose of pyridostigmine occurs, a flaccid paralysis similar to that seen with a myasthenic crisis may be observed. However, such a cholinergic crisis is usually accompanied by autonomic symptoms such as bronchospasm, vasodilation, and increased salivary secretions. Autonomic symptoms are not associated with inadequately treated MG. Perioperative discontinuation will certainly lead to increased sensitivity to nondepolarizing muscle relaxants, whereas continuation may be associated with failure of bowel anastomosis.[69] Many anesthesiologists avoid nondepolarizing neuromuscular blockers on these patients intraoperatively.

Associated illness MG can coexist with a variety of other autoimmune diseases, which should be screened for perioperatively, including thyroid dysfunction,[70] rheumatoid arthritis, and systemic lupus erythematosus.[71]

Cardiac Patients with MG may have cardiac abnormalities, including ST and T-wave changes and rhythm disturbances.[72] Routine screening is not recommended in all patients, but physicians should have a low threshold in obtaining an electrocardiogram in patients with poor exercise tolerance or fatigue.[73] A small percentage of patients may also have symptoms of autonomic instability, including gastroparesis and blood-pressure lability.[74]

Respiratory Patients with MG are at increased risk of respiratory insufficiency in the postoperative period. The classic risk factors for this include disease duration longer than 6 years, history of chronic respiratory disease, daily pyridostigmine dose greater than 750 mg, and vital capacity less than 2.9 L,[75] but these have been refuted in subsequent studies. Aside from the obvious respiratory muscle weakness, patients with a large thymoma may be at risk of airway collapse with induction of anesthesia. a computed tomography and/or MRI scan should be obtained to evaluate for tracheal compression, as well as pulmonary function tests, which may help evaluate for dynamic airway collapse. In addition, myasthenic patients with observed weakness of the oral and pharyngeal muscles may have symptoms that mimic a bulbar palsy. This condition is often accompanied by ocular symptoms, and more aggressive treatment of the patient's underlying myasthenia is indicated lest collapse of the upper airway take place in the perioperative period.

Immunosuppressant therapy Steroids may put patients at higher risk for poor wound healing and perioperative infections, but several studies have shown benefits in postoperative respiratory function when compared with patients who did not receive steroids.[76,77] There is evidence that chronic steroid use blunts the hypothalamic-pituitary-adrenal axis response to surgical stress, but studies evaluating the benefits of perioperative stress-dose steroids are lacking. It is the authors' practice to provide supplementation in the perioperative period, as the benefits greatly outweigh the risks.[78]

Lambert-Eaton Syndrome

Lambert-Eaton syndrome is a neuromuscular disorder that causes weakness secondary to antibodies to voltage-gated calcium channels.[79] Patients often have lower extremity weakness, autonomic dysfunction such as dry mouth, and may have other autoimmune diseases such as thyroiditis, juvenile-onset diabetes, and pernicious anemia. Lambert-Eaton syndrome is associated with underlying malignancy in a majority of cases.[80] Patients may have bulbar dysfunction, putting them at risk for aspiration, and develop respiratory dysfunction after anesthesia, requiring optimization of pulmonary status in the preoperative period.

DISORDERS OF MYOCYTES
Muscular Dystrophies

Muscular dystrophy is a term given to a mixed group of disorders that are inherited and characterized by variable degrees of muscle wasting and weakness. The group is subdivided into 6 types: Duchenne, Becker, Emery-Dreifuss, oculopharyngeal, limb-girdle, and fascioscapulohumeral. Duchenne and Becker muscular dystrophy are the most common and are X-linked. Duchenne muscular dystrophy (DMD) has an incidence of approximately 1 in 3500 live male births.

DMD presents during early childhood, with difficulty running and climbing stairs. Most children are wheelchair bound by age 12 years, and die of pneumonia or cardiac dysfunction in their second decade. Becker muscular dystrophy presents later (around age 12), and most patients survive to their fourth or fifth decade. In both DMD and Becker muscular dystrophy, female carriers may have a slight to modest degree of weakness, and may also develop a dilated cardiomyopathy.[81]

There is no cure for the muscular dystrophies and treatment is supportive, with emphasis on respiratory care and treatment of cardiac complications. Respiratory interventions include aggressive chest physiotherapy, nocturnal intermittent positive pressure ventilation, and elective tracheostomy. Patients may require surgical interventions for contracture releases and scoliosis repair. Patients with muscular dystrophy are at elevated risk of perioperative complications, and should have an extensive workup before elective surgery (**Table 4**).[82]

Preoperative considerations
Preoperative counseling Patients are at increased risk of perioperative complications including cardiac arrest[83,84] and rhabdomyolysis, and should undergo preoperative counseling to address these risks. In addition, the patient's desires regarding resuscitation measures and advanced directive should be delineated and well documented.

Cardiac Cardiac involvement is common in patients with DMD[85] and manifests in a variety of forms, including rhythm abnormalities and cardiomyopathy. There have been many case reports of sudden death and congestive heart failure during surgery in this population. It is now recommended that patients undergo routine cardiac surveillance (including echocardiography) as soon as they receive a diagnosis of muscular dystrophy, as many times they develop cardiac dysfunction before symptoms are recognized.[86] Before surgery patients should undergo a thorough cardiac

Table 4
Preanesthetic and presedation considerations for patients with Duchenne muscular dystrophy

Initiation of noninvasive respiratory aids	1. Preoperative training in noninvasive positive pressure ventilation (NPPV) 2. Training in manual and mechanically assisted cough
Cardiac assessment and optimization	Consultation with cardiologist highly recommended because cardiac involvement can exist despite minimal respiratory involvement and normal resting electrocardiogram
Nutrition and gastrointestinal issues	1. Obtain serum albumin and prealbumin 2. Early use of NPPV to decrease work of breathing 3. Early therapy for dysphagia
Advanced directives	1. Clear understanding of risk of prolonged intubation or tracheostomy by patient 2. Consider temporary suspension of Do Not Resuscitate order

Data from Birnkrant DJ, Benditt JO, Carter ER, et al. American College of Chest Physicians consensus statement on the respiratory and related management of patients with Duchenne muscular dystrophy undergoing anesthesia or sedation. Chest 2007;132(6):1977–86.

workup, including dobutamine stress echocardiogram if cardiac abnormalities are present. The patient's medical therapy should also be optimized.[87]

Respiratory Patients should undergo preoperative assessment with a pulmonologist. Assessment should include measurement of FVC, maximum inspiratory pressure, maximum expiratory pressure, peak cough flow, and oxyhemoglobin saturation in room air. For patients who are deemed to be high risk, consideration should be made toward preoperative training in NPPV and manual and mechanically assisted cough.[88]

Gastrointestinal Patients with DMD often have smooth muscle dysfunction, which results in gastroparesis and delayed gastric emptying time. This dysmotility may also increase the risk of distention with mask ventilation. Gastric decompression with a nasogastric tube might be advisable following mask ventilation.

Myotonic Dystrophy

Myotonia is a clinical symptom characterized by persistent contraction of a muscle fiber after voluntary contraction or stimulation has stopped. Myotonic dystrophy is a group of heterozygous musculoskeletal disorders characterized by weakness.[89] The adult-onset form usually presents between the ages of 15 and 35 years. Ptosis and facial weakness are common manifestations. There may also be multisystem involvement including balding, defects in cardiac conduction, cataracts, and endocrine abnormalities.[90]

Preoperative considerations
Respiratory These patients may have diaphragmatic and accessory muscle atrophy, which predisposes them to postoperative respiratory complications.[91] Myotonic patients have impaired swallowing, putting them at higher risk of aspiration. Moreover, they are at increased risk of drug-induced central respiratory depression. Therefore, premedication and intraoperative narcotics should be carefully titrated.[92]

Cardiac Myotonic dystrophy can cause histologic alterations to the cardiac conduction system, such as fatty infiltration, fibrosis, and atrophy.[93] Therefore, they are at risk for conduction abnormalities, with first-degree heart block being the most common. There are also reports of paroxysmal complete heart block. Patients with myotonic dystrophy should receive an ECG at least annually, and especially before surgery.[94]

Gastrointestinal Patients with myotonic dystrophy have delayed gastric emptying, and this has been shown even in patients without gastrointestinal symptoms. Delayed gastric emptying has been shown to correlate with the duration of the disease.[95] Along with pharyngeal muscle weakness, this puts patients with myotonic dystrophy at higher risk for aspiration, and precautions should be taken.

Endocrine Patients often have concurrent endocrine abnormalities, including thyroid disease and diabetes. Both types of myotonic dystrophy are associated with insulin resistance. These illnesses should be screened for in the preoperative period and treated if necessary.

SUMMARY

Neuromuscular disorders are a heterogeneous group of diseases that often have systemic manifestations that coincide with their neurologic symptoms. There are anesthetic implications for both the primary neurologic disorder and the systemic disease, which may include increased risk of complications secondary to the actual anesthetic such as rhabdomyolysis, idiopathic reactions to muscle relaxants, and sensitivity to a variety of sedatives. There may also be an increased risk of arrhythmias, respiratory dysfunction, and aspiration secondary to comorbid pulmonary or cardiac disease. Patients with neuromuscular disorders should undergo preoperative evaluation in a multidisciplinary setting. Ideally the patient's primary care provider will take the lead role and seek input from a variety of perioperative physicians including anesthesiologists, surgeons, cardiologists, and neurologists. As many of these illnesses may be terminal, adequate preoperative assessment should include a discussion regarding end-of-life wishes.

REFERENCES

1. Bertorini TE. Introduction: evaluation of patients with neuromuscular disorders. In: Bertorini T, editor. Clinical evaluation and diagnostic tests for neuromuscular disorders: treatment and management. Philadelphia: Elsevier Saunders; 2011. p. 3–19.
2. Mitchell JD, Borasio GD. Amyotrophic lateral sclerosis. Lancet 2007;369(9578): 2031–41.
3. Miller RG, Mitchell JD, Moore DH. Riluzole for amyotrophic lateral sclerosis (ALS)/motor neuron disease (MND). The Cochrane Library 2012.
4. Short SO, Hillel AD. Palliative surgery in patients with bulbar amyotrophic lateral sclerosis. Head Neck 1989;11(4):364–9.
5. Hillel AD, Miller R. Bulbar amyotrophic lateral sclerosis: patterns of progression and clinical management. Head Neck 1989;11:51–9.
6. Miller RG, Jackson CE, Kasarskis EJ, et al. Practice parameter update: the care of the patient with amyotrophic lateral sclerosis: drug, nutritional, and respiratory therapies (an evidence-based review) Report of the Quality Standards Subcommittee of the American Academy of Neurology. Neurology 2009;73:1218–26.

7. Bach JR. Amyotrophic lateral sclerosis: prolongation of life by noninvasive respiratory AIDS. Chest 2002;122:92–8.
8. Sancho J, Servera E, Díaz J, et al. Efficacy of mechanical insufflation-exsufflation in medically stable patients with amyotrophic lateral sclerosis. Chest 2004;125: 1400–5.
9. Gallagher JP. Pathologic laughter and crying in ALS: a search for their origin. Acta Neurol Scand 1989;80:114–7.
10. Schiffer RB, Herndon RM, Rudick RA. Treatment of pathologic laughing and weeping with amitriptyline. N Engl J Med 1985;312:1480–2.
11. Andersen PM, Borasio GD, Dengler R, et al. Good practice in the management of amyotrophic lateral sclerosis: clinical guidelines. An evidence-based review with good practice points. EALSC Working Group. Amyotroph Lateral Scler 2007;8:195–213.
12. Huyse FJ, Touw DJ, Van Schijndel RS, et al. Psychotropic drugs and the perioperative period: a proposal for a guideline in elective surgery. Psychosomatics 2006;47:8–22.
13. Lunn MR, Wang CH. Spinal muscular atrophy. Lancet 2008;371:2120–33.
14. Phillips DP, Roye DP Jr, Farcy JP, et al. Surgical treatment of scoliosis in a spinal muscular atrophy population. Spine (Phila Pa 1976) 1990;15:942–5.
15. Samaha FJ, Buncher CR, Russman BS, et al. Pulmonary function in spinal muscular atrophy. J Child Neurol 1994;9:326–9.
16. Chng SY, Wong YQ, Hui JH, et al. Pulmonary function and scoliosis in children with spinal muscular atrophy types II and III. J Paediatr Child Health 2003;39: 673–6.
17. Heier CR, Satta R, Lutz C, et al. Arrhythmia and cardiac defects are a feature of spinal muscular atrophy model mice. Hum Mol Genet 2010;19:3906–18.
18. Tanaka H, Uemura N, Toyama Y, et al. Cardiac involvement in the Kugelberg-Welander syndrome. Am J Cardiol 1976;38:528–32.
19. Roos M, Sarkozy A, Chierchia GB, et al. Malignant ventricular arrhythmia in a case of adult onset of spinal muscular atrophy (Kugelberg-Welander disease). J Cardiovasc Electrophysiol 2009;20:342–4.
20. Palladino A, Passamano L, Taglia A, et al. Cardiac involvement in patients with spinal muscular atrophies. Acta Myol 2011;30:175–8.
21. Flachenecker P. Epidemiology of neuroimmunological diseases. J Neurol 2006; 253:2–8.
22. Rudick RA, Cohen JA, Weinstock-Guttman B, et al. Management of multiple sclerosis. N Engl J Med 1997;337:1604–11.
23. Dorotta IR, Schubert A. Multiple sclerosis and anesthetic implications. Curr Opin Anaesthesiol 2002;15:365–70.
24. Koff MD, Cohen JA, McIntyre JJ, et al. Severe brachial plexopathy after an ultrasound-guided single-injection nerve block for total shoulder arthroplasty in a patient with multiple sclerosis. Anesthesiology 2008;108:325–8.
25. Bader AM, Hunt CO, Datta S, et al. Anesthesia for the obstetric patient with multiple sclerosis. J Clin Anesth 1988;1:21–4.
26. Vita G, Carolina Fazio M, Milone S, et al. Cardiovascular autonomic dysfunction in multiple sclerosis is likely related to brainstem lesions. J Neurol Sci 1993;120: 82–6.
27. Howard RS, Wiles CM, Hirsch NP, et al. Respiratory involvement in multiple sclerosis. Brain 1992;115:479–94.
28. Smeltzer SC, Utell MJ, Rudick RA, et al. Pulmonary function and dysfunction in multiple sclerosis. Arch Neurol 1988;45:1245.

29. Scanzello CR, Figgie MP, Nestor BJ, et al. Perioperative management of medications used in the treatment of rheumatoid arthritis. HSS J 2006;2:141–7.
30. Available at: http://www.fscip.org/facts.htm. Accessed December 28, 2012.
31. Hambly PR, Martin B. Anaesthesia for chronic spinal cord lesions. Anaesthesia 1998;53:273–89.
32. Stevens RD, Bhardwaj A, Kirsch JR, et al. Critical care and perioperative management in traumatic spinal cord injury. J Neurosurg Anesthesiol 2003;15: 215–29.
33. Fehlings MG, Tator CH. An evidence-based review of decompressive surgery in acute spinal cord injury: rationale, indications, and timing based on experimental and clinical studies. J Neurosurg 1999;91:1–11.
34. Schonwald G, Fish KJ, Perkash I. Cardiovascular complications during anesthesia in chronic spinal cord injured patients. Anesthesiology 1981;55:550–8.
35. McKinley WO, Jackson AB, Cardenas DD, et al. Long-term medical complications after traumatic spinal cord injury: a regional model systems analysis. Arch Phys Med Rehabil 1990;80:1402–10.
36. Dumont RJ, Okonkwo DO, Verma S, et al. Acute spinal cord injury, part I: pathophysiologic mechanisms. Clin Neuropharmacol 2001;24:254–64.
37. Dumont RJ, Verma S, Okonkwo DO, et al. Acute spinal cord injury, part II: contemporary pharmacotherapy. Clin Neuropharmacol 2001;24:265–79.
38. Colachis SC 3rd. Autonomic hyperreflexia with spinal cord injury. J Am Paraplegia Soc 1992;15:171–86.
39. Brown BT, Carrion HM, Politano VA. Guanethidine sulfate in the prevention of autonomic hyperreflexia. J Urol 1979;122:55–7.
40. Lambert DH, Deane RS, Mazuzan JE. Anesthesia and the control of blood pressure in patients with spinal cord injury. Anesth Analg 1982;61:344–8.
41. Brown R, DiMarco AF, Hoit JD, et al. Respiratory dysfunction and management in spinal cord injury. Respir Care 2006;51(8):853–68.
42. Kao CH, Ho YJ, Changlai SP, et al. Gastric emptying in spinal cord injury patients. Dig Dis Sci 1999;44:1512–5.
43. Segal JL, Milne N, Brunnemann SR, et al. Metoclopramide-induced normalization of impaired gastric emptying in spinal cord injury. Am J Gastroenterol 1987;82:1143–8.
44. Maynard FM, Karunas RS, Waring WP III. Epidemiology of spasticity following traumatic spinal cord injury. Arch Phys Med Rehabil 1990;71:566–9.
45. Penn RD, Savoy SM, Corcos D, et al. Intrathecal baclofen for severe spinal spasticity. N Engl J Med 1989;320:1517–21.
46. Green LB, Nelson VS. Death after acute withdrawal of intrathecal baclofen: case report and literature review. Arch Phys Med Rehabil 1999;80:1600–4.
47. Grider JS, Brown RE, Colclough GW. Perioperative management of patients with an intrathecal drug delivery system for chronic pain. Anesth Analg 2008;107:1393–6.
48. Pareyson D, Marchesi C. Diagnosis, natural history, and management of Charcot-Marie-Tooth disease. Lancet Neurol 2009;8:654–67.
49. Antognini JF. Anaesthesia for Charcot-Marie-Tooth disease: a review of 86 cases. Can J Anaesth 1992;39:398–400.
50. Aboussouan LS, Lewis RA, Shy ME. Disorders of pulmonary function, sleep, and the upper airway in Charcot-Marie-Tooth disease. Lung 2007;185:1–7.
51. Tetzlaff JE, Schwendt I. Arrhythmia and Charcot-Marie-Tooth disease during anesthesia. Can J Anaesth 2000;47:829.
52. Isner JM, Hawley RJ, Weintraub AM, et al. Cardiac findings in Charcot-Marie-Tooth disease: a prospective study of 68 patients. Arch Intern Med 1979;139:1161–5.

53. Yuki N, Hartung HP. Guillain-Barré syndrome. N Engl J Med 2012;366:2294–304.
54. Hughes RA, Wijdicks E, Barohn RJ, et al. Practice parameter: immunotherapy for Guillain-Barré syndrome: report of the Quality Standards Subcommittee of the American Academy of Neurology. Neurology 2003;61:736–40.
55. Sharshar T, Chevret S, Bourdain F, et al. Early predictors of mechanical ventilation in Guillain-Barré syndrome. Crit Care Med 2003;31:278–83.
56. Hahn AF. The challenge of respiratory dysfunction in Guillain-Barré syndrome. Arch Neurol 2001;58:871–2.
57. Hughes RC, Wijdicks EM, Benson E, et al. Supportive care for patients with Guillain-Barré syndrome. Arch Neurol 2005;62:1194–8.
58. Lichtenfeld P. Autonomic dysfunction in the Guillain-Barré syndrome. Am J Med 1971;50:772–80.
59. Moulin DE, Hagen N, Feasby TE, et al. Pain in Guillain-Barré syndrome. Neurology 1997;48:328–31.
60. Pandey CK, Bose N, Garg G, et al. Gabapentin for the treatment of pain in Guillain-Barré syndrome: a double-blinded, placebo-controlled, crossover study. Anesth Analg 2002;95:1719–23.
61. Pandey CK, Raza M, Tripathi M, et al. The comparative evaluation of gabapentin and carbamazepine for pain management in Guillain-Barré syndrome patients in the intensive care unit. Anesth Analg 2005;101:220–5.
62. Hughes RA, Anthony VS, van Doorn PA. Corticosteroids for Guillain-Barré syndrome. Cochrane Database Syst Rev 2010;(2):CD001446.
63. Drachman DB. Myasthenia gravis. N Engl J Med 1994;330:1797–810.
64. Mantegazza R, Bonanno S, Camera G, et al. Current and emerging therapies for the treatment of myasthenia gravis. Neuropsychiatr Dis Treat 2011;7:151.
65. Mulder DG, Herrmann C, Keesey J, et al. Thymectomy for myasthenia gravis. Am J Surg 1983;146:61–6.
66. Pinching AJ, Peters DK, Newsom-Davis J. Remission of myasthenia gravis following plasma-exchange. Lancet 1976;308:1373–6.
67. Gajdos P, Chevret S, Clair B, et al. Clinical trial of plasma exchange and high-dose intravenous immunoglobulin in myasthenia gravis. Ann Neurol 2004;41:789–96.
68. Juel VC. Myasthenia gravis: management of myasthenic crisis and perioperative care. Semin Neurol 2004;24:74–81.
69. Herz BL. Colonic anastomotic disruption in myasthenia gravis. Dis Colon Rectum 1987;30:809–11.
70. Boelaert K, Newby PR, Simmonds MJ, et al. Prevalence and relative risk of other autoimmune diseases in subjects with autoimmune thyroid disease. Am J Med 2010;123:183.
71. Bhinder S, Majithia V, Harisdangkul V. Myasthenia gravis and systemic lupus erythematosus: truly associated or coincidental—two case reports and review of the literature. Clin Rheumatol 2006;25:555–6.
72. Kohn PM, Tucker HJ, Kozokoff NJ. The cardiac manifestations of myasthenia gravis with particular reference to electrocardiographic abnormalities. Am J Med Sci 1965;249:561–9.
73. Guglin M, Campellone JV, Heintz K, et al. Cardiac disease in myasthenia gravis: a literature review. J Clin Neuromuscul Dis 2003;4:199–203.
74. Vernino S, Cheshire WP, Lennon VA. Myasthenia gravis with autoimmune autonomic neuropathy. Auton Neurosci 2001;88:187–92.
75. Leventhal SR, Orkin FK, Hirsh RA. Prediction of the need for postoperative mechanical ventilation in myasthenia gravis. Anesthesiology 1980;53:26–30.

76. Kaneda H, Saito Y, Saito T, et al. Preoperative steroid therapy stabilizes postoperative respiratory conditions in myasthenia gravis. Gen Thorac Cardiovasc Surg 2008;56:114–8.

77. Endo S, Yamaguchi T, Saito N, et al. Experience with programmed steroid treatment with thymectomy in nonthymomatous myasthenia gravis. Ann Thorac Surg 2004;77:1745.

78. Brown CJ, Donald Buie W. Perioperative stress dose steroids: do they make a difference? J Am Coll Surg 2001;193:678–86.

79. Adams DC, Heyer EJ. Problems of anesthesia in patients with neuromuscular disease. Anaesthesiol Clin 1997;15:673–89.

80. O'neill JH, Murray NM, Newsom-Davis J. The Lambert-Eaton myasthenic syndrome. A review of 50 cases. Brain 1998;111:577–96.

81. Emery AE. The muscular dystrophies. Lancet 2002;359:687–95.

82. Morris P. Duchenne muscular dystrophy: a challenge for the anesthetist. Paediatr Anaesth 1997;7:1–4.

83. Sethna N, Rockoff MA, Worthen M, et al. Anesthesia-related complications in children with Duchenne muscular dystrophy. Anesthesiology 1988;68:462–4.

84. Larsen UT, Juhl B, Hein-Sørensen O, et al. Complications during anaesthesia in patients with Duchenne's muscular dystrophy (a retrospective study). Can J Anaesth 1989;36:418–22.

85. Gilroy JH, Gahalan JL, Berman R, et al. Cardiac and pulmonary complications in Duchenne's progressive muscular dystrophy. Circulation 1963;27:484–93.

86. Nigro G, Comi LI, Politano L, et al. The incidence and evolution of cardiomyopathy in Duchenne muscular dystrophy. Int J Cardiol 1990;26:271–7.

87. Cripe LH, Klitnzer TT, Beekman RH, et al. Cardiovascular health supervision for individuals affected by Duchenne or Becker muscular dystrophy. Pediatrics 2005;116:1569–73.

88. Birnkrant DJ, Panitch HB, Benditt JO, et al. American College of Chest Physicians consensus statement on the respiratory and related management of patients with Duchenne muscular dystrophy undergoing anesthesia or sedation. Chest 2007;132:1977–86.

89. Russell SH, Hirsch NP. Anaesthesia and myotonia. Br J Anaesth 1994;72:210–7.

90. Aldridge LM. Anaesthetic problems in myotonic dystrophy: a case report and review of the Aberdeen experience comprising 48 general anaesthetics in a further 16 patients. Br J Anaesth 1985;57:1119–30.

91. Mathieu J, Allard P, Gobeil G, et al. Anesthetic and surgical complications in 219 cases of myotonic dystrophy. Neurology 1997;49:1646–50.

92. Mudge BJ, Taylor PB, Vanderspek AF. Perioperative hazards in myotonic dystrophy. Anaesthesia 2007;35:492–5.

93. Nguyen HH, Wolfe JT III, Holmes DR Jr, et al. Pathology of the cardiac conduction system in myotonic dystrophy: a study of 12 cases. J Am Coll Cardiol 1988; 11:662–71.

94. Griggs RC, Davis RJ, Anderson DC, et al. Cardiac conduction in myotonic dystrophy. Am J Med 1975;59:37–42.

95. Bellini M, Alduini P, Costa F, et al. Gastric emptying in myotonic dystrophic patients. Dig Liver Dis 2002;34:484–8.

Patients with Ischemic Heart Disease

Patrick N. Odonkor, MB, ChB, Alina M. Grigore, MD, MHS*

KEYWORDS

- Perioperative management of ischemic heart disease
- Perioperative cardiac risk assessment • Noncardiac surgery • Coronary stents
- Myocardial ischemia • Coronary artery disease

KEY POINTS

- Major clinical factors associated with perioperative cardiac events (PCEs) are: (1) unstable coronary syndromes, (2) decompensated heart failure, (3) significant dysrhythmias, and (4) severe valvular heart disease.
- Major aortic and peripheral vascular surgeries are associated with high risk for PCEs.
- Perioperative use of antiplatelet agents in patients with coronary stents involves a multi-disciplinary approach that depends on the type of stent and the type of surgical procedure.
- Preoperative initiation of β-blocker therapy in high- and intermediate-risk patients reduces the incidence of PCEs.
- Preoperative optimization of coexisting disease modifies the risk for morbidity and improves postoperative outcomes.

Ischemic heart disease (IHD) occurs when myocardial oxygen supply is not adequate for myocardial oxygen demand. It is most commonly caused by coronary artery disease (CAD), and the 2 terms are often used interchangeably. In the United States as many as 15.4 million Americans aged 20 years and older suffer from CAD, which represents a major cause of morbidity and mortality. In 2009, about 1 in every 6 deaths in the United States was caused by CAD.[1] According to some estimates, close to one-third of patients undergoing noncardiac surgery in the United States have either CAD or risk factors associated with CAD.[2] IHD is an independent predictor of cardiac complications after major noncardiac surgery.[3] Major perioperative cardiac events (PCEs) that occur in patients with IHD include perioperative myocardial infarction (MI), heart failure (HF), ventricular dysrhythmias, cardiac arrest, and death. The occurrence of PCEs is associated with increased costs of health care. The detection of CAD before surgery makes it possible to initiate appropriate interventions before elective

Department of Anesthesiology, University of Maryland School of Medicine, Suite S8D12 22 South Greene Street, Baltimore, MD 21201, USA
* Corresponding author.
E-mail address: agrigore@anes.umm.edu

Med Clin N Am 97 (2013) 1033–1050
http://dx.doi.org/10.1016/j.mcna.2013.05.006
0025-7125/13/$ – see front matter © 2013 Elsevier Inc. All rights reserved.

noncardiac surgical procedures and to limit the occurrence of PCEs. In patients undergoing emergent procedures that cannot be delayed, perioperative interventions that reduce the incidence of major cardiac complications can be initiated. Appropriate perioperative surveillance for ischemia must be instituted, with patients being managed in the intensive care setting if necessary.

PERIOPERATIVE RISK ASSESSMENT

Multiple clinical indices are available for the assessment of perioperative cardiac risk. The revised cardiac risk index by Lee and colleagues[3] is easy to use and consists of 6 independent predictors for perioperative complications in stable patients undergoing elective noncardiac surgery. These predictive factors are: (1) history of IHD, (2) high-risk surgery, (3) history of congestive heart failure (CHF), (4) history of cerebrovascular disease, (5) preoperative treatment of diabetes with insulin, and (6) preoperative serum creatinine level greater than 2.0 mg/dL (**Box 1**). During the development of the revised cardiac risk index, the factors that defined preoperative IHD, with the highest correlation to major cardiac complications, were: (1) current chest pain caused by myocardial ischemia, (2) use of nitrate therapy, (3) pathologic Q wave on electrocardiogram (ECG), (4) history of MI, or (5) history of positive exercise test for ischemia. There was no significant difference in the incidence of major cardiac complications in patients who did not exhibit any of these factors, even if they had undergone prior revascularization procedures with coronary artery bypass graft (CABG) surgery or percutaneous coronary intervention (PCI). To minimize perioperative risk, the decision about which patients with IHD need further evaluation before elective surgical procedures should be considered carefully.

In the 2007 American College of Cardiology/American Heart Association (ACC/AHA) guidelines for perioperative cardiovascular evaluation for noncardiac surgery, clinical risk factors for PCEs were grouped into high-, intermediate-, and low-risk categories (**Table 1**). High-risk or major clinical risk factors that predicted PCEs were: (1) active cardiac conditions such as unstable coronary syndromes, including unstable angina, severe angina, or recent MI; (2) decompensated HF; (3) significant dysrhythmias; and (4) severe valvular heart disease. The major clinical risk factors include: (1) a history of MI within 1 month, (2) the presence of clinical symptoms of myocardial ischemia, (3) a

---

Box 1
Six independent variables from the revised cardiac risk index associated with increased incidence of major cardiac complications after major nonemergent nonvascular surgery

1. History of ischemic heart disease

2. High-risk surgery

3. History of congestive heart failure

4. History of cerebrovascular disease

5. Preoperative treatment of diabetics with insulin

6. Preoperative serum creatinine level greater than 2.0 mg/dL

The presence of 2 or more of these variables was associated with significantly higher complication rates.

Data from Lee TH, Marcantonio ER, Mangione CM, et al. Derivation and prospective validation of a simple index for prediction of cardiac risk of major noncardiac surgery. Circulation 1999;100:1043–9.

Table 1 Association of clinical conditions with risk for perioperative cardiac events	
High-risk or major risk factors (active cardiac conditions)	Unstable coronary syndromes Unstable angina Severe angina Recent myocardial infarction Decompensated heart failure Significant dysrhythmias Uncontrolled supraventricular dysrhythmias Symptomatic ventricular dysrhythmias Severe valvular heart disease
Intermediate-risk factors (independent clinical risk factors from revised cardiac risk index)	History of ischemic heart disease History of congestive heart failure History of cerebrovascular disease Preoperative treatment of diabetics with insulin Preoperative serum creatinine level greater than 2.0 mg/dL
Minor risk factors	Minor conduction or rhythm abnormalities Left ventricular hypertrophy on resting electrocardiogram Uncontrolled systemic hypertension Advanced age

positive stress test, and (4) a history of decompensated HF caused by IHD. In patients who present with any of these major clinical risk factors for PCEs, delay or cancellation of elective surgical procedures allows time for appropriate management and optimization of these active cardiac conditions before surgery. The category of intermediate clinical risk factors consisted of the factors from the revised cardiac risk index. Even though the type of surgery was included in the revised cardiac risk index, the risk for PCEs associated with type of surgery was discussed separately. This intermediate-risk group includes patients with a history of IHD, such as a history of MI more than 1 month before surgery or a Q wave on their ECG. In such patients, the risk for PCEs is low if they have a negative myocardial stress test. In addition, in the 2007 ACA/AHA guidelines, the following conditions were classified as minor risk factors for PCEs: (1) minor conduction or rhythm abnormalities, (2) left ventricular hypertrophy (LVH) on resting ECG, (3) uncontrolled systemic hypertension, and (4) advanced age.[4] The presence of multiple risk factors confers greater risk for PCEs than the presence of only 1 factor. For example, multiple minor risk factors in an asymptomatic 70-year-old patient with poorly controlled hypertension, with evidence of LVH on preoperative ECG and who also has a harsh murmur in the second right-intercostal space, may be predictive of high risk for PCEs. This patient may need further evaluation for IHD and valvular abnormality before proceeding with surgery. Increased risk for PCEs associated with multiple risk factors also occurs in patients with intermediate and major clinical risk factors.

Another factor that should be considered during preoperative risk assessment is the type of surgical procedure and its association with the occurrence of major cardiac complications (**Table 2**).[4] High-risk surgery is one of the independent predictors for major cardiac complications after noncardiac surgery in the revised cardiac risk index.[3] High-risk surgical procedures include major vascular surgery, because patients who undergo major vascular procedures have underlying cardiovascular diseases that predispose them to perioperative cardiovascular complications. Severe or symptomatic large-vessel peripheral arterial disease has been associated with an

Table 2	
Cardiac risk[a] stratification for noncardiac surgical procedures	
Risk Stratification	**Procedure Examples**
Vascular (reported cardiac risk often more than 5%)	Aortic and other major vascular surgery Peripheral vascular surgery
Intermediate (reported cardiac risk generally 1%–5%)	Intraperitoneal and intrathoracic surgery Carotid endarterectomy Head and neck surgery Orthopedic surgery Prostate surgery
Low[b] (reported cardiac risk generally <1%)	Endoscopic procedures Superficial procedures Cataract surgery Breast surgery Ambulatory surgery

[a] Combined incidence of cardiac death and nonfatal myocardial infarction.
[b] These procedures do not generally require further preoperative cardiac testing.
    Data from Fleisher LA, Beckman JA, Brown KA, et al. ACC/AHA 2007 Guidelines on perioperative cardiovascular evaluation and care for noncardiac surgery: a report of the American College of Cardiology/American Heart Association Task Force on Practice Guidelines (Writing Committee to revise the 2002 guidelines on perioperative cardiovascular evaluation for noncardiac surgery). Circulation 2007;116:e429.

increased risk for death from cardiovascular causes, including IHD.[5] This risk may be independent of whether such patients have surgery or not. Major open-thoracic, head and neck, abdominal, and orthopedic procedures, as well as other prolonged surgical procedures associated with significant stress response, major blood loss, pain, and significant hemodynamic changes, are intermediate-risk surgical procedures, with a reported 1% to 5% risk for PCEs. Low-risk procedures for PCEs are less invasive, for example: (1) laparoscopic and endoscopic procedures, (2) ambulatory and superficial surgical procedures, and (3) ophthalmologic procedures such as cataract surgery. Relatively short procedures not associated with significant bleeding or major fluid shifts also carry a low risk for perioperative cardiac complications.

The following recommendations were taken from the 2007 ACC/AHA guidelines for perioperative cardiovascular evaluation and care for noncardiac surgery.[4] Preoperative assessment of functional status serves as a guide for perioperative risk assessment and the need for further evaluation by stress tests before elective surgery. Patients who are asymptomatic at high levels of exertion are at low risk for PCEs; therefore, they are unlikely to benefit from further testing before elective surgery. Poor exercise tolerance, defined as inability to walk 4 blocks or climb 2 flights of stairs, has been associated with serious perioperative complications.[6] Functional activity can also be expressed as metabolic equivalents (METs), with 4 METs being equivalent to poor functional tolerance. **Fig. 1** shows an algorithm for cardiac evaluation and care for patients 50 years or older who are undergoing noncardiac surgery based on active clinical conditions, known cardiovascular disease, or cardiac risk factors.[4] In patients with poor or unknown functional capacity, the need for further evaluation may be determined by the presence of clinical risk factors and type of surgery (see **Tables 1** and **2**). In patients with 3 or more clinical risk factors undergoing high-risk surgery, such as open vascular surgery whereby patients may already have underlying cardiovascular disease, testing should be done if it will change management. In patients with 1 or 2 clinical risk factors who are undergoing high-risk or intermediate-risk surgery, it is reasonable to proceed with the surgery, either maintaining heart rate control with β-blocker therapy, where

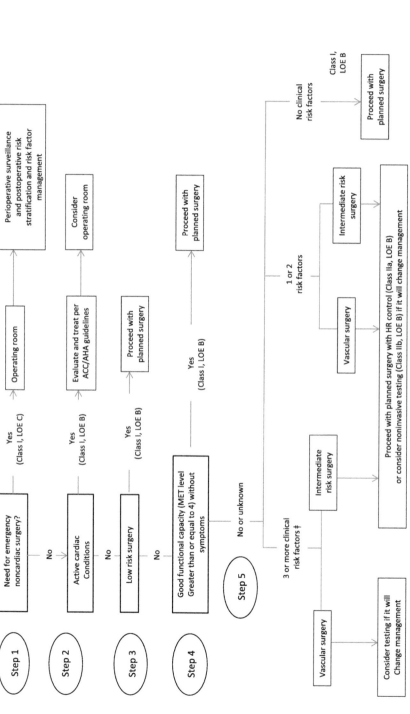

Fig. 1. Cardiac evaluation and care algorithm for noncardiac surgery based on active clinical conditions, known cardiovascular disease, or cardiac risk factors for patients 50 years of age or older. ACC/AHA, American College of Cardiology/American Heart Association; HR, heart rate; LOE, level of evidence; MET, metabolic equivalent. (*From* Fleisher LA, Beckman JA, Brown KA, et al. ACC/AHA 2007 Guidelines on perioperative cardiovascular evaluation and care for noncardiac surgery: a report of the American College of Cardiology/American Heart Association Task Force on Practice Guidelines (Writing Committee to revise the 2002 guidelines on perioperative cardiovascular evaluation for noncardiac surgery). Circulation 2007;116:e428; with permission.)

appropriate, or considering further specific testing if it will change management. The management strategy is less clear for patients who are undergoing intermediate-risk surgery with poor or unknown functional capacity and 3 or more clinical factors.

In patients who need acute emergent surgical procedures, delay is not possible. Such patients should proceed to surgery, but with more vigilant perioperative monitoring (continuous blood pressure monitoring via arterial access, central venous access, cardiac output monitoring, transesophageal echocardiography) and pharmacologic interventions that have been associated with lower risk for PCEs, such as appropriate perioperative use of β-blockers. High-risk patients may be transferred for emergency surgery in a center that has a cardiac catheterization laboratory, to facilitate early evaluation and management of perioperative ischemic events if they do occur. Postoperative care should be undertaken in a setting such as an intensive care unit, where evidence of myocardial ischemia can be promptly detected and managed appropriately. Appropriate interventions and management must be continued in the postoperative and post-hospitalization period. For example, long-term use of β-blockers and lipid-lowering therapy should be encouraged, with plans in place for long-term follow-up by a cardiologist.

PREOPERATIVE ASSESSMENT OF PATIENTS WITH ISCHEMIC HEART DISEASE

Preoperative clinical assessment of noncardiac surgery is usually performed a few days before the scheduled day of surgery. For patients with IHD, this assessment should generally follow along the lines of the perioperative risk assessment already described; however, it cannot be done in isolation, because patients with IHD tend to have other coexisting medical conditions. The most common symptoms encountered in patients presenting with IHD are: (1) angina, (2) dyspnea, (3) cough, (4) edema, (5) palpitations, and (6) syncopal episodes. As part of the natural progression of the disease, patients with advanced, chronic, ischemic heart conditions often present with a history of: (1) prior angina, (2) unstable coronary syndromes, (3) MI, (4) arrhythmias, (5) decompensated HF, (6) presence of pacemaker (PM) or implantable cardioverter-defibrillator (ICD) (a topic discussed in the article by Shulman and colleagues elsewhere in this issue), (7) severe valvular disease, and (8) pulmonary hypertension. A thorough history, physical examination, and appropriate preoperative testing allow for the identification and subsequent optimization of coexisting diseases, which could modify risk for morbidity and affect the postoperative outcome. Examples of coexisting diseases include: (1) clinical conditions from the revised cardiac risk index, (2) peripheral vascular disease, (3) hepatic dysfunction, (4) chronic pulmonary disease, (5) pulmonary hypertension, (6) systemic hypertension, and (7) obesity. The results of preoperative testing in these patients can then be used to assess the need for interventions before scheduled surgery. For example, a preoperative echocardiogram can reveal the cause of valvular heart disease, and quantitatively assess valvular function as well as left ventricular and right ventricular function.

Current medications must be accurately recorded. Medications that are used in the management of IHD include: (1) β-blockers, (2) antiplatelet agents, (3) renin-angiotensin-aldosterone antagonists, (4) lipid-lowering agents, (5) nitrates, and (6) α2-agonists. Their indications, interaction with other medications (including anesthetic agents), and side-effect profiles must be taken into consideration in formulating plans for perioperative management. Appropriate management of commonly used medications (including phosphodiesterase-5 [PDE5] inhibitors, alcohol, tobacco, and over-the-counter, herbal, and illicit drugs) and awareness about drug interactions are also important. For example, administration of intravenous nitroglycerin is contraindicated in patients receiving a PDE5 inhibitor (sildenafil) for the treatment of erectile dysfunction or pulmonary hypertension.

Perioperative risk assessment and guidelines should be viewed as valuable tools in formulating and implementing an individual plan for perioperative management in individual patients. Guidelines and recommendations for perioperative management of other clinical conditions such as pulmonary diseases may also be blended into the plan for perioperative management.

PATHOPHYSIOLOGY OF PERIOPERATIVE MYOCARDIAL ISCHEMIA

The underlying pathophysiologic mechanisms that cause perioperative myocardial ischemia (PMI) and infarction are not well understood. When myocardial oxygen demand is greater than myocardial oxygen supply, myocardial ischemia occurs. During the perioperative period, multiple factors related to stress, such as neurohormonal changes, pain, dehydration, bleeding, hypertension, hypotension, and tachycardia, potentiate this imbalance, leading to PMI. Stress-induced PMI associated with MI (1) is preceded most often by ST-segment depression on ECG; (2) is most often a non–Q-wave MI; (3) is mostly silent (>50%); and (4) most commonly occurs in the early postoperative period, usually within the first 48 hours after surgery. It occurs more commonly in patients with stable CAD who also have significant narrowing of their coronary vessels.[7] Plaque rupture and coronary thrombosis associated with acute coronary syndromes usually occur in coronary vessels that are not severely narrowed by atherosclerotic plaque, and are associated with an acute obstruction in blood flow in coronary vessels, secondary to thrombus formation. Acute coronary syndromes may also occur in the perioperative period. In patients who have had PCIs, with or without stenting, predisposition to thrombosis at the intervention site depends on whether healing and endothelialization have occurred. This risk is discussed further in the section on PCI and coronary stents.

PERIOPERATIVE TESTING FOR ISCHEMIC HEART DISEASE

Preoperative resting 12-lead ECG is a low-cost screening tool for cardiac diseases such as IHD, dysrhythmias, and LVH. It is frequently obtained during preoperative evaluation of patients undergoing noncardiac surgery. Although there is evidence that ischemic changes on preoperative resting ECG may be predictive of increased risk for perioperative morbidity and mortality secondary to coronary events,[8] an abnormal preoperative resting 12-lead ECG test does not necessarily predict postoperative cardiac complications.[9] Conversely, the absence of abnormalities on the preoperative resting ECG does not imply the absence of IHD. For example, patients with stable angina may only manifest ischemic changes on their ECG when they are experiencing angina. Preoperative resting ECG may be helpful in determining which patients require further evaluation before elective surgical procedures. During the development of the revised cardiac risk index, pathologic Q waves on the ECG were associated with a high correlation for major cardiac complications.[3] Changes on the ECG associated with ischemia (eg, Q waves, ST-T wave changes, and LVH) can alert the physician to patients who risk developing PMI complications. Other changes related to conduction and rhythm abnormalities can also help predict which patients risk progressing to more malignant dysrhythmias that may progress to PMI complications. As an example, patients who have bundle branch block on their preoperative resting ECG should be carefully evaluated for IHD, because this finding may be associated with the occurrence of postoperative ischemic events.[10] However, the decision to further test a patient with an abnormal resting 12-lead ECG must take into account both the type of surgery and the patient's functional capacity. Further testing is only useful if it leads to a change in management that will reduce the risk for perioperative cardiac complications.

The 2007 ACC/AHA guidelines recommend checking the resting 12-lead ECG in patients with at least 1 clinical risk factor (intermediate risk factors from **Table 1**) who are undergoing vascular surgical procedures, and also in patients with known IHD, peripheral arterial disease, and cerebrovascular disease who are undergoing intermediate-risk surgical procedures (see **Table 2**). Patients who have a good functional capacity and who are undergoing a low-risk surgical procedure may not need further testing before surgery. An ECG within 30 days of the date of surgery is generally accepted as adequate.[4]

Exercise ECG testing is a noninvasive stress test for assessing risk for ischemic response in patients with known or suspected IHD. It also provides information about the patient's functional capacity. A negative exercise ECG test at high workload points to good functional capacity with a low risk for PCEs. A positive test at low workload is associated with high risk for perioperative and long-term cardiac events. Exercise ECG testing is not a highly specific or sensitive test for IHD, and test results are influenced by other factors such as baseline myocardial function, the age of the patient, and the severity of underlying coronary disease. In patients who are unable to exercise because of physical limitations unrelated to heart disease, a pharmacologic stress ECG may be done by administering dobutamine to increase the heart rate while monitoring for ischemic ECG changes.

Other noninvasive stress tests may be done on patients who have evidence of IHD such as stable or unstable angina, recent history of MI, and/or evidence of ischemia on resting ECG or exercise ECG, as well as on patients who are unable to exercise to adequate workloads. Preoperative stress testing is commonly done by either dobutamine stress echocardiography (DSE) or adenosine or dipyridamole myocardial perfusion imaging, using either thallium-201 or technetium-99m. The detection of new or worsening wall-motion abnormalities on DSE is associated with increased risk for PCEs, and DSE appears to be even better at predicting risk for PCEs in patients with clinical risk factors such as IHD, HF, and diabetes.[4] The myocardial perfusion test is highly sensitive in the detection of risk for PCEs in patients with reversible perfusion defects, and it appears that risk for PCEs is directly proportional to the size of the reversible defect. Myocardial perfusion tests may also predict long-term cardiac events in patients with fixed perfusion defects. Because of its overall low positive predictive value, these tests are probably best used in patients at high clinical risk for PCEs.[4] Patients who test positive during noninvasive stress tests may undergo further evaluation with coronary angiography to assess the coronary vasculature for both the site and the severity of disease.

Coronary angiography makes it possible to delineate the presence and extent of disease in the coronary vessels of patients with IHD. A decision can then be made about need for coronary revascularization either by PCI and stenting or by cardiac surgery before elective noncardiac surgery. The 2007 ACC/AHA guidelines recommend coronary revascularization before noncardiac surgery in patients with stable angina who also have either significant left main CAD or 3-vessel CAD, and in patients with stable angina who have 2-vessel CAD with significant stenosis of the proximal left anterior descending artery and either an ejection fraction of less than 50% or demonstrable ischemia on noninvasive testing. Coronary revascularization before elective noncardiac surgery is also recommended in patients presenting with high-risk unstable angina, non–ST-segment elevation MI, or acute ST-elevation MI. In general, the indication for preoperative revascularization is similar to that for coronary revascularization, irrespective of the need for noncardiac surgery.[4] The decision about revascularization should generally follow ACC/AHA guidelines for surgery or PCI. Appropriate timing for elective noncardiac surgery after revascularization is not clearly defined. Some studies have advocated waiting 1 month after CABG surgery before proceeding with major vascular surgery.[11]

PERCUTANEOUS CORONARY INTERVENTION AND CORONARY STENTS

The use of balloon angioplasty or atherectomy to relieve obstruction in coronary vessels is usually referred to as PCI, and is typically done simultaneously with the introduction of coronary stents. Balloon angioplasty, when done alone, confers a relatively higher risk for restenosis of the coronary vessel, as well as an increased propensity toward additional revascularization procedures in the coronary vessel when compared with the concomitant use of coronary stents.[12] Application of coronary stents at the time of PCI is now more routinely done in patients whose lesions can be appropriately managed with stents.

There are 2 main types of coronary stent currently in clinical use in the United States. The first type is the bare-metal stent (BMS), made of either stainless steel or cobalt chromium. The introduction of BMS in clinical practice resulted in a decline in both the incidence of acute coronary obstruction during PCI and the rate at which patients required subsequent interventions to treat restenosis after PCI. The second type consists of drug-eluting stents (DES), which are made of the same material but are designed to deliver drugs, such as paclitaxel, sirolimus, everolimus and zotarolimus, into the coronary vessels. The introduction of DES into clinical practice resulted in an even greater decline in restenosis rates. One significant problem with DES is late-stent thrombosis, which is caused by delayed stent endothelialization and usually occurs more than 30 days after PCI. The risk for late-stent thrombosis may still be present several years after stent implantation.

In-stent thrombus formation is a potential complication associated with the use of stents, and is a major cause of significant morbidity and mortality. Administration of antiplatelet medications, usually in the form of dual-antiplatelet therapy (DAPT) until the stent has been completely endothelialized, can prevent stent thrombosis.

Recent data have shown that discontinuation of DAPT beyond 6 months in patients with DES does not appear to have a large impact on the risk of adverse cardiac events.[13,14] However, it is unclear whether these findings can be extrapolated to patients undergoing surgery. The perioperative period is associated with neurohormonal and inflammatory changes that cause a hypercoagulable state, characterized by increased platelet reactivity, decreased fibrinolysis, conditions that promote shear stress on arterial plaque, and enhanced vascular reactivity predisposing the patient to vasospasm. All these factors, along with the tendency toward withdrawal of antiplatelet agents before surgery for fear of predisposing patients to excessive perioperative hemorrhagic complications, increase the risk for perioperative stent thrombosis. Other risk factors associated with perioperative stent thrombosis in patients with DES are shown in **Box 2**.[15]

During the preoperative assessment of patients who have had PCI and stenting, it is important to determine which coronary lesions were treated, which type of stent was used, which antiplatelet therapy was initiated, and the time interval between PCI and the planned surgical procedure, to plan for appropriate perioperative management. Risk for excessive perioperative hemorrhage associated with the surgical procedure also needs to be considered. The clinical consequences of perioperative hemorrhage should be weighed against those of perioperative stent thrombosis and MI when making a decision about management of perioperative antiplatelet therapy. Recognition of

> **Box 2**
> **Risk factors for perioperative stent thrombosis with drug-eluting stents**
>
> Stent(s) implanted in the left main coronary artery
>
> Stent(s) implanted in bifurcations or crossing arterial branch points
>
> Greater total stent length (multiple stents and/or overlapping stents)
>
> Heightened platelet activity (surgery, malignancies, diabetes)
>
> In-stent restenosis
>
> Left ventricular dysfunction
>
> Localized hypersensitivity vasculitis (possibly to the stent polymer or antiproliferative drug)
>
> Penetration by stent into necrotic core
>
> Plaque disruption into nonstented segment
>
> Renal failure/insufficiency
>
> Diabetes
>
> Resistance to antiplatelet medications
>
> Inappropriate discontinuation of antiplatelet drug therapy
>
> *Data from* Newsome LT, Weller RS, Gerancher JC, et al. Coronary artery stents: II. Perioperative considerations and management. Anesth Analg 2008;107:577.

the potential risks associated with premature discontinuation of antiplatelet therapy in patients who have coronary stents led to the publication of a 2007 AHA/ACC/Society for Cardiovascular Angiography and Interventions/American College of Surgeons/American Dental Association Science Advisory, which recommends treatment of patients with DAPT, which is usually a combination of thienopyridine (eg, clopidogrel and ticlopidine) and aspirin for a minimum of 4 to 6 weeks for BMS, and a minimum of 12 months for DES. It also recommends that patients should not stop taking their DAPT without contacting their cardiologist and that in patients who are likely to require invasive or surgical procedures within the subsequent 12 months, consideration should be given to implantation of a BMS, or performance of balloon angioplasty with provisional stent implantation, instead of the routine use of a DES.[16]

In patients who have had only balloon angioplasty without stenting, it is appropriate to delay elective surgery for 2 to 4 weeks to allow healing to occur at the site of angioplasty. However, elective surgery should be done within 8 weeks after angioplasty because the risk of restenosis at the injury site increases after this period. Perioperative aspirin therapy should be continued in these patients if possible. The current recommendation is to postpone elective surgical procedures for 4 to 6 weeks after PCI with BMS to reduce the likelihood of stent thrombosis in the perioperative period. In patients who have had PCI with DES, elective surgery should be postponed until the patient has completed 1 year of DAPT. Beyond these recommended time limits for patients with stents, the Science Advisory recommends holding clopidogrel while continuing aspirin, then resuming clopidogrel as soon as possible after noncardiac surgery.[16] However, the 2007 ACC/AHA guidelines recommend continuing DAPT perioperatively when clinical implications of stent thrombosis are significantly worse than of perioperative hemorrhage.[4] Therefore, DAPT may be continued during the perioperative period in patients who are at low risk for perioperative hemorrhage and in patients with either multiple stents or left main coronary artery stenting. It may be beneficial to continue DAPT beyond the recommended durations in these high-risk groups, whose outcomes may be significantly worse in the event of a thrombosed stent. For urgent procedures that cannot be delayed, the current recommendation is to continue aspirin, if practicable, and resume clopidogrel as soon as possible after the procedure because of the heightened risk for late-stent thrombosis.[4,16] **Fig. 2** shows a management algorithm for patients with DES presenting for noncardiac surgery. This topic is discussed further in the section on perioperative management of medications in patients with IHD.

In acute surgical emergencies where there is very high risk for both stent thrombosis and perioperative hemorrhage, some patients have been managed with a bridging therapy, consisting of a short-acting intravenous antiplatelet drug such as tirofiban or eptifibatide, which are glycoprotein IIb/IIIa inhibitors, after the discontinuation of clopidogrel. However, the benefits of this kind of therapy have not been proved.[17]

MEDICATIONS USED IN THE MANAGEMENT OF ISCHEMIC HEART DISEASE

Goals of medical therapy for IHD include symptom relief and prevention of MI or death, with appropriate use of medications such as: (1) antiplatelet drugs, (2) β-blockers, (3) renin-angiotensin-aldosterone blockers, (4) calcium-channel blockers (CCBs), (5) nitrates, (6) lipid-lowering agents, and (7) α2-agonists.

Antiplatelet therapy is recommended for the prevention of MI and death in patients with IHD. Aspirin is a cyclooxygenase inhibitor that inhibits platelet aggregation occurring as part of the physiologic response to plaque disruption in the progression to obstruction of coronary vessels in acute coronary syndromes. Aspirin is used in the

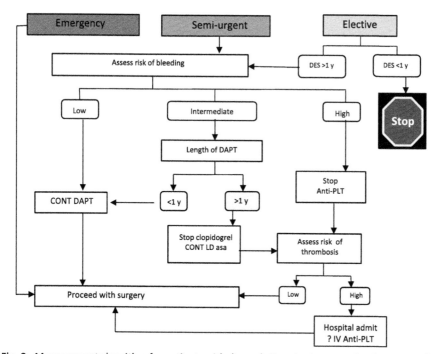

Fig. 2. Management algorithm for patients with drug-eluting stents presenting for noncardiac surgery. asa, aspirin; CONT, continue; DAPT, dual-antiplatelet therapy; DES, drug-eluting stent; IV, intravenous; LD, low-dose; PLT, platelet. (*From* Popescu WM. Perioperative management of the patient with a coronary stent. Curr Opin Anaesthesiol 2010;23:113; with permission.)

clinical management of patients with stable angina, unstable angina, and MI, as well as in patients who have had PCIs, with and without stents, and after CABG surgery.[18] Another antiplatelet agent commonly used in the clinical management of IHD to prevent coronary thrombosis is clopidogrel, a thienopyridine derivative that inhibits platelet adenosine diphosphate receptors to prevent platelet activation and aggregation; it is used both in the management of acute ischemic syndromes and after coronary stenting as part of DAPT.[19] Other thienopyridine derivatives that may be used in both the management of acute ischemic syndromes and after stenting are prasugrel and ticlopidine. Currently in clinical use, prasugrel is a relatively newer oral thienopyridine that is associated with greater risk for hemorrhagic complications; therefore, it is not recommended in patients who may require surgery. Ticlopidine use has been associated with the development of thrombotic thrombocytopenic purpura and low white blood cell count.

β-Blockers are recommended for the relief of symptoms and the prevention of death or MI in patients with stable IHD.[20] These agents reduce myocardial oxygen demand by reducing heart rate, ventricular contractility, and systemic blood pressure; they may also be used in the management of patients during acute ischemic syndromes. β-Blockers have been shown to improve survival in patients with both ischemic and nonischemic HF,[21] and to reduce the occurrence of perioperative cardiac mortality and nonfatal MI after major vascular surgery.[22,23]

Renin-angiotensin-aldosterone blocker therapy is recommended for the prevention of MI or death in patients with IHD. This group of drugs includes: (1) angiotensin-converting enzyme inhibitors (ACEIs), such as captopril and enalapril, (2) angiotensin receptor blockers (ARBs), such as losartan and valsartan, and (3) the aldosterone antagonists, spironolactone and eplerenone. In patients with CHF, ACEIs have been shown to reduce both mortality and hospitalization.[24] Captopril is an ACEI that was shown to improve survival and reduce morbidity and mortality secondary to major cardiovascular effects in patients with asymptomatic left ventricular dysfunction after MI.[25] ACEIs are currently recommended for all patients with stable IHD who also have hypertension, diabetes, left ventricular ejection fraction less than 40%, or chronic kidney disease. ARBs may be used in patients who are intolerant to ACEIs.[20] The aldosterone antagonists eplerenone and spironolactone are both potassium-sparing diuretics that have been shown to reduce the risk of cardiovascular death in patients with both HF and left ventricular dysfunction after MI.[26]

Most dihydropyridine CCBs cause vasodilation associated with reflex tachycardia and, therefore, are not used in the management of patients with IHD. However, some dihydropyridine CCBs, such as amlodipine, nicardipine and nifedipine, do not cause reflex tachycardia, and are therefore used in the treatment of chronic stable angina and vasospastic angina. Verapamil and diltiazem are nondihydropyridine CCBs that are recommended for relief of symptoms when β-blockers are contraindicated in patients with stable IHD.[20] Verapamil may also be used in the treatment of vasospastic angina, and diltiazem may be used in the management of supraventricular dysrhythmias.

Long-acting nitrates are another recommended possibility for relief of symptoms when β-blockers are contraindicated in patients with stable IHD.[20] Isosorbide dinitrate and isosorbide mononitrate belong to this category of drugs. Sublingual nitroglycerin tablets or spray are used for immediate relief in patients with angina, and nitroglycerin may also be administered as a transdermal patch or an intravenous infusion.

In addition, ranolazine is a sodium-channel blocker that is used for symptom relief when β-blockers are contraindicated.[20] It was approved by the Food and Drug Administration for use in the United States in 2006. Ranolazine has been shown to have antidysrhythmic properties that may be beneficial in the management of patients with IHD.

The reduction of serum lipid levels is a goal of therapy in the management of patients with IHD, because high serum lipid levels are a recognized risk factor for the development of CAD. This therapy includes both lifestyle modification and administration of lipid-lowering medications such as 3-hydroxy-3-methylglutaryl coenzyme A reductase inhibitors (statins), which inhibit the production of cholesterol in the liver. Use of statins has been shown to decrease mortality in patients who are at risk for developing CAD.[27] There is some published evidence about improved postoperative survival associated with preoperative statin therapy in patients undergoing noncardiac surgery.[28,29] A retrospective study on patients undergoing vascular surgery also showed a reduction in perioperative cardiovascular complications in those who were placed on preoperative statins.[30] Short-term statin use has also been associated with improvement in both cardiac function and symptoms in patients with dilated cardiomyopathy.[30] The exact mechanisms leading to these benefits are unclear and may not solely involve lipid-lowering effects. Some other proposed mechanisms, including atherosclerotic plaque stabilization, improved endothelial function, and anti-inflammatory properties, may be involved.

α2-Adrenergic agonists (eg, clonidine, dexmedetomidine, and mivazerol) act both centrally and peripherally by inhibiting the release of catecholamines from neurons. These agents also have sedative and analgesic properties and may be used clinically in the management of hypertension, or for sedation. A meta-analysis on the perioperative use of α2-agonists showed a reduction in both MI and mortality after vascular surgery.[31]

PERIOPERATIVE MANAGEMENT OF MEDICATIONS IN ISCHEMIC HEART DISEASE

Perioperative management of medications in ischemic heart disease is shown in **Table 3**. Perioperative decisions about the management of antiplatelet medications in IHD must weigh the sequelae arising from perioperative hemorrhage associated with their use against the risk for perioperative ischemic events associated with their withdrawal. For surgical procedures that are associated with low risk for perioperative hemorrhage, antiplatelet medications may be continued in the perioperative period. One review on the perioperative use of aspirin recommends discontinuing aspirin only if the severity of hemorrhagic complications associated with its use are comparable with the potential cardiovascular effects of its withdrawal, as may occur in intracranial surgery and, possibly, transurethral prostatectomy.[32] Addition of clopidogrel or other thienopyridines to aspirin (ie, DAPT) confers an increased risk for perioperative hemorrhagic complications; however, it may only be associated with an increased risk for perioperative mortality from excessive hemorrhage in surgical procedures involving enclosed spaces, such as intracranial surgery.[33] The decision about the continuation or discontinuation of antiplatelet medications in the perioperative period should not be taken lightly, and is best made after discussions between the surgeon, cardiologist, and anesthesiologist who are involved in the care of the patient. As discussed earlier, in patients with coronary stents who are on clopidogrel and whose surgical procedure cannot be postponed, clopidogrel should be reinitiated as soon as possible after surgery if the risk associated with bleeding is significant enough to warrant holding clopidogrel and, thereby, exposing the patient to the risk of stent thrombosis. When appropriate, it is recommended to hold clopidogrel for 5 to 7 days before surgery because the anticoagulant effects of thienopyridines may extend for about a week after discontinuation. Perioperative aspirin therapy should be continued in these patients, if possible.

β-Blocker administration must be continued during the perioperative period in patients who are already taking β-blockers. Patients who are undergoing high-risk and

Table 3
Perioperative management of medications used in treatment of patients with ischemic heart disease undergoing noncardiac surgery

Medication	Perioperative Management
Antiplatelet agents	Continue in perioperative period. Hold only if severity of hemorrhagic complications is comparable with potential cardiovascular effects of withdrawal. When appropriate in patients on DAPT, hold clopidogrel 5 d before elective noncardiac surgery
β-Blockers	Continue throughout perioperative period. Initiate in patients with CAD or multiple risk factors for CAD undergoing high- and intermediate-risk surgery. Hold if patient is hypotensive or bradycardic
Renin-angiotensin-aldosterone blocker therapy	Continue ACEIs and ARBs throughout perioperative period. Hold if patient is hypotensive. Monitor serum electrolytes for hyperkalemia in patients on aldosterone blockers
Calcium-channel blockers	Continue throughout perioperative period. Hold if patient is hypotensive
Nitrates	Continue throughout perioperative period. Intravenous nitroglycerine may be used in the perioperative period to manage ischemia. Hold if patient is hypotensive
Statins	Continue throughout perioperative period. Statin therapy may be initiated in the perioperative period in patients who meet criteria for initiation of lipid-lowering therapy
α2-Adrenergic agonists	Continue throughout perioperative period. Hold if patient is hypotensive. Avoid sudden withdrawal of clonidine

Abbreviations: ACEIs, angiotensin-converting enzyme inhibitors; ARBs, angiotensin-II receptor blockers; CAD, coronary artery disease; DAPT, dual-antiplatelet therapy.

intermediate-risk surgical procedures may benefit from the perioperative administration of β-blockers titrated to heart rate and blood pressure if they are found on preoperative evaluation to have CAD or multiple clinical risk factors for the development of ischemic cardiac complications. When possible, β-blockers should be initiated from days to weeks before scheduled noncardiac surgery,[34] but the routine use of perioperative β-blockers in noncardiac surgery is not recommended. A large randomized trial that used a fixed dose of extended-release metoprolol in the perioperative period during noncardiac surgery showed an increased incidence of nonfatal stroke associated with hypotension, in addition to the prevention of nonfatal MI.[35] Therefore, β-blockers should not be administered to patients who are hypotensive and/or bradycardic during the perioperative period. β-Blockers should also not be withdrawn suddenly in patients who are on chronic β-blocker therapy, because of an increased risk for myocardial ischemia. An underlying cause of tachycardia, such as hypovolemia, anemia, or pain, should be treated appropriately when present. Perioperative β-blockers should be titrated to a heart-rate goal of 60 to 80 beats/min in the absence of hypotension, and they may be administered throughout the perioperative period and up to 1 month after surgery.

Perioperative use of renin-angiotensin-aldosterone blocker therapy may be associated with intraoperative hypotension, leading to significant perioperative complications. Under anesthesia and surgery, ACEIs and ARBs cause a reduction in both preload and cardiac output. Some investigators have recommended temporarily withdrawing ACEIs and ARBs preoperatively in patients predisposed to hypotension, or continuing the medication while maintaining an appropriate intravascular volume status in these patients. Hypotensive episodes may be managed with intravascular fluid administration and vasopressors such as phenylephrine, ephedrine, and/or vasopressin.[36] The aldosterone blockers are potassium-sparing diuretics, and may cause electrolyte abnormalities such as hyperkalemia; therefore, serum electrolytes should be monitored during the perioperative period.

Perioperative use of CCBs was shown in a meta-analysis to reduce the incidence of ischemia and supraventricular tachycardia, with the majority of such benefit being associated with diltiazem, which also caused a reduction in PCEs.[37] CCBs should be continued in the perioperative period in the absence of hypotension.

Nitrates are vasodilators that, when used in the perioperative period, may be associated with hypotension, which can be exacerbated at induction of anesthesia or in association with hypovolemia, secondary to excessive blood loss. There are some clinical reports citing the successful use of intravenous nitroglycerin in the management of perioperative ischemia during noncardiac surgery[38]; however, this finding has not been corroborated by all reports.[39] In the absence of hypotension, nitrate use should be continued in the perioperative period.

Although preoperative use of statins has been associated with improved survival and reduction of cardiovascular complications, this association has not been well defined for goals of therapy before surgery. The current recommendation is to continue statin therapy in patients who are already on statins and undergoing noncardiac surgery.[34] Perioperative initiation of statin therapy may be considered in patients who meet the criteria for initiating lipid-lowering therapy, without any adverse effects on the perioperative outcomes. Long-term postoperative statin therapy should follow recommended guidelines.

$\alpha 2$-Adrenergic agonists reduce the adrenergic response to major surgery and also have analgesic and sedative properties, all desirable effects in the perioperative period for patients with IHD who are undergoing major surgical procedures. Perioperative administration may be continued in the absence of hypotension, especially in patients undergoing high-risk surgery who also have clinical risk factors for PCEs. Sudden withdrawal of clonidine should be avoided, because this is known to cause rebound hypertension.

SUMMARY

Patients with IHD who are undergoing surgery are at risk for development of PCEs, and this risk depends on the type of surgery, the presence of clinical risk factors, and the functional status of patients. Appropriate perioperative management of medications such as DAPT and β-blocker therapy has a significant impact on outcomes. Perioperative management decisions should be communicated clearly between the surgeon, cardiologist, and anesthesiologist involved in the care of the patient. Appropriate perioperative management reduces the incidence of PCEs.

REFERENCES

1. Go AS, Mozaffarian D, Roger VL, et al. Heart disease and stroke statistics—2013 update. A report from the American Heart Association. Circulation 2013;127: e6–245.
2. Mackey WC, Fleisher LA, Haider S, et al. Perioperative myocardial ischemic injury in high-risk vascular surgery patients: incidence and clinical significance in a prospective clinical trial. J Vasc Surg 2006;43:533–8.

3. Lee TH, Marcantonio ER, Mangione CM, et al. Derivation and prospective valida-tion of a simple index for prediction of cardiac risk of major noncardiac surgery. Circulation 1999;100:1043–9.

4. Fleisher LA, Beckman JA, Brown KA, et al. ACC/AHA 2007 guidelines on peri-operative cardiovascular evaluation and care for noncardiac surgery: a report of the American College of Cardiology/American Heart Association Task Force on Practice Guidelines (Writing Committee to revise the 2002 guidelines on peri-operative cardiovascular evaluation for noncardiac surgery). Circulation 2007; 116:e418–500.

5. Criqui MH, Langer RD, Fronek A, et al. Mortality over a period of 10 years in patients with peripheral arterial disease. N Engl J Med 1992;326:381.

6. Reilly DF, McNeely MJ, Doerner D, et al. Self-reported exercise tolerance and the risk of serious perioperative complications. Arch Intern Med 1999;159:2185–92.

7. Landesberg G. The pathophysiology of perioperative MI: facts and perspectives. J Cardiothorac Vasc Anesth 2003;17:90–100.

8. Tervahauta M, Pekkanen J, Punsar S, et al. Resting electrocardiographic abnor-malities as predictors of coronary events and total mortality among elderly men. Am J Med 1996;100:641–5.

9. Liu LL, Dzankic S, Leung JM. Preoperative electrocardiogram abnormalities do not predict postoperative cardiac complications in geriatric surgical patients. J Am Geriatr Soc 2002;50:1186–91.

10. van Klei WA, Bryson GL, Yang H, et al. The value of routine preoperative electro-cardiography in predicting MI after noncardiac surgery. Ann Surg 2007;246: 165–70.

11. Breen P, Lee JW, Pomposelli F, et al. Timing of high-risk vascular surgery following coronary artery bypass surgery: a 10-year experience from an academic medical centre. Anaesthesia 2004;59:422–7.

12. Fischman DL, Leon MB, Baim SD, et al. A randomized comparison of coronary-stent placement and balloon angioplasty in the treatment of coronary artery dis-ease. N Engl J Med 1994;331:496–501.

13. Valgimigli M, Campo G, Monti M, et al. Short- versus long-term duration of dual-antiplatelet therapy after coronary stenting: a randomized multicenter trial. Circu-lation 2012;125(16):2015–26.

14. Ferreira-Gonzalez I, Marsal J, Ribera A, et al. Double antiplatelet therapy after drug-eluting stent implantation: risk associated with discontinuation with the first year. J Am Coll Cardiol 2012;60(15):1333–9.

15. Newsome LT, Weller RS, Gerancher JC, et al. Coronary artery stents: II. Perioper-ative considerations and management. Anesth Analg 2008;107:570–90.

16. Grines CL, Bonow RO, Casey DE Jr, et al. Prevention of premature discontinuation of dual-antiplatelet therapy in patients with coronary artery stents: a science advi-sory from the American Heart Association, American College of Cardiology, Society for Cardiovascular Angiography and Interventions, American College of Surgeons, and American Dental Association, with representation from the American College of Physicians. Circulation 2007;115:813–8.

17. Popescu WM. Perioperative management of the patient with a coronary stent. Curr Opin Anaesthesiol 2010;23:109–15.

18. Willard JE, Lange RA, Hillis LD. The use of aspirin in IHD. N Engl J Med 1992;327: 175–81.

19. Galla JM, Lincoff GM. The role of clopidogrel in the management of IHD. Curr Opin Cardiol 2007;22:273–9.

20. Fihn SD, Gardin JM, Abrams J, et al. 2012 ACCF/AHA/ACP/AATS/PCNA/SCAI/ STS guideline for the diagnosis and management of patients with stable IHD. A report of the American College of Cardiology Foundation/American Heart Association Task Force on Practice Guidelines, and the American College of Physicians, American Association for Thoracic Surgery, Preventive Cardiovascular Nurses Association, Society for Cardiovascular Angiography and Interventions, and Society of Thoracic Surgeons. J Am Coll Cardiol 2012;60:2564–603.

21. Cruickshank JM. Beta-blockers continue to surprise us. Eur Heart J 2000;21: 354–64.

22. Poldermans D, Boersma E, Bax JJ, et al. Bisoprolol reduces perioperative cardiac death and MI in high-risk patients undergoing major vascular surgery. N Engl J Med 1999;341:1789–95.

23. Lindenauer PK, Pekow P, Wang K, et al. Perioperative beta-blocker therapy and mortality after major noncardiac surgery. N Engl J Med 2005;353:349–61.

24. Garg R, Yusuf S. Overview of randomized trials of angiotensin-converting enzyme inhibitors on mortality and morbidity in patients with HF. Collaborative Group on ACE Inhibitor Trials. JAMA 1995;273:1450–6.

25. Pfeffer MA, Braunwald E, Moye LA, et al. Effect of captopril on mortality and morbidity in patients with left ventricular dysfunction after MI. Results of the survival and ventricular enlargement trial. The SAVE Investigators. N Engl J Med 1992;327:669–77.

26. Catena C, Colussi G, Brosolo G, et al. Aldosterone and aldosterone antagonists in cardiac disease: what is known, what is new. Am J Cardiovasc Dis 2012;2: 50–7.

27. Grundy SM, Cleeman JI, Merz CN, et al. Implications of recent clinical trials for the National Cholesterol Education Program Adult Treatment Panel III guidelines. Circulation 2004;110:227–39.

28. Hindler K, Shaw AD, Samuels J, et al. Improved postoperative outcomes associated with preoperative statin therapy. Anesthesiology 2006;105:1260–72.

29. Poldermans D, Bax JJ, Kertai MD, et al. Statins are associated with a reduced incidence of perioperative mortality in patients undergoing major noncardiac vascular surgery. Circulation 2003;107:1848–51.

30. O'Neil-Callahan K, Katsimaglis G, Tepper MR, et al. Statins decrease perioperative cardiac complications in patients undergoing noncardiac vascular surgery. The Statins for Risk Reduction in Surgery (StaRRS) study. J Am Coll Cardiol 2005;45:336–42.

31. Wijeysundera DN, Naik JS, Beattie WS. Alpha-2 adrenergic agonists to prevent perioperative cardiovascular complications: a meta-analysis. Am J Med 2003; 114:742–52.

32. Burger W, Chemnitius JM, Kneissl GD, et al. Low-dose aspirin for secondary cardiovascular prevention: cardiovascular risks after its perioperative withdrawal versus bleeding risks with its continuation—review and meta-analysis. J Intern Med 2005;257:399–414.

33. Chassot PG, Delabays A, Spahn DR. Perioperative antiplatelet therapy: the case for continuing therapy in patients at risk of MI. Br J Anaesth 2007;99(3): 316–28.

34. Fleisher LA, Beckman JA, Brown KA, et al. 2009 ACCF/AHA focused update on perioperative beta blockade incorporated into the ACC/AHA 2007 guidelines on perioperative cardiovascular evaluation and care for noncardiac surgery. Circulation 2009;120:e169–276.

35. Devereaux PJ, Yang H, Yusuf S, et al. Effects of extended-release metoprolol succinate in patients undergoing non-cardiac surgery (POISE trial): a randomised controlled trial. Lancet 2008;371:1839–47.

36. Colson P, Ryckwaert F, Coriat P. Renin angiotensin system antagonists and anesthesia. Anesth Analg 1999;89:1143–55.

37. Wijeysundera DN, Beattie WS. Calcium channel blockers for reducing cardiac morbidity after noncardiac surgery: a meta-analysis. Anesth Analg 2003;97: 634–41.

38. Coriat P, Daloz M, Bousseau D, et al. Prevention of intraoperative myocardial ischemia during noncardiac surgery with intravenous nitroglycerin. Anesthesiology 1984;61:193.

39. Dodds TM, Stone JG, Coromilas J, et al. Prophylactic nitroglycerin infusion during noncardiac surgery does not reduce perioperative ischemia. Anesth Analg 1993; 76:705.

Patients with Pacemaker or Implantable Cardioverter-Defibrillator

Peter M. Schulman, MD[a],*, Marc A. Rozner, PhD, MD[b],
Valerie Sera, MD[a], Eric C. Stecker, MD, MPH[c]

KEYWORDS

- Pacemaker • Cardioverter-Defibrillator • Preoperative • Perioperative
- Management

KEY POINTS

- Providers charged with preoperative management frequently encounter patients with a cardiac implantable electronic device (CIED). Safe and efficient perioperative management of this complex patient population requires specific knowledge and the development of a comprehensive system-based approach to care.
- Before surgery, the CIED physician should be contacted for records and a perioperative prescription. Documentation of CIED interrogation and appropriate function (maximum 6 months [implantable cardioverter-defibrillator (ICD)], 1 year [pacemaker]) should be confirmed before induction of anesthesia.
- Electromagnetic interference (EMI) remains the principal intraoperative issue. If EMI is likely, ICD antitachycardia therapy should be disabled and external defibrillation pads applied. Reprogramming to an asynchronous pacing mode should be considered for any pacing-dependent patient.
- Magnet behavior should be confirmed if magnet use is planned. Some rate enhancements might require disabling. Optimizing oxygen delivery for major surgery might require increasing the lower rate limit. Appropriate positioning of the electrosurgery unit dispersive electrode can minimize EMI from electrosurgery.
- Postoperatively, CIEDs often require reinterrogation to confirm appropriate function, restore rate enhancements, and optimize pacing parameters. The ICD patient must have continuous cardiac monitoring until antitachycardia therapy is restored.
- Any interrogation and reprogramming must be documented in the medical record.

[a] Department of Anesthesiology & Perioperative Medicine, Oregon Health & Science University, Mail Code: UHS-2, 3181 S.W. Sam Jackson Park Road, Portland, OR 97239, USA; [b] Departments of Cardiology, Anesthesiology and Perioperative Medicine, University of Texas MD Anderson Cancer Center, 1400 Holcombe Blvd, Mail Code 0409, Houston, TX 77030, USA; [c] Cardiac Electrophysiology, Knight Cardiovascular Institute, Oregon Health & Science University, Mail Code: UHN-62, 3181 S.W. Sam Jackson Park Road, Portland, OR 97239, USA
* Corresponding author.
E-mail address: peterschulman@gmail.com

Med Clin N Am 97 (2013) 1051–1075
http://dx.doi.org/10.1016/j.mcna.2013.05.004
0025-7125/13/$ – see front matter © 2013 Elsevier Inc. All rights reserved.

INTRODUCTION

Four years after invention of the transistor in 1954, C. W. Lillehei, a cardiothoracic surgeon, and Earl Bakken, an electrical technician, developed the first battery-operated system to pace the heart. The first completely implantable, battery-powered pacemaker (PM) followed just 2 years later, and by 1985 the US Food and Drug Administration (FDA) had approved the implantable cardioverter-defibrillator (ICD) for clinical use.[1] In 1997, ICDs were approved for permanent antibradycardia pacing functions in addition to antitachycardia therapies. Further technological innovations have resulted in sophisticated 3-chamber pacing (right atrium [RA], right ventricle [RV], and left ventricle [LV]) to provide cardiac resynchronization therapy (CRT, also called biventricular [BiV] pacing) from both PMs (CRT-P) and ICDs (CRT-D); available in the United States since 2001. In 2012, a subcutaneous leadless ICD (that uses a subcutaneous electrode instead of traditional transvenous or epicardial leads) received FDA approval.

In North America, at least 3 million patients have a cardiac implantable electronic device (CIED),[2] with more than 400,000 PMs and 120,000 ICDs implanted annually in the United States.[3] An aging population, new indications for device use, and continued technological enhancements will likely increase the number of patients with a CIED. Consequently, clinicians involved in perioperative care should expect to encounter and manage such patients.

Although modern CIEDs have excellent functionality, this functionality comes at the cost of complexity. The sophistication of these devices, the multitude of complex issues surrounding effective perioperative management of the CIED patient, and changing patient conditions can increase the difficulty of providing care for these patients, especially for clinicians (including family physicians, internists, hospitalists, anesthesiologists, and surgeons) who are not CIED experts. Particular challenges for clinicians include evolving technology, specialized function of the devices, manufacturer-specific proprietary features, lack of standardization among device manufacturers, and an array of published literature that is often outdated and sometimes incorrect. In addition, electrical equipment (especially monopolar electrosurgical devices) often used when caring for these patients can interfere with CIED function, because no testing of interference with CIEDs is required before bringing a medical device to market. Perioperative planning often requires consideration of intraoperative electromagnetic interference (EMI), because it can lead to pacing inhibition (and asystole in a pacing-dependent patient), an inappropriate shock from an ICD, or induce a pacing-system driven tachycardia. Sometimes, surgical plans can be altered to substitute equipment that creates minimal or no EMI (such as bipolar electrosurgery) to mitigate these issues.

Certain procedures that are not part of the surgical event, but become required as a result of the surgery, can affect a CIED patient or interfere with CIED operation. Nerve stimulators, which introduce electricity and are used during some regional anesthetic procedures, can result in EMI and pacing inhibition[4] as well as interfere with electrocardiographic (ECG) monitoring.[5] For certain patients and operations, central venous cannulation is necessary, but placement of a thoracic central venous cannula in a patient with fresh leads (less than 3 months since implant)[6] might cause lead dislodgement, and any metal guide wire inserted into the thorax of a patient with an ICD can create false ventricular signals, leading to an ICD high-voltage discharge and possible patient injury.[7]

In response to these challenges, the American Society of Anesthesiologists (ASA), the Heart Rhythm Society (HRS), the Canadian Society, and others have published documents intended to guide clinicians in the perioperative management of CIED patients.[2,6,8]

Practitioners involved in the preparation of CIED patients for surgery or the perioperative management of these patients should be familiar with the recommendations put forth by these organizations. They should also understand the indications for implantation, as well as the basic functions, operations, and limitations of these devices. Furthermore, to maximize CIED patient safety, practitioners should be facile in understanding and detecting potential problems in order to avert iatrogenic complications at a stage before the surgical procedure, including the need to triage to an expert in perioperative management of CIEDs.

This review begins by addressing the basic function of CIEDs, indications for implantation, and modes of operation. It then outlines the main considerations and controversies involved in the preoperative preparation and perioperative management of these patients. At the conclusion of this review, the reader will understand the considerations involved in the safe and effective perioperative management of the patient with a CIED.

DEVICE FUNCTION

Traditional CIED systems consist of a pulse generator and 1 to 3 leads. The earliest systems contained a large pulse generator that required abdominal implantation. Over time, technology has allowed for miniaturization of the pulse generator, which is now almost always implanted underneath the clavicle in a subcutaneous pectoral pocket. Modern pulse generators contain complex circuitry capable of analyzing and responding to incoming information; memory, so that information can be stored and later analyzed; and a battery (typically the largest single element within the device).

Technological advancements in lead technology have mirrored those of pulse generators. Although the earliest leads had to be affixed to the outside of the heart (epicardial leads) via thoracotomy, modern transvenous leads are inserted directly into the cardiac chambers through the superior vena cava. Modern transvenous leads offer several advantages over epicardial leads, including less trauma, lower pacing threshold (which lengthens battery life), and lower defibrillation threshold (DFT) (which improves ICD efficacy). Because of the aforementioned advantages of transvenous leads as well as the fact that epicardial lead placement is more invasive, epicardial leads are used only when transvenous lead placement is either not possible or is contraindicated (ie, mechanical tricuspid valve or adverse venous anatomy). Transvenous leads may be inserted into the RA, RV, or coronary sinus (CS), and all leads are capable of sensing and pacing in their respective chambers. For transvenous ICDs, the RV lead includes electrodes to provide high-voltage defibrillation therapy. Therefore, in contradistinction to conventional PMs, transvenous ICDs have 1 or 2 shock coils on the RV lead, allowing these CIEDs to be easily distinguished from one another via chest radiograph (**Fig. 1**). In most CRT systems, a CS lead is used to pace the LV, and the position of the CS lead is best determined by lateral chest radiograph (**Fig. 2**). Whether the patient receives 1, 2, or all 3 of these leads depends on the indications for implantation and device type selected. Subcutaneous ICDs do not have traditional transvenous or epicardial leads (**Fig. 3**) and have more limited functionality.

Transvenous leads can be either unipolar or bipolar. With a bipolar lead, the cathode and anode are both present on the lead itself, whereas with a unipolar lead, only the cathode is present on the lead, and the pulse generator functions as the anode. Thus, the distance between the cathode and anode is smaller with a bipolar lead,

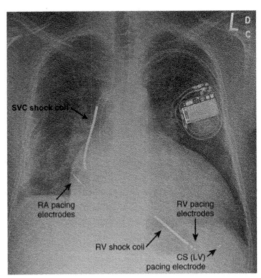

Fig. 1. A defibrillator system with biventricular antibradycardia pacemaker capability. This chest film was taken from a 50-year-old man with head and neck cancer, coronary artery disease, and ischemic cardiomyopathy with ejection fraction of 15%. The ICD generator is in the left pectoral position with 3 leads: a conventional, bipolar lead to the RA, a quadripolar lead to the RV, and a unipolar lead to the CS. (CS lead is in an unusual location: inferior and apical, close to RV lead). This system is designed to provide resynchronization (antibradycardia) therapy in the setting of a dilated cardiomyopathy with a prolonged QRS (and frequently with a prolonged P-R interval as well). The bipolar lead in the RA performs both sensing and pacing functions. The lead in this RV is a true bipolar lead with ring and tip electrodes for pacing and sensing. The presence of a shock conductor (termed a shock coil) on the RV lead in the RV distinguishes a defibrillation system from a conventional pacemaking system. The lead in the CS depolarizes the LV, and the typical current pathway includes the anode (ring electrode) in the RV. Because of the typically wide QRS complex in a left bundle branch pattern, failure to capture the LV can lead to ventricular oversensing (and inappropriate antitachycardia therapy) in an ICD system. Many defibrillation systems (including this one) also have a shock coil in the superior vena cava (*SVC*), which usually is electrically identical to the defibrillator case (called the can). When the defibrillation circuit includes the ICD case, it is called an active can configuration. (*From* Rozner MA, Schulman PM. How should we prepare the patient with a pacemaker/implantable cardioverter-defibrillator? In: Fleisher LA, ed. Evidence-based practice of anesthesiology, 3rd edition. Philadelphia: Elsevier, 2013; with permission.)

reducing susceptibility to EMI during sensing. PM systems (but not ICD systems) with bipolar leads can be programmed to the unipolar mode for pacing, sensing, or both. Sometimes, a PM automatically switches from bipolar to unipolar pacing and sensing if a lead fault is detected.

Differences between bipolar and unipolar pacing include: bipolar pacing usually produces lower amplitude spikes recorded during analogue-recorded ECG compared with unipolar pacing; digitally processed ECG systems often fail to show spikes if programmed to filter high-frequency signals (typical for any bedside ECG monitor); and unipolar spikes can be misinterpreted as QRS complexes by observers unfamiliar with pacing issues. In addition, ECG monitors can undercount or overcount the ECG pulse rate. Thus, both the ASA and HRS recommend monitoring every patient with some form of mechanical pulse display and rate counter whenever patient ECG monitoring is required, whether it is the pulse oximeter plethysmogram or an

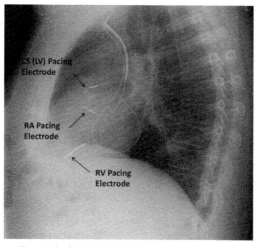

Fig. 2. Lateral chest radiograph showing position of CS lead.

invasive arterial line. An example of ECG rate overcounting is shown in **Fig. 4**, and a simulation showing rate undercounting is shown in **Fig. 5**. Many automated ECG analyzers report "pacing, no further analysis" even in the setting of clear pacing system malfunction (**Fig. 6**).

During implant (and at every follow-up visit), lead impedance values and thresholds for sensing and pacing are measured. Some CIEDs automatically perform daily threshold and impedence tests, which can be reviewed at the time of device interrogation. Values outside the acceptable range, or that wildly fluctuate, may suggest a faulty connection, dislodged lead tip, fractured coil, or insulation breach.[9] For ICDs, the DFT, which is the lowest amount of energy required to defibrillate the heart, may also be tested during the implant procedure. Some physicians use empirical energy

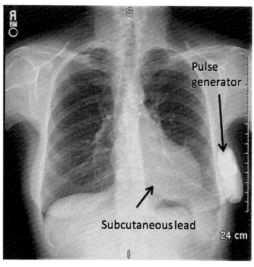

Fig. 3. Subcutaneous ICD.

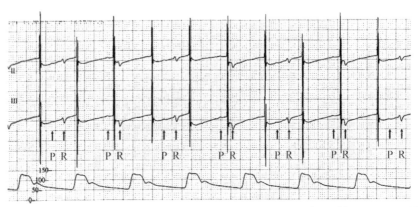

Fig. 4. Improper placement of a transesophageal PM, resulting in pacing without capture. ECG lead II (*top*), the middle recording is ECG lead III (*middle*), and the bottom recording is the invasive arterial pressure waveform (*bottom*). This 72-year-old man developed sinus bradycardia with evidence of tissue underperfusion intraoperatively. A transesophageal PM was placed (fixed mode AOO), and the monitor reported an ECG heart rate of 75 bpm in the setting of non-capture and a sinus rate of 50 bpm. The patient's native atrial (*P*) and ventricular (*R*) depolarizations showing first-degree A-V block (P-R interval of 280 milliseconds) have been marked. The arterial pressure waveform confirms pacing noncapture. (*From* Rozner MA. Implantable cardiac pulse generators: pacemakers and cardioverter-defibrillators. In: Miller RD, Eriksson LI, Fleisher LA, et al, eds. Miller's Anesthesia, 7th edition. Philadelphia: Elsevier, 2009; with permission.)

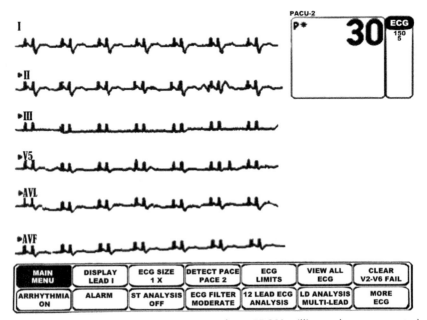

Fig. 5. A PM simulator set to AV pacing, rate 75 bpm, PR 200 milliseconds was connected to a Dash monitor (GE Healthcare, Milwaukee, WI), which had been appropriately configured to display pacing artifacts (Detect Pace = Pace 2) and lead analysis set to lead I. However, the monitor is reporting an ECG heart rate of 30 bpm, likely because of the low-voltage signals sensed on leads 3, V5, aVL, and aVF. This phenomenon can frequently be observed clinically but has not been investigated to any great extent.

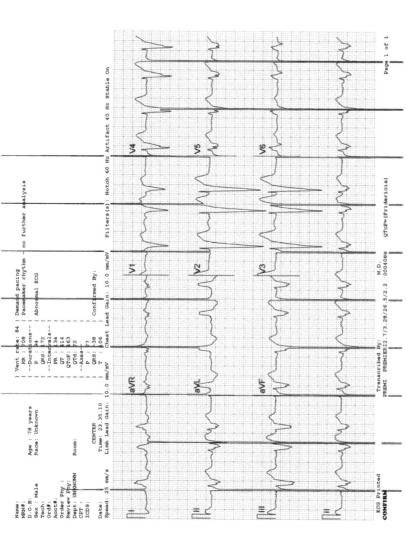

Fig. 6. A critically ill 78-year-old man (with presumed transfusion-related lung injury) with a single-chamber ICD (tachytherapy disabled, pacing VVI 50 bpm) underwent transesophageal PM placement for sinus bradycardia at 52 bpm with frequent PVCs, resulting in frequent ventricular-only pacing with the creation of retrograde P waves and poor perfusion. (The cycle length of the underlying sinus rhythm was 1154 milliseconds. With a PVC at 450 milliseconds from the QRS [see 3rd and 10th QRS above], along with the 134-millisecond PR interval, the next P wave following the compensatory pause would occur at 1724 milliseconds after the PVC. As a result, the ICD would issue a pace at 1200 milliseconds from the PVC, resulting in continued AV dyssynchrony.) The transesophageal pacing device was initially set to 80 bpm, but it was reduced to 60 bpm. This 12-lead ECG clearly shows inappropriate atrial pacing at the second, fourth, fifth, seventh, and ninth pace, but the automated interpretation (and the ECG reader) reported no analysis because of the pacing.

settings and forgo DFT testing to avoid the need for induction of ventricular fibrillation (VF), which has been associated with patient injury.

All PMs and transvenous ICDs have sophisticated pacing, sensing, and electrical storage capabilities. Subcutaneous ICDs have no permanent pacing capability. ICDs use R-R intervals (heart rate) to detect tachyarrhythmias. Each cardiac R-R interval is measured and the rate categorized as normal, too fast (short R-R interval), or too slow (long R-R interval). When enough short R-R intervals are detected, an antitachycardia event begins. ICDs then attempt to distinguish between malignant (ventricular tachycardia [VT] or VF) and nonmalignant (SVT, atrial fibrillation with rapid ventricular response) tachyarrhythmia based on programmable discriminators (such as QRS morphology, R-R interval variability, P-R relationship [when available]). When therapy becomes indicated, transvenous ICDs can deliver antitachycardia pacing (ATP) (less painful, so better tolerated; less battery consumption) or shock, depending on the presentation and device programming.[1] Most newer transvenous ICDs deliver ATP while charging the capacitor for shock if no previous ATP had been delivered. ATP has about an 85% success rate at terminating episodes of hemodynamically stable VT[10]; it is often programmed as the first therapy option for VT because it is painless and requires less energy than defibrillation.[9] However, the use of ATP can delay the time to first shock, because each ATP cycle requires 8 to 15 seconds. ATP can also accelerate stable VT into unstable VT or VF. Other reasons for prolonged time to defibrillation include low battery voltage, frequent ICD discharges, EMI (which can increase the capacitor charge time), or cold temperature.[1] ICD shocks terminate VF in more than 98% of episodes.[11] Subcutaneous ICDs cannot deliver ATP, and DFTs for subcutaneous ICDs are about twice those for transvenous ICDs.

Although ATP can be used as a first-line therapy for VT in lieu of shock, it still might be associated with myocardial injury. The recently published MADIT-RIT (Multicenter Automatic Defibrillator Implantation Trial-Reduce Inappropriate Therapy) trial reported that any inappropriate therapy (for rhythm other than VT or VF), whether ATP or shock, is associated with higher mortality.[12] Despite improvements in detection of ventricular tachyarrhythmias, on average more than 10% of shocks are inappropriate.[1]

To prevent an inappropriate shock, most ICDs are programmed to reconfirm VT or VF after charging. Once a shock has been delivered, no further ATP can take place. Like PMs, transvenous ICDs begin antibradycardia pacing when the R-R interval is too long. The extent of pacing dependency in ICD patients remains unknown.[13] Subcutaneous ICDs provide ventricular-only pacing support for a brief period after therapy.

Arguably, the most profound advances in CIED technology have been in the area of CRT. Heart failure from impaired LV systolic function accounts for roughly 1 million hospitalizations and more than 58,000 deaths annually.[14] Despite maximum medical therapy, many patients continue to be symptomatic. Advanced heart failure is well known to be accompanied by conduction defects and arrhythmias caused by sinus or atrioventricular (AV) node dysfunction and intraventricular conduction delays or bundle branch block (QRS>120 milliseconds).[11] In turn, slowed transmission of LV depolarization delays activation of the LV lateral and inferolateral walls, leading to dyssynchronous ventricular contraction and decreased stroke volume. This intraventricular and interventricular dyssynchrony has been shown to increase the risk of death in this population.

The goal of CRT is to restore synchronous LV activation by pacing both ventricles in order to approximate more normal ventricular conduction. As opposed to AV sequential dual-chamber (RA and RV only) pacing, CRT devices pace both the LV and RV to coordinate, or resynchronize LV contraction and RV/LV ejection. Atrial-synchronized

BiV pacing can improve myocardial mechanics and energy utilization, resulting in improved cardiac output, hemodynamics, heart failure symptoms, and quality of life and mortality in patients with heart failure.[15]

IMPLANT INDICATIONS

The American College of Cardiology (ACC) and the American Heart Association (AHA) in conjunction with the HRS have issued guidelines on indications for CIED placement.[16] A summary of indications for implantation is shown in **Table 1**. Most patients with a need for a PM have sinus or AV nodal disease. In addition, an increasing percentage of patients with dilated cardiomyopathy now undergo BiV pacing. BiV pacing from a conventional pacemaker (CRT-P) is discussed in more detail later.

Indications for implantation of a transvenous ICD are summarized in **Table 1**. Transvenous ICDs significantly reduce all-cause mortality and mortality caused by arrhythmias when compared with antiarrhythmic drugs alone.[17,18] Initially, transvenous ICDs were indicated only for secondary prevention of sudden cardiac death after VF arrest or sustained VT. Studies suggesting prophylactic placement in patients without history of tachyarrhythmia have significantly increased the number of patients for whom ICD therapy is indicated. MADIT, completed in 1996, proved benefit in primary prevention of sudden cardiac arrest in patients with heart failure, impaired left ventricular function (LV ejection fraction [LVEF] <35%) caused by previous myocardial infarction, clinical nonsustained VT, and VT inducible by electrophysiology study.[18]

Two additional seminal trials have confirmed the benefit of implanting ICDs for primary prevention. (1) MADIT-II (ischemic cardiomyopathy, LVEF <30%, and heart failure functional class I, II, or III),[19] and (2) SCD-HeFT (Sudden Cardiac Death–Heart Failure Trial) (LVEF <35% regardless of the cause and heart failure class II or III)[20] significantly increased the number of patients eligible for ICD implantation without showing previous ventricular tachyarrhythmia.

Table 1
Indications for PM or ICD implantation

	Left Ventricular Ejection Fraction at Time of Implant (%)[a]	QRS Duration	Heart Failure Functional Class[b]	Coronary Artery Disease	Bradycardia and Possible Pacer Dependence
Conventional PM	>35	Any	Any	+/–	+
Transvenous ICD	<35	Any	I, II, III	+/–	+/–
Subcutaneous ICD	<35	Any	I, II, III	+/–	– (no permanent pacing)
CRT-D	<35	>120 ms	III, IV (recently some I and II)	+/–	+/–
CRT-P	<35 preferring no ICD	>120 ms	III, IV (recently some I and II)	+/–	+/–

[a] Left ventricular ejection fraction (LVEF) often changes after implant, particularly in setting of CRT. Most patients requiring pacing who have LVEF <35% receive an ICD, although patient preference or other circumstances could affect this decision.
[b] Patients with class IV heart failure generally receive only ICD in the setting of CRT. CRT was initially restricted to patients with class III or IV heart failure, but recently indications have expanded to class I and II in certain clinical scenarios.

Additional ACC/AHA indications for ICD placement regardless of LVEF include previous cardiac arrest from a nonreversible cause, hypertrophic cardiomyopathy, long QT or Brugada syndrome with syncope, arrhythmogenic RV dysplasia, or infiltrative cardiomyopathy (sarcoidosis, amyloidosis).[9]

For patients with symptomatic heart failure despite optimal medical therapy, the 2008 ACC/AHA/HRS Guidelines for CRT include LVEF less than 35%, QRS duration greater than 120 milliseconds, sinus rhythm, and New York Heart Association (NYHA) class III or ambulatory class IV symptoms (**Table 1**).[16] As most CRT patients also meet criteria for ICD implantation, a CRT-D rather than CRT-P is more frequently selected. In 2012, the ACC/AHA/HRS issued a focused update in this area; class I indications were expanded to include patients with NYHA class II, extending the message that CRT is now indicated for patients with milder symptoms. However, the 2012 update restricted the class I recommendation to patients with left bundle branch block (LBBB) morphology and QRS duration greater than 150 milliseconds (LBBB with QRS 120–149 milliseconds or non-LBBB pattern with QRS >150 milliseconds has been downgraded to a class IIa recommendation).[21]

Up to 30% of patients meeting standard criteria for CRT do not show improvement (CRT nonresponders).[9,22] These most recent guideline revisions represent an effort to better define patients who are likely to benefit from CRT pacing.

PACING MODES

The Pacemaking Code of the North American Society of Pacing and Electrophysiology and the British Pacing and Electrophysiology Group (NBG) was first published in 1983 and last revised in 2002 (**Table 2**).[23] This code provides a generic understanding of the antibradycardia programming of any CIED. The code has 5 positions: position I describes the chamber(s) paced; position II describes the chamber(s) sensed; position III describes how the CIED responds to a sensed event; position IV adds an R for rate modulation; and position V describes the presence or absence of multisite pacing (such as for BiV pacing or CRT).

As described by the code, and depending on the number of leads and device programming and features, pacing may be delivered to and sensing may occur from a single chamber, 2 chambers, or multiple chambers. The most common single-chamber and dual-chamber pacing modes in the United States are VVI and DDD, respectively.[24] In the VVI mode, pacing and sensing take place only in the ventricle. Ventricular pacing occurs at the programmed lower rate limit; the I in the third position indicates that pacing output is inhibited by a sensed ventricular event. Chronic atrial fibrillation with a slow ventricular response reflects a common reason to select VVI pacing.

Table 2
NASPE/BPEG Generic PM Code (NBG) (revised 2002)

Position I	Position II	Position III	Position IV	Position V
Chambers paced	Chambers sensed	Response to sensing	Programmability	Multisite pacing
O = none	O = none	O = none	O = none	O = none
A = atrium	A = atrium	I = inhibited	R = rate modulation	A = atrium
V = ventricle	V = ventricle	T = triggered		V = ventricle
D = dual (A+V)	D = dual (A+V)	D = dual (T+I)		D = dual (A+V)

In the DDD mode, sensing and pacing take place in both the RA and RV. The D in the third position indicates that atrial events are either sensed or paced, and the CIED then ensures that ventricular events are synchronized to this atrial activity. In the absence of rate modulation (discussed later) and several advanced programmable features, atrial pacing in the DDD mode should occur at the programmed lower rate limit.

Because of its ability to maintain AV synchrony, multiple studies have shown the DDD mode to be superior to VVI for preventing PM syndrome (symptoms from AV dissociation) for patients requiring significant ventricular pacing.[24–26] Other pacing modes that can preserve AV synchrony include atrial pacing in patients with intact AV nodal function (eg, AAI, DDI) and those modes in which sensed atrial activity triggers ventricular pacing (eg, VDD) in patients with AV nodal block. Preserving AV synchrony usually optimizes LV filling and cardiac output and minimizes AV valvular insufficiency and retrograde atrial depolarization, which can occur with isolated RV pacing.[24]

Although preserving AV synchrony can be important when RV pacing is required, unnecessary RV pacing has been associated with detrimental effects such as atrial fibrillation, LV dysfunction, and congestive heart failure.[27] In the late 1990s, the DAVID (Dual Chamber and VVI Implantable Defibrillator) trial compared DDD pacing with VVI pacing in ICD patients without proven need of pacing.[28] Patients were randomized to 1 of 2 groups: 1 group had the pacing component of the ICD programmed to VVI at 40 beats per minute (bpm) (backup pacing only), whereas the other group had the pacing component programmed to DDD at 70 bpm. The study was stopped prematurely because of an increase in the primary composite end point of death or worsened heart failure in the DDD group. As a consequence of this and other studies,[27] pacing algorithms to minimize ventricular pacing have been developed and widely implemented for patients who require pacing (discussed later). Patients not requiring regular pacing, such as those undergoing primary ICD implant for protection against VT or VF or those undergoing CIED implant in the setting of infrequent sinus pauses, often receive single-chamber devices programmed to VVI pacing at a rate of 40 to 50 bpm.

Although DDD is the most common pacing mode, it is not appropriate for all circumstances. For the patient with paroxysmal atrial arrhythmia, this mode requires enabling of the mode switch feature to prevent forced ventricular pacing in the setting of high atrial rates. DDD pacing without a functioning atrial lead can result in R-on-T pacing and VF.[29]

The AAI mode requires intact AV nodal function, because sensing and pacing take place only in the atrium. Because patients with SA node disease have a 0.6% to 5% annual risk of developing AV block[24,30] AAI pacing is rarely used in the United States. However, because of the desire to minimize RV pacing, special hybrid pacing modes now exist that incorporate the use of AAI, allowing a device to switch back and forth between AAI and DDD depending on the presence or absence of intrinsic AV conduction.[31] Sometimes, these algorithms allow significantly prolonged AV delays or a dropped QRS, which can mimic pacing system malfunction.

The modes VDD and DDI warrant mentioning. VDD allows for dual-chamber sensing but ventricular-only pacing. It can be used in the case of AV nodal dysfunction but intact and appropriate sinus node behavior. This pacing strategy requires only a single lead incorporating atrial sensing electrodes as well as ventricular conductors that can both sense and pace, which reduces the overall diameter and blood flow obstruction of the lead (**Fig. 7**). However, this mode lacks the ability to provide atrial pacing. DDI pacing is used for the patient with a dual-chamber device suffering from paroxysmal rapid atrial arrhythmias such as atrial fibrillation. This mode prevents high ventricular pacing rates, which could result from attempted ventricular tracking of an atrial

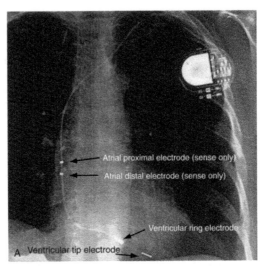

Fig. 7. A VDD pacing system. This configuration is placed into patients with abnormal AV conduction but normal sinus node function, as it cannot be used to depolarize the atrium. This device has 2 electrodes positioned within the RA that can provide sensing to detect intrinsic atrial activity. The ventricular portion of the lead shows the classic bipolar pattern with a ring electrode just proximal to the tip electrode, and these electrodes can be used for sensing intrinsic ventricular activity, as well as depolarizing the ventricle. Because the surface ECG often shows ventricular pacing that tracks the atrial activity, inspection of the surface ECG often produces an erroneous diagnosis of a dual-chamber (DDD) PM. (*From* Rozner MA. Implantable cardiac pulse generators: pacemakers and cardioverter-defibrillators. In: Miller RD, Eriksson LI, Fleisher LA, et al, eds. Miller's Anesthesia, 7th edition. Philadelphia: Elsevier, 2009; with permission.)

arrhythmia, but offers AV synchrony only in the setting of atrial pacing. Most DDD devices have a programmable feature allowing for automatic switching to DDI on detection of a high atrial rate. Depending on the manufacturer, this feature is called mode switch, automatic mode switch, or atrial tachy response.

Asynchronous modes (e.g. AOO, VOO, and DOO) pace their respective chambers without regard to underlying electrical activity. Asynchronous ventricular pacing can result in R-on-T phenomena, so asynchronous pacing modes are used primarily for temporary pacing applications (eg. emergency situations) or during procedures in which EMI might cause pacing inhibition. Asynchronous pacing is often used in the operating room, particularly in the pacing-dependent patient when EMI from monopolar electrocautery is deemed likely.[6]

In the fourth position, the NBG code uses an R to denote the presence of rate modulation. Because some patients cannot increase their heart rate in response to increased oxygen demand (termed chronotropic incompetence), CIED manufacturers have devised several mechanisms to detect patient exercise, such as sensors that detect vibration, respiration, or changes in RV pressure. However, activation of rate response sensors from vigorous chest wall skin preparation, pressure on the generator, vibration from a bone saw, or EMI from a minute ventilation device, resulting in an increased paced rate, has led to inappropriate in-hospital treatment and patient harm.[32–35]

The fifth position of the NBG code denotes multisite pacing, meaning the presence of more than 1 lead in a single cardiac chamber, biatrial, or BiV pacing. Although classically, CRT pacing takes place with discrete leads for each ventricle, multisite atrial and biatrial pacing to prevent atrial fibrillation[36] as well as multisite ventricular pacing to achieve CRT without access to the LV[37] have been reported. Some implanters have used a standard dual-chamber pacing device in an off-label setting for multisite ventricular pacing, in which 1 RV lead (typically in the outflow tract) is connected to the atrial port and the other RV lead (typically in the apex) is connected to the ventricular port.

Like PMs, transvenous ICDs have a 4-place generic NBD code (see **Table 3**) to indicate lead placement and device function, although this code is rarely used outside the research application. Position I indicates the chamber(s) shocked, position II indicates the chamber(s) in which ATP is administered, position III identifies the detection method, and position IV indicates the chamber(s) delivering antibradycardia pacing.[24] Because all transvenous ICDs can perform pacing for bradycardia, the most comprehensive description includes the first 3 characters of the NBD, followed by a dash (-), then the 5-character PM NBG.[38] Many PMs and ICDs now have antiatrial tachycardia, which includes ATP and low-energy cardioversion. Most devices providing antiatrial tachycardia therapy require at least 1 minute of atrial arrhythmia before delivering any therapy.

CIEDS AND PERIOPERATIVE RISK

Although CIEDs are reliable, system malfunction or failure can result from several factors: (1) generator issues; (2) lead issues; or (3) external issues such as EMI. Although the scope of perioperative problems directly related to the CIED is limited, the presence of a CIED may be a general marker for patients at higher risk of cardiovascular or general medical complications in the operative and postoperative period.

An FDA database analysis provides information on the general failure rate of these devices. Maisel and colleagues[39] evaluated the database over a 12-year period and found that, per 1000 implants, 4.6 PMs and 20.7 ICDs had been explanted for issues other than battery depletion. Between 1990 and 2002 (the study period), 2.25 million PMs and 415,780 ICDs were implanted, and 30 PM and 31 ICD patients died as a direct result of device malfunction. Subsequently, Laskey and colleagues[40] analyzed FDA records for transvenous ICD explantations for 2003 to 2007 (459,000 transvenous ICDs and 256,000 CRT-D implanted) and found 10,593 (2.3%) transvenous-ICD and 1925 (0.8%) CRT-D failures. Death might be the first indication of a failed ICD system.[41]

Alerts exist for premature ICD lead failure, which can result in inappropriate shock or failure of shock delivery.[42,43] In addition, several PMs and ICDs remain on alert for silent premature battery depletion,[44,45] and an entire line of Boston Scientific devices have their magnetic mode permanently disabled because of a switch malfunction.[46]

Although it is not known whether the presence of a CIED portends increased perioperative morbidity and mortality, scenarios frequently associated with device failure

Table 3
North American Society of Pacing and Electrophysiology (now the Heart Rhythm Society)/ British Pacing and Electrophysiology Group generic defibrillator code (NBD)

Position I	Position II	Position III	Position IV (or Use PM Code)
Shock chambers	ATP chambers	Tachycardia detection	Antibradycardia pacing chambers
O = none	O = none	E = electrogram	O = none
A = atrium	A = atrium	H = hemodynamic	A = atrium
V = ventricle	V = ventricle		V = ventricle
D = dual (A+V)	D = dual (A+V)		D = dual (A+V)

occur with some regularity in the operating room. For example, failure to capture can result from myocardial ischemia/infarction, acid-base disturbance, electrolyte abnormalities, or abnormal antiarrhythmic drug level(s).[47] Although outright generator or lead failure is rare under routine circumstances, the exposure to EMI that frequently occurs in the operating room presumably places these patients at significantly higher risk for both of these adverse events.

Although well-controlled studies are lacking, specific evidence in the literature suggests that CIED patients may be at increased perioperative risk. Badrinath and colleagues[48] retrospectively reviewed ophthalmic surgery cases at a single center in India from 1979 to 1988 (14,787 cases) and found that the presence of a PM was associated with a significantly increased mortality within 6 weeks postoperatively. The causes of death in this study were predominantly caused by cardiorespiratory failure or cardiac arrest. Pili-Floury and colleagues[49] reported that 2 of 65 PM (3.1%) patients undergoing significant noncardiac surgery died postoperatively of cardiac causes over a 30-month study period. CIED-specific perioperative issues may adversely affect outcomes. Pili-Floury and colleagues[49] reported that 12% of patients required preoperative modification of PM programming and 7.8% required postoperative modification. Levine and colleagues[50] reported increases in pacing thresholds (the amount of energy required to sustain myocardial depolarization) in some thoracic operations. In abstract form, Rozner and colleagues[51] reported a 2-year retrospective review of 172 PM patients evaluated at a preoperative anesthesia clinic, showing that 27 of 172 (16%) needed a preoperative intervention (9 of 27 were generator replacement for newly discovered battery depletion). In addition, follow-up of 149 of these patients who went on to have a surgical procedure showed 5 ventricular pacing threshold increases, 1 atrial pacing threshold increase, and 1 PM electrical reset (all of which occurred during nonthoracic surgery in which monopolar electrocautery was used). Cheng and colleagues[52] prospectively evaluated 92 patients with PMs or ICDs undergoing noncardiac surgery or endoscopic procedures. There was no change in pacing or sensing thresholds but significantly decreased lead impedance in all chambers. One ICD reported an elective reset caused by battery depletion during the case, and several devices reported EMI but no therapy was delivered.

Multiple factors have been reported to cause confusion regarding effective perioperative care of this patient group. First, all ICDs have bradycardia pacing capabilities, so the presence of pacing artifacts on an ECG might lead a clinician to mistake a transvenous ICD for a PM. Second, magnet application to an ICD never produces asynchronous pacing. Instead, magnet application to an ICD usually, but not always, suspends antitachycardia therapies, because some ICDs can be programmed to ignore magnet placement.[47] Third, although some ICDs emit a tone on magnet application to confirm that antitachycardia therapies have been suspended, most ICDs do not emit tones or have any other mechanism to allow for confirmation of appropriate magnet placement. Fourth, ICDs process and respond to EMI differently than a PM. Electronic devices that may be mistaken for cardiac pulse generators are being implanted with increasing frequency for various reasons such as pain control, management of Parkinson disease, phrenic nerve stimulation of the diaphragm, or vagus nerve stimulation (as part of epilepsy therapy).

PRACTICE RECOMMENDATIONS AND EXPERT CONSENSUS STATEMENTS

Based on the information presented earlier, as well as additional case reports describing perioperative CIED-related complications,[47,53,54] many experts consider CIED patients to be at higher perioperative risk and strongly advocate treating them accordingly.

To promote safe perioperative management and mitigate risk in these patients, the ASA published an updated Practice Advisory in 2011 providing expert recommendations for perioperative management of patients with a CIED.[8] This advisory was followed by an Expert Consensus Statement from the HRS in collaboration with the ASA and other organizations.[6] The HRS document in particular emphasizes an individualized approach to patient management, effective multidisciplinary communication before the procedure, a team approach throughout the perioperative period, and reduced reliance on industry representatives to independently manage CIED patients. These documents acknowledge that many providers, including anesthesiologists, surgeons, and internists lack the knowledge, experience and requisite technological devices to independently manage CIED patients. The HRS document further states that the best perioperative care of a patient with a CIED generally comes from the recommendations of a physician or designated CIED team member with specific expertise and experience in monitoring and managing these devices.

Although the importance of these recommendations cannot be overstated, the reality is that not every surgical patient with a CIED is triaged to a CIED expert; especially in the case of a surgical urgency or emergency, in which engaging a CIED expert may not be feasible. Furthermore, because the frequency of patients with CIEDs presenting for surgery seems to be increasing, clinicians who are not CIED experts are being increasingly asked to contribute to the effective preoperative preparation or perioperative management of these patients. Therefore, it is incumbent on clinicians to develop an understanding of how these devices function, as well as the relevant perioperative management considerations as described in this document.

PREOPERATIVE CONSIDERATIONS

Important features of the preoperative CIED evaluation are summarized under preoperative key points in **Box 1**. For the non-CIED expert involved in preoperative preparation of a CIED patient, identifying the generator manufacturer and model provides the first step in perioperative risk reduction and care of these patients. The next step is to establish proper device function, which can be accomplished by determining the most recent device interrogation and analyzing a copy of the interrogation report. A CIED report should provide detailed information regarding the type of device, the indication for its implantation, battery status, current settings (including whether magnet response has been deactivated), pacing dependency, and an overall indication of whether the device was functioning properly at the time of the assessment. Typically, CIEDs should be evaluated every 3 to 12 months, with shorter intervals recommended for patients with more complicated devices or medical conditions and devices under alert notification.[55] However, as mentioned earlier, considerable evidence indicates that PM failure rates are estimated at 5 per 1000 per year and ICD failure rates approach 2.5%.[39,40] Thus, review of the patient's CIED performance, or a de novo interrogation if the device has not been recently interrogated, seems prudent, especially for hemodynamically challenging surgery or cases in which EMI (ie, the need for monopolar electrosurgery) is likely to occur. Although there are no data conclusively showing the need to perform a comprehensive preoperative evaluation of a CIED, anecdotal evidence and case series suggest that incomplete evaluation can result in intraoperative problems and patient harm.[47] In any situation wherein a preoperative device evaluation cannot take place, one should be prepared for perioperative device malfunction or failure.

Although the presence of a CIED generally does not indicate the need for specific preoperative laboratory tests (including chest radiograph, cardiac stress test, or

Box 1
Perioperative recommendations for the patient with a cardiac generator

Preoperative Key Points

The clinician involved in preparing patients for surgery should:

1. Identify the presence of a CIED

2. Identify the generator manufacturer and model (PM, transvenous ICD, subcutaneous ICD) of the CIED

3. Establish contact with the patient's CIED physician/clinic to establish appropriate device function, obtain records, and a specific perioperative prescription (HRS)

4. Have the CIED interrogated by a competent authority shortly before the anesthetic (ASA). HRS recommends an interrogation within 6 months for an ICD and within 1 year for a PM

5. Obtain a copy of this interrogation. Ensure that ICD detection and treatment settings are appropriate and that the CIED paces the heart with an adequate safety margin

In collaboration with a CIED expert:

1. Consider replacing any device near its elective replacement period in a patient scheduled to undergo either a major surgery or surgery within 25 cm of the generator

2. Determine the patient's underlying rate and rhythm to determine the need for backup (external) pacing support

3. Identify the magnet rate and rhythm for a PM, if a magnet mode is present and magnet use is planned

4. Program minute ventilation rate responsiveness off, if present

5. Consider programming all rate enhancements off to prevent rhythm misinterpretation

6. Consider increasing the pacing rate to optimize oxygen delivery to tissues for major cases

7. If EMI is likely: (a) disable antitachycardia therapy if an ICD; (b) consider asynchronous pacing for some pacing-dependent patients. Magnet application might be acceptable for some PMs (provide asynchronous pacing) or ICDs (disable antitachycardia therapy). Asynchronous pacing from an ICD requires reprogramming

Intraoperative Key Points

- Monitor cardiac rhythm/peripheral pulse with pulse oximeter plethysmogram or arterial waveform

- Consider disabling the artifact filter on the ECG monitor

- Whenever possible, avoid use of monopolar electrosurgery (ESU)

- Use bipolar ESU if possible; if not possible, pure cut (monopolar ESU) is better than blend or coag

- Position the ESU dispersive electrode to divert electricity away from the generator-heart circuit, even if the pad must be placed on the distal forearm and the wire covered with sterile drape

- If the ESU causes ventricular oversensing, pacing quiescence, or inappropriate tachycardia, limit the effect by suspending the use of monopolar electrocautery, reprogramming the cardiac generator, or placing a magnet over the PM (not indicated for ICD)

Postoperative Key Points

- Many patients require postoperative interrogation or reprogramming. In particular, any CIED that underwent preoperative or intraoperative reprogramming should be reinterrogated and restored to appropriate parameters. Postoperative CIED interrogation should always be prompted by intraoperative hemodynamic instability or any concern for inappropriate CIED function. In many cases, rate enhancements may need to be reinitiated, and optimum heart rate and pacing parameters should be determined and programmed. The ICD patient must remain in a fully monitored setting (postanesthesia care unit or intensive care unit) until antitachycardia therapy is restored.

echocardiogram), preoperative management of the patient with a CIED must include evaluation and optimization of coexisting disease(s). Special attention to underlying medical issues should be given to the patient with an ICD (which often indicates the presence of cardiomyopathy or other coexisting cardiac disease) as well as the patient with CRT. Patients with heart failure should be evaluated with respect to heart failure guidelines.[56]

Although, as a general principle, tests should be ordered based on usual non-CIED factors such as the history of the patient and the stability of underlying disease, some situations specifically related to the presence of a CIED might necessitate certain testing. For instance, a chest radiograph might be useful for the patient with an LV lead expected to undergo central line placement, because the CS lead dislodges in at least 4.7% of patients at a rate of 2.3% per year.[57] In addition, for cases in which previous records are not available or it is not possible to obtain a de novo interrogation or consultation with a CIED expert, a chest radiograph can provide device type identification, including PM versus ICD versus CRT as well as device manufacturer (**Fig. 8**). The chest film can also provide information about lead configuration and possibly a lead fracture. Additional steps that might provide information about the device include (1) reviewing the implant card that CIED patients are instructed to carry with them at all times and (2) calling the device manufacturer. **Table 4** contains a list of device manufacturers and their phone numbers.

After confirming appropriate device function, the next step in safely preparing a CIED patient for surgery should be identifying the patient's underlying rate and rhythm, which can identify pacing dependence. In general, pacing dependence implies the lack of spontaneous ventricular activity when the CIED is programmed to the VVI mode (AAI for single-chamber atrial devices) at the lowest programmable rate. In the absence of an interrogation, pacing dependency might be established through history or by examining the ECG. A history of AV nodal ablation or a previous placement of a temporary pacing wire confirms likely pacing dependence, and implantation for symptomatic bradyarrhythmia or syncope suggests possible pacing dependence. On the surface ECG, pacing dependence might be present if every complex is paced, except in the case of QRS complexes for CRT, because the goal of CRT programming is to achieve 100% BiV pacing. Pacing dependency represents a key consideration for intraoperative management, as discussed in more detail later.

Other considerations include: ensuring that magnet behavior is appropriate (asynchronous pacing, proper rate and acceptable AV delay for PM, suspension of antitachycardia therapies for ICD) if magnet use is planned (discussed in detail later); programming minute ventilation rate response (and possibly other pacing features that can mimic pacing system malfunction) to off when present; and increasing the lower pacing rate to optimize oxygen delivery for major surgery.

INTRAOPERATIVE CONSIDERATIONS

Although recommendations for intraoperative management usually remain beyond the scope of the preoperative consultant, some key points deserve mention, because consultants may be asked to advise perioperative care team members, especially in urgent or emergent situations. Important intraoperative key points are summarized in **Box 1**).

Patient monitoring (discussed earlier) and protection of the patient and the pulse generator against the effects of EMI (most commonly from monopolar electrosurgery) remain the principal intraoperative issues. For ICDs, the ASA and HRS differ in their specific recommendations. The ASA states that all ICDs should have antitachycardia therapy disabled whenever monopolar electrosurgical unit (ESU) use is planned,

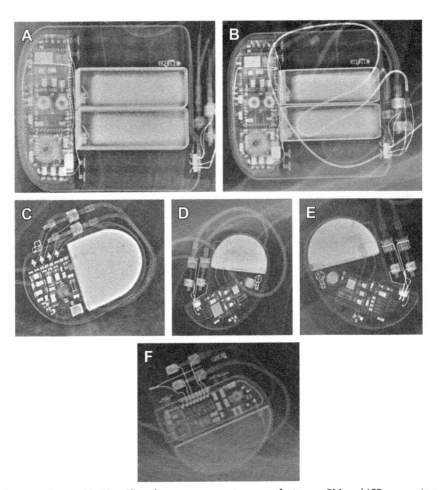

Fig. 8. Radiographic identifiers for some generator manufacturers. PM and ICD generators can be identified from operative dictations, patient cards, or some chest radiographs. Using digital radiograph equipment with postprocessing zoom capability, corporate radiograph logo identifiers from CPI (*A*), Guidant (*B*), Medtronic (*C*), Pacesetter (*D*), St Jude Medical (*E*), and Boston Scientific (*F*) are shown. (*From* Rozner MA. Implantable cardiac pulse generators: pacemakers and cardioverter-defibrillators. In: Miller RD, Eriksson LI, Fleisher LA, et al, eds. Miller's Anesthesia, 7th edition. Philadelphia: Elsevier, 2009; with permission.)

whereas the HRS states that ICD deactivation might not be needed for monopolar ESU application inferior to the umbilicus. Both the ASA and HRS documents agree that consideration should be given to reprogramming the CIED to an asynchronous pacing mode for a pacing-dependent patient undergoing a procedure likely to cause EMI, and both statements caution that magnet application to an ICD does not accomplish this goal.

Further, significant controversy exists regarding the use of a magnet to achieve asynchronous pacing (in the case of a PM) or temporarily suspend antitachycardia therapy (in the case of an ICD). Although many centers routinely place a magnet on a CIED to contend with the issue of EMI, this approach may be unreliable, and several investigators have warned against substituting magnet application for individualized

Table 4	
Device manufacturers and phone numbers	
AM Pacemaker (Guidant Medical)	800-227-3422
Angeion	800-264-2466
Arco Medical (Boston Scientific)	800-227-3422
Biotronik	800-547-0394
Boston Scientific	800-227-3422
Cardiac Control Systems	Unavailable
Cardiac Pacemakers–CPI (Boston Scientific)	800-227-3422
Cardio Pace Medical (Novacon)	Unavailable
Cook Pacemaker	800-245-4715
Coratomic (Biocontrol Technology)	Unavailable
Cordis (St Jude Medical)	800-722-3774
Diag/Medcor (St Jude Medical)	800-722-3774
Edwards Pacemaker Systems (Medtronic)	800-325-2518
ELA Medical (Sorin)	877-669-7674
Intermedics (Boston Scientific)	800-227-3422
Medtronic	800-505-4636
Pacesetter (St Jude Medical)	800-722-3774
Siemans-Elema (St Jude Medical)	800-722-3774
Sorin	877-669-7674
Telectronics Pacing (St Jude Medical)	800-722-3774
Ventritex (St Jude Medical)	800-722-3774
Vitatron (Medtronic)	800-328-2518

Note: In general, manufacturer telephone support is available from a technician/specialist 24 hours per day, 365 days per year. Information that can be obtained includes device type, model and serial number, and data available at the time of implant. More specific information about CIED function (such as programmed parameters, battery, and lead status) may or may not be available from the manufacturer depending in part on whether the patient has remote (home) monitoring.

treatment. In a recently published series describing cases from 3 institutions, inadequate preoperative assessment of CIED function coupled with erroneous assumptions about the effects of magnet application contributed to or caused inappropriate ICD therapy, premature CIED battery depletion, and patient injury.[47] The investigators concluded that practitioners should exercise caution when applying magnets to PMs or defibrillators for surgery. Although magnet application to control CIED function might represent an appropriate management strategy in some cases, the practice of blindly placing a magnet over an ICD is discouraged by both the ASA and HRS. In lieu of blind magnet application, both the ASA and HRS advise practitioners to either obtain knowledge of device functionality and magnet effects before surgery or obtain a timely preoperative CIED interrogation.

For an ICD patient whose antitachycardia therapies are disabled (whether by programming or magnet placement), ECG monitoring and the ability to deliver external cardioversion or defibrillation must always be present; an approach often recommended includes application of external defibrillation pads before surgery until antitachycardia therapies have been restored. When applying external pads, an effort should be made to exclude the pulse generator from the current path to the extent possible. However, one should always remember that the patient, and not the ICD, is being

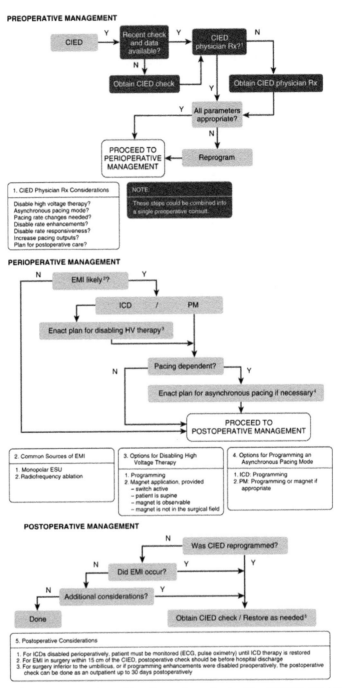

Fig. 9. Operative management considerations of a patient with a PM/ICD. HV, high voltage. (*From* Rozner MA, Schulman PM. How should we prepare the patient with a pacemaker/ implantable cardioverter-defibrillator? In: Fleisher LA, ed. Evidence-based practice of anesthesiology, 3rd edition. Philadelphia: Elsevier, 2013; with permission.)

treated. After any cardioversion/defibrillation, the CIED should be reinterrogated to ensure that normal function is maintained.

To mitigate the risk of EMI from monopolar electrosurgery, both the ASA and HRS concur that the ESU dispersive electrode should be placed so that the presumed ESU current path is directed away from the pulse generator and leads and does not cross the chest.

POSTOPERATIVE CONSIDERATIONS

Key postoperative considerations are summarized under postoperative key points in **Box 1**. Any CIED that underwent preoperative or intraoperative reprogramming should be reinterrogated and restored to appropriate parameters. Patients who have undergone hemodynamically significant surgery, encountered significant EMI issues, or whose ICD high-voltage therapies were disabled by programming must be monitored until the device is interrogated and proper function is confirmed or restored. For nonreprogrammed devices, consideration should be given to ensuring appropriate programming for the patient's postoperative course, which might entail the need to increase the pacing rate or disable features that allow prolonged AV times. The HRS states that stable patients who did not require perioperative reprogramming can be checked after patient discharge within a month of the surgery, rather than the immediate postoperative period. The ASA states that postoperative interrogation might be unnecessary if no monopolar ESU was used, no blood was transfused, there was limited fluid administered, and there were no untoward issues. The postoperative CIED plan, as well as any interrogation or reprogramming, should be recorded into the patient's chart.

Specific recommendations regarding preoperative, intraoperative, and postoperative considerations have been summarized as an algorithm (**Fig. 9**).

SUMMARY

The growing number of patients who present for surgery with a PM or ICD in place necessitates development of a knowledge base on the part of clinicians involved in perioperative care who are not CIED experts. This knowledge base, which should include understanding indications for CIED implantation, basic CIED function, and differences between conventional PMs and ICDs, allows the creation of a management plan tailored to each patient and their surgery. Both the ASA and HRS have published advisory statements, and although the methodology differs, both documents state that proper CIED function should be verified and a specific CIED prescription should be obtained before the surgery. In addition to acquiring general knowledge about CIED function, practitioners caring for patients in the preoperative environment should address the following specific issues in all patients presenting for surgery:

- Is a CIED in place?
- Has a CIED specialist been informed of the surgery and asked to provide recommendations about perioperative management?
- Is the CIED a PM or ICD, and which company manufactured it (so that the appropriate programming machine can be used)?
- Is EMI likely to occur during the surgery? In general, surgeries involving monopolar electrosurgery superior to the inguinal ligament are likely to cause EMI, and those involving monopolar electrosurgery inferior to the inguinal ligament, or only bipolar electrosurgery are unlikely to cause EMI.
- If EMI is likely and the patient has an ICD, antitachycardia therapies must be turned off immediately before surgery and then restored in the immediate

postoperative period. Continuous telemetry monitoring must be maintained and the capability for backup external cardioversion and defibrillation must be immediately available while antitachycardia therapies are suspended. If the plan for suspending antitachycardia therapies involves magnet application in lieu of formal device reprogramming, magnet function must be verified as enabled, easy access to the magnet must exist to allow for its observation and removal, and magnet placement must not interfere with the surgery.

- If EMI is likely and the patient is dependent on CIED pacing (with either a PM or ICD), the CIED should generally be programmed to an asynchronous pacing mode (AOO, VOO, or DOO) before surgery. For PMs, when appropriate, it is often possible to use a magnet for this purpose. In general, magnets do not affect the bradycardia pacing mode or rate of an ICD, meaning that formal device reprogramming is required when an asynchronous pacing mode is desired.

For clinicians involved in preoperative care of the patient with a CIED, acquiring a knowledge base and developing a systematic approach for these patients ensures safe and efficient perioperative care.

REFERENCES

1. Rozner MA. Implantable cardiac pulse generators: pacemakers and cardioverter-defibrillators. Miller's Anesthesia textbook. 7th edition. Elsevier; 2009.
2. Healey JS, Merchant R, Simpson C, et al. Society position statement: Canadian Cardiovascular Society/Canadian Anesthesiologists' Society/Canadian Heart Rhythm Society joint position statement on the perioperative management of patients with implanted pacemakers, defibrillators, and neurostimulating devices. Can J Anaesth 2012;59:394–407.
3. Castillo JG, Silvay G, Viles-Gonzalez J. Perioperative assessment of patients with cardiac implantable electronic devices. Mt Sinai J Med 2012;79:25–33.
4. Engelhardt L, Große J, Birnbaum J, et al. Inhibition of a pacemaker during nerve stimulation for regional anaesthesia. Anaesthesia 2007;62:1071–4.
5. Rozner MA. Peripheral nerve stimulators can inhibit monitor display of pacemaker pulses. J Clin Anesth 2004;16:117–20.
6. Crossley GH, Poole JE, Rozner MA, et al. The Heart Rhythm Society (HRS)/American Society of Anesthesiologists (ASA) Expert Consensus Statement on the perioperative management of patients with implantable defibrillators, pacemakers and arrhythmia monitors: facilities and patient management this document was developed as a joint project with the American Society of Anesthesiologists (ASA), and in collaboration with the American Heart Association (AHA), and the Society of Thoracic Surgeons (STS). Heart Rhythm 2011;8:1114–54.
7. Varma N, Cunningham D, Falk R. Central venous access resulting in selective failure of ICD defibrillation capacity. Pacing Clin Electrophysiol 2001;24:394–5.
8. American Society of Anesthesiologists. Practice advisory for the perioperative management of patients with cardiac implantable electronic devices: pacemakers and implantable cardioverter-defibrillators: an updated report by the American Society of Anesthesiologists task force on perioperative management of patients with cardiac implantable electronic devices. Anesthesiology 2011;114:247–61.
9. Chua J, Patel K, Neelankavil J, et al. Anesthetic management of electrophysiology procedures. Curr Opin Anaesthesiol 2012;25:470–81.
10. Sweeney MO. Antitachycardia pacing for ventricular tachycardia using implantable cardioverter defibrillators. Pacing Clin Electrophysiol 2004;27:1292–305.

11. Stone ME, Salter B, Fischer A. Perioperative management of patients with cardiac implantable electronic devices. Br J Anaesth 2011;107:i16–26.
12. Moss AJ, Schuger C, Beck CA, et al. Reduction in inappropriate therapy and mortality through ICD programming. N Engl J Med 2012;367:2275–83.
13. Korantzopoulos P, Letsas KP, Grekas G, et al. Pacemaker dependency after implantation of electrophysiological devices. Europace 2009;11:1151–5.
14. Ho JK, Mahajan A. Cardiac resynchronization therapy for treatment of heart failure. Anesth Analg 2010;111:1353–61.
15. Rivero-Ayerza M, Theuns DA, Garcia-Garcia HM, et al. Effects of cardiac resynchronization therapy on overall mortality and mode of death: a meta-analysis of randomized controlled trials. Eur Heart J 2006;27:2682–8.
16. Epstein AE, DiMarco JP, Ellenbogen KA, et al. ACC/AHA/HRS 2008 Guidelines for Device-Based Therapy of Cardiac Rhythm Abnormalities: a report of the American College of Cardiology/American Heart Association Task Force on Practice Guidelines (Writing Committee to Revise the ACC/AHA/NASPE 2002 Guideline Update for Implantation of Cardiac Pacemakers and Antiarrhythmia Devices): developed in collaboration with the American Association for Thoracic Surgery and Society of Thoracic Surgeons. Circulation 2008;117:e350–408.
17. Buxton AE, Lee KL, Fisher JD, et al. A randomized study of the prevention of sudden death in patients with coronary artery disease. Multicenter Unsustained Tachycardia Trial Investigators. N Engl J Med 1999;341:1882–90.
18. Moss AJ, Hall WJ, Cannom DS, et al. Improved survival with an implanted defibrillator in patients with coronary disease at high risk for ventricular arrhythmia. Multicenter Automatic Defibrillator Implantation Trial Investigators. N Engl J Med 1996;335:1933–40.
19. Moss AJ, Zareba W, Hall WJ, et al. Prophylactic implantation of a defibrillator in patients with myocardial infarction and reduced ejection fraction. N Engl J Med 2002;346:877–83.
20. Bardy GH, Lee KL, Mark DB, et al. Amiodarone or an implantable cardioverter-defibrillator for congestive heart failure. N Engl J Med 2005;352:225–37.
21. Tracy CM, Epstein AE, Darbar D, et al. 2012 ACCF/AHA/HRS focused update of the 2008 guidelines for device-based therapy of cardiac rhythm abnormalities: a report of the American College of Cardiology Foundation/American Heart Association Task Force on Practice Guidelines and the Heart Rhythm Society [corrected]. Circulation 2012;126:1784–800.
22. Diaz-Infante E, Mont L, Leal J, et al. Predictors of lack of response to resynchronization therapy. Am J Cardiol 2005;95:1436–40.
23. Bernstein AD, Daubert JC, Fletcher RD, et al. The revised NASPE/BPEG generic code for antibradycardia, adaptive-rate, and multisite pacing. North American Society of Pacing and Electrophysiology/British Pacing and Electrophysiology Group. Pacing Clin Electrophysiol 2002;25:260–4.
24. Allen M. Pacemakers and implantable cardioverter defibrillators. Anaesthesia 2006;61:883–90.
25. Skanes AC, Krahn AD, Yee R, et al. Progression to chronic atrial fibrillation after pacing: the Canadian Trial of Physiologic Pacing. CTOPP Investigators. J Am Coll Cardiol 2001;38:167–72.
26. Lamas GA, Lee KL, Sweeney MO, et al. Ventricular pacing or dual-chamber pacing for sinus-node dysfunction. N Engl J Med 2002;346:1854–62.
27. Quesada A, Botto G, Erdogan A, et al. Managed ventricular pacing vs. conventional dual-chamber pacing for elective replacements: the PreFER MVP study: clinical background, rationale, and design. Europace 2008;10:321–6.

28. Wilkoff BL, Cook JR, Epstein AE, et al. Dual-chamber pacing or ventricular backup pacing in patients with an implantable defibrillator: the Dual Chamber and VVI Implantable Defibrillator (DAVID) Trial. JAMA 2002;288:3115–23.

29. Schulman PM, Stecker EC, Rozner MA. R-on-T and cardiac arrest from dual-chamber pacing without an atrial lead. Heart Rhythm 2012;9:970–3.

30. Trohman RG, Kim MH, Pinski SL. Cardiac pacing: the state of the art. Lancet 2004;364:1701–19.

31. Subramanian A, Selvaraj RJ, Cameron D. A tale of four atrioventricular intervals. Europace 2010;12:441–2.

32. Altose MD, Leon-Ruiz E. Etomidate-induced pacemaker-mediated ventricular tachycardia. Anesthesiology 2007;106:1059–60.

33. Schwartzenburg CF, Wass CT, Strickland RA, et al. Rate-adaptive cardiac pacing: implications of environmental noise during craniotomy. Anesthesiology 1997;87: 1252–4.

34. Rozner MA. The patient with a cardiac pacemaker or implanted defibrillator and management during anaesthesia. Curr Opin Anaesthesiol 2007;20:261–8.

35. Lau W, Corcoran SJ, Mond HG. Pacemaker tachycardia in a minute ventilation rate-adaptive pacemaker induced by electrocardiographic monitoring. Pacing Clin Electrophysiol 2006;29:438–40.

36. Fitts SM, Hill MR, Mehra R, et al. Design and implementation of the Dual Site Atrial Pacing to Prevent Atrial Fibrillation (DAPPAF) clinical trial. DAPPAF Phase 1 Investigators. J Interv Card Electrophysiol 1998;2:139–44.

37. Chudzik M, Piestrzeniewicz K, Klimczak A, et al. Bifocal pacing in the right ventricle: an alternative to resynchronization when left ventricular access is not possible in end-stage heart failure patients. Cardiol J 2010;17:35–41.

38. Rozner MA, Schulman PM. How should we prepare the patient with a pacemaker/implantable cardioverter-defibrillator?. In: Fleisher LA, editor. Evidence-Based Practice Of Anesthesiology. 3rd edition. Philadelphia: Saunders; 2013. p. 88–97.

39. Maisel WH, Moynahan M, Zuckerman BD, et al. Pacemaker and ICD generator malfunctions: analysis of Food and Drug Administration annual reports. JAMA 2006;295:1901–6.

40. Laskey W, Awad K, Lum J, et al. An analysis of implantable cardiac device reliability. The case for improved postmarketing risk assessment and surveillance. Am J Ther 2012;19:248–54.

41. Gornick CC, Hauser RG, Almquist AK, et al. Unpredictable implantable cardioverter-defibrillator pulse generator failure due to electrical overstress causing sudden death in a young high-risk patient with hypertrophic cardiomyopathy. Heart Rhythm 2005;2:2681–3.

42. Ellenbogen KA, Wood MA, Shepard RK, et al. Detection and management of an implantable cardioverter defibrillator lead failure: incidence and clinical implications. J Am Coll Cardiol 2003;41:73–80.

43. Urgent medical device information: Sprint Fidelis lead patient management recommendations. Medtronic; 2007. Available at: http://www.medtronic.com/fidelis/physician-letter.html. Accessed March 19, 2013.

44. Product advisories. Boston Scientific; 2013. Available at: http://www.bostonscientific.com/templatedata/imports/HTML/PPR/ppr/support/current_advisories.pdf. Accessed March 23, 2013.

45. Potential rapid battery depletion EnTrust® VR/DR/AT ICDs. Medtronic; 2012. Available at: http://wwwp.medtronic.com/productperformance/document.html?id=300068. Accessed March 23, 2013.

46. Guidant Contak Renewal 3, 4 RF ICD magnet switch. Product Advisories. Published 6/23/05. Available at: http://www.bostonscientific.com/templatedata/imports/HTML/PPR/ppr/support/current_advisories.pdf. Accessed March 19, 2013.

47. Schulman PM, Rozner MA. Use caution when applying magnets to pacemakers or defibrillators for surgery. Anesthesia Analgesia. http://dx.doi.org/10.1213/ANE.0b013e31829003a1.

48. Badrinath SS, Bhaskaran S, Sundararaj I, et al. Mortality and morbidity associated with ophthalmic surgery. Ophthalmic Surg Lasers 1995;26:535–41.

49. Pili-Floury S, Farah E, Samain E, et al. Perioperative outcome of pacemaker patients undergoing non-cardiac surgery. Eur J Anaesthesiol 2008;25:514–6.

50. Levine PA, Balady GJ, Lazar HL, et al. Electrocautery and pacemakers: management of the paced patient subject to electrocautery. Ann Thorac Surg 1986;41:313–7.

51. Rozner MA, Roberson JC, Nguyen AD. Unexpected high incidence of serious pacemaker problems detected by pre-and postoperative interrogations: a two-year experience. J Am Coll Cardiol 2004;43(5):113A.

52. Cheng A, Nazarian S, Spragg DD, et al. Effects of surgical and endoscopic electrocautery on modern-day permanent pacemaker and implantable cardioverter-defibrillator systems. Pacing Clin Electrophysiol 2008;31:344–50.

53. Streckenbach SC. Intraoperative pacemaker rate changes associated with the rest mode. Anesthesiology 2008;109:1137–9.

54. Izrailtyan I, Schiller RJ, Katz RI, et al. Case report: perioperative pacemaker-mediated tachycardia in the patient with a dual chamber implantable cardioverter-defibrillator. Anesth Analg 2013;116:307–10.

55. Wilkoff BL, Auricchio A, Brugada J, et al. HRS/EHRA Expert Consensus on the Monitoring of Cardiovascular Implantable Electronic Devices (CIEDs): description of techniques, indications, personnel, frequency and ethical considerations. Heart Rhythm 2008;5:907–25.

56. Hunt SA, Abraham WT, Chin MH, et al. 2009 Focused update incorporated into the ACC/AHA 2005 Guidelines for the Diagnosis and Management of Heart Failure in Adults A Report of the American College of Cardiology Foundation/American Heart Association Task Force on Practice Guidelines Developed in Collaboration With the International Society for Heart and Lung Transplantation. J Am Coll Cardiol 2009;53:e1–90.

57. Landolina M, Gasparini M, Lunati M, et al. Long-term complications related to biventricular defibrillator implantation: rate of surgical revisions and impact on survival: insights from the Italian Clinical Service Database. Circulation 2011;123:2526–35.

Patients with Vascular Disease

Ann-Marie Manley, MD*, Sarah E. Reck, MD

KEYWORDS

- Preoperative evaluation • Vascular disease • Noncardiac surgery • Anesthesia

KEY POINTS

- Patients with vascular disease often have multiple medical comorbidities, such as cardiovascular disease, diabetes, chronic renal disease, and cerebrovascular disease.
- The preoperative evaluation is an opportunity to optimize a patient before elective surgery and coordinate care among the perioperative care team.
- Vascular surgery is high risk for perioperative cardiac complications.

INTRODUCTION

On conducting a preoperative evaluation of a patient with vascular disease, it is crucial to compile a detailed history and perform a thorough physical examination. One must assess for other comorbidities as well as the extent of the vascular disease. Patients with vascular disease often have coexisting ischemic heart disease, hypertension, cerebrovascular disease, or chronic renal insufficiency. The goal of the preoperative evaluation is to identify modifiable risk factors, coordinate a treatment plan with other members of the perioperative care team (**Fig. 1**), and optimize the patient's medical condition to shift the balance of risk/benefit ratio before proceeding with nonemergent surgery (**Fig. 2**).

The preoperative evaluation is also an opportunity to educate the patient about preoperative medication instructions, and has been shown to reduce patient anxiety and improve satisfaction.[1] The primary care provider may also prepare the patient for the discussion they will have with their anesthesiologist. For example, "the anesthesiologist may talk to you about an additional blood pressure monitor called an arterial line." With this approach, the patient does not hear for the first time about additional invasive monitoring as late as the night before or on the morning of surgery. In a recent population-based study of anesthesia consultation before major noncardiac

Funding Sources and Conflict of Interest: Nil.

Department of Anesthesiology, Medical College of Wisconsin, Froedtert Memorial Lutheran Hospital, 9200 West Wisconsin Avenue, Milwaukee, WI 53226, USA

* Corresponding author.

E-mail address: amanley@mcw.edu

Med Clin N Am 97 (2013) 1077–1093

http://dx.doi.org/10.1016/j.mcna.2013.05.008

0025-7125/13/$ – see front matter © 2013 Elsevier Inc. All rights reserved.

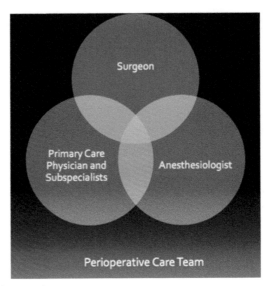

Fig. 1. Perioperative care team.

surgery, preanesthetic consultation was associated with reduced length of stay in hospital.[2]

EVALUATION OF COEXISTING DISEASES

It can be argued that a detailed history and thorough physical examination are more helpful and cost effective than any laboratory or diagnostic test. This section briefly discusses common coexisting diseases in the patient with vascular disease. The reader is referred to an article elsewhere in this issue for more information on disease-specific recommendations.

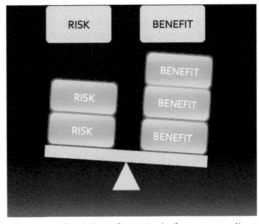

Fig. 2. Shifting the balance of risk/benefit ratio before proceeding with nonemergent surgery.

Ischemic Heart Disease

Risk assessment

Vascular surgery has a high risk for perioperative cardiac morbidity and mortality (>5%).[3] The current American College of Cardiology/American Heart Association (ACC/AHA) guidelines stratify patient risk based on 3 factors[3]:

- Procedure-related risks
  - Low (endoscopic procedures, superficial procedures not requiring general anesthesia)
  - Intermediate (intraperitoneal, intrathoracic, carotid endarterectomy (CEA), orthopedic surgery)
  - High (aortic and other major vascular surgery)
- Functional capacity
  - Greater than 4 metabolic equivalents (METS)
  - Less than 4 METS
- Presence of patient clinical predictors
  - Ischemic heart disease
  - Compensated or prior heart failure
  - Cerebrovascular disease
  - Diabetes mellitus
  - Renal insufficiency

Depending on the patient's risk profile, additional testing may be indicated if it will change management (**Box 1, Table 1**). If the decision is made to proceed with further workup, the most appropriate test will depend on the patient's underlying medical disease, ability to exercise, baseline electrocardiogram (ECG), and institution resources. The 2012 Updated American Society of Anesthesiologists Advisory on Preoperative Evaluation states that age alone may not be an indication for preoperative ECG; instead a patient's risk factors for cardiovascular disease may be a more appropriate indication for an ECG.[4] It should be noted than an abnormal preoperative ECG does not closely correlate with perioperative cardiovascular complications. The ACC/AHA guidelines recommend preoperative resting ECG in patients with at least 1 clinical risk factor (see list of patient clinical predictors above) undergoing vascular surgical procedures and in patients with known ischemic heart disease, peripheral arterial disease, and cerebrovascular disease undergoing intermediate-risk surgery (see list of procedure-related risks above).[3]

Preoperative B-type natriuretic peptide (NP) may be considered for the vascular patient scheduled for noncardiac surgery. A recent meta-analysis reported that the preoperative NP levels can be used to independently predict cardiovascular events in the 30 days after vascular surgery.[5] Although there are no guidelines recommending the routine testing of NP levels before surgery, it is an additional tool that may help identify high-risk patients.

Box 1
Examples of when perioperative cardiac testing will change management

- A less invasive or nonsurgical treatment option would be considered if the patient is deemed high risk

- Elective surgery will be canceled

- Additional invasive monitoring will be considered

Table 1
Risk assessment

Functional Capacity	Surgery	Clinical Risk Factors	Recommendations
>4 METS	Any	0–4	Proceed with no additional testing
<4 METS or unable to assess	Low risk	0–4	Proceed with no additional testing
<4 METS or unable to assess	Intermediate or high risk	0	Proceed with no additional testing
<4 METS or unable to assess	Intermediate or high risk	1–2	Proceed with heart-rate control or consider testing if it will change your management
<4 METS or unable to assess	Intermediate risk	≥3	Proceed with heart-rate control or consider testing if it will change your management
<4 METS or unable to assess	High risk	≥3	Consider testing if it will change your management

Perioperative β-blockade

The patient with vascular disease should be considered for perioperative β-blockade. This decision should take into consideration the patient's clinical risk factors for ischemic heart disease and the cardiac burden of the planned surgery. Initiation of high-dose β-blockade immediately before surgery can cause serious complications such as bradycardia, hypotension, and stroke.[6] For patients not currently on a β-blocker, a gradual titration to hemodynamic effect started several weeks before surgery is generally recommended. The following are the guidelines used by the authors' institution, which are adapted from the 2009 ACC/AHA update[3]:

Inclusion Criteria
1. Patients undergoing surgical procedures of moderate to high risk
   - All vascular surgical procedures: aortic, carotid, peripheral
   - Major orthopedic: total joints, open spine surgery
   - Open abdominal, pelvic, gastrointestinal, urologic, gynecologic
   - Major head and neck

   AND
2a. Patients with known coronary artery disease (CAD)

   OR
2b. Patients with at least 2 of the following risk factors for CAD:
   - Diabetes mellitus
   - Peripheral vascular disease
   - Renal insufficiency (Cr >2.0)
   - Cerebrovascular disease (stroke, transient ischemic attack [TIA])

Exclusion Criteria:
   - Acute or recent (<1 month) exacerbation of heart failure
   - Severe left ventricular dysfunction (<30% ejection fraction) unless already taking β-blocker
   - Significant bradycardia
   - Second- or third-degree heart block

- Reactive airway disease and dependence on daily β-agonists or bronchospasm exacerbation
- Allergy to β-blockers
- Systolic blood pressure less than 100 mm Hg or heart rate less than 50 beats/min

If a patient is to be started on a β-blocker, atenolol or metoprolol, 25 to 50 mg daily is recommended, titrating to a heart rate lower than 65 beats/min. If a patient is on a β-blocker, this should be continued uninterrupted perioperatively. Further discussion regarding the use of β-blockers in patients with heart disease can be found in an article elsewhere in this issue.

Perioperative anticoagulation

Patients with vascular disease are often on chronic anticoagulants. The most common drugs encountered are:

- Vitamin K antagonists: warfarin
- Antiplatelet therapy: aspirin, clopidogrel
- Direct thrombin inhibitors: dabigatran

Each patient's situation will need to be evaluated on an individual basis. A plan will need to be made in coordination with the prescribing physician (usually the cardiologist or primary care physician) and the surgeon. The risk of surgical bleeding will need to be weighed against the risk of in-stent thrombosis, venous thromboembolism, or stroke. It is recommended that patients at high risk for thromboembolic events receive bridging anticoagulation while warfarin is held (**Table 2**).[7,8] For patients with coronary stents, the ACC/AHA guidelines recommend the following[3]:

- Bare-metal stent (BMS):
  - Delay elective surgery for 30 to 45 days
  - Continue aspirin perioperatively
- Drug-eluting stent (DES):
  - Delay elective surgery for 365 days
  - Continue aspirin perioperatively

Table 2
Thromboembolic risk stratification

High Risk (>10%/y)	Moderate Risk (4%–10%/y)	Low Risk (<4%/y)

Mechanical valve
  In mitral valve position
  Older aortic valve prosthesis
  Stroke or TIA within 6 mo
	Aortic prosthesis
	  Hypertension
	  Atrial fibrillation
	  Age >75 y
	  Stroke or TIA
	  Heart failure
		Aortic prosthesis without
		  atrial fibrillation and no
		  other risk factors for stroke

Atrial fibrillation
  CHADS$_2$ score = 5–6
  Stroke or TIA within 3 mo
  Rheumatic heart disease
	Atrial fibrillation
	  CHADS$_2$ score = 3–4
		Atrial fibrillation
		  CHADS$_2$ score = 0–2

VTE within 3 mo
  Severe thrombophilia
	VTE within past 3–12 mo
	  Recurrent VTE
	  Active cancer
		VTE (single event >12 mo ago
		  and no other risk factors

Abbreviations: CHADS$_2$: C = congestive heart failure, H = hypertension, A = age >75 y, D = diabetes, S$_2$ = prior stroke/TIA/thromboembolism; TIA, transient ischemic attack; VTE, venous thromboembolism.

Recent data have shown that discontinuation of dual-antiplatelet therapy beyond 6 months in patients with DES does not appear to have a large impact on risk of adverse cardiac events.[9,10] It is probably safe to proceed with elective surgery 6 months after DES placement with the continuation of aspirin perioperatively; however, this decision should be made on an individual basis is consultation with the patient's cardiologist. According to the ACC/AHA guidelines, consideration should be made to continue dual-antiplatelet therapy perioperatively beyond the recommend time frame in patients at high risk for the consequences of stent thrombosis.[3]

Hypertension

Blood pressure goals will differ depending on the type of surgery the patient is undergoing and any underlying vascular disease (see later discussion on blood pressure management).

Pulmonary

Risk assessment

Perioperative pulmonary complications can lead to unexpected admissions to the intensive care unit (ICU), prolonged length of hospital stay, and death. Pulmonary complications are the second most common serious perioperative morbidity after cardiovascular events.[11] Risk factors for pulmonary complications include[12]:

- Cigarette smoking
- Advanced age (>70 years)
- Chronic obstructive pulmonary disease
- Prolonged surgery (>2 hours)
- Poor nutrition (albumin <3 g/dL)
- Poor exercise capacity
- Obesity (body mass index >30 kg/m^2) particularly when associated with restrictive lung disease
- General anesthesia
- Type of surgery (upper abdominal, thoracic, aortic)

For the patient with stable chronic lung disease, there is little utility in preoperative pulmonary function testing or chest radiography. However, this does not apply to the patient being evaluated for lung resection. The patient's clinical history and physical examination findings are more valuable than any test result. If a patient is not acutely decompensating owing to infection or another cause, it is unlikely that the result of any pulmonary function test will alter the anesthetic management. This is not to say that the underlying disease process does not affect surgical and anesthetic decisions (for further discussion of the patient with pulmonary disease, see the article elsewhere in this issue). For example, a patient with severe restrictive lung disease, pulmonary hypertension, and right heart failure may not be a suitable candidate for the physiologic changes induced during a lengthy robotic procedure in the steep Trendelenburg position.

For the anesthesiologist, the preoperative visit is also an opportunity to develop a plan for postoperative pain management. For the primary care physician, the preoperative visit is an opportunity to discuss patient expectations for postoperative pain management and help coordinate a plan with the surgeon and anesthesiologist. Such planning is especially important for the patient with chronic pain. Thoracic epidural for postoperative pain management has been shown to reduce pulmonary complications.[13] As with all procedures, the risks and benefits of neuraxial anesthesia need to be weighed and discussed with the patient. Absolute contraindications to thoracic epidural are:

- Patient refusal
- Coagulopathy or use of anticoagulants (with the exception of nonsteroidal anti-inflammatory drugs [NSAIDs])
- Local anesthetic allergy
- Infection at the site of insertion

Smoking

Patients with chronic pulmonary disease should be assessed for medical optimization. Of the aforementioned risk factors for perioperative pulmonary complications, smoking and nutritional status are modifiable. It is now becoming recognized that the preoperative visit provides an opportunity to intervene at a teachable moment. Most patients are aware of the general health hazards of smoking; however, they may not be aware of the specific risks in the perioperative period. Although it is optimal for patients to quit smoking 8 weeks before surgery, it has been shown that even brief periods of abstinence or "fasting" from smoking can provide benefits such as normalization of CO levels and decreased frequency of intraoperative ischemia.[14] The American Society of Anesthesiologists has developed a Stop Smoking Initiative, with tools available at www.asahq.org/stopsmoking. The greatest benefit to the patient is the possibility of successful smoking cessation and the long-term health benefits.

Diabetes

According to the Centers for Disease Control and Prevention, diabetes is the seventh leading cause of death in the United States. It is a risk factor for vascular disease and CAD, among multiple other microvascular and macrovascular complications. With the obesity epidemic in the United States there has been an associated increased incidence in the diagnosis of diabetes (**Fig. 3**). In 2010, it was estimated that 8.3% of the population have diabetes.[15]

For a more accurate assessment of the patient's control of blood sugar, a hemoglobin A_{1C} panel should be ordered, which provides the patient's average blood glucose level over the past several months. Because of the risks associated with hypoglycemia, intensive perioperative glucose management is no longer recommended.[16] A glycohemoglobin of less than 8% is reasonable for patients with extensive comorbidities, but less than 7% is preferable (**Table 3**).[17] There are no specific guidelines for intraoperative glucose goals; however, it is probably reasonable to set a goal of less than 180 mg/dL based on data from ICU patients. As always, blood pressure control, lipid control, and smoking cessation will decrease perioperative complications.

Renal

Chronic renal insufficiency (CRI) is a clinical risk factor for perioperative cardiac complications.[3] Patients with vascular disease may have CRI secondary to a variety of pathologic processes such as diabetic nephropathy, hypertensive nephropathy, or renal artery stenosis. Patients with CRI are at risk for perioperative decline in renal function. Nephrotoxic drugs, such as NSAIDs, should be avoided perioperatively. These patients do not tolerate renal hypoperfusion, which can occur with hypotension and decreased cardiac output or with vasoconstriction from endogenous or exogenous sources.

Close attention needs to be paid to the patient's fluid status and electrolytes. An ECG is recommended, because of the ischemic risk in addition to the conduction disturbances that occur with electrolyte imbalances such as hyperkalemia. Patients with CRI not only have chronic anemia but also likely have platelet dysfunction. Depending

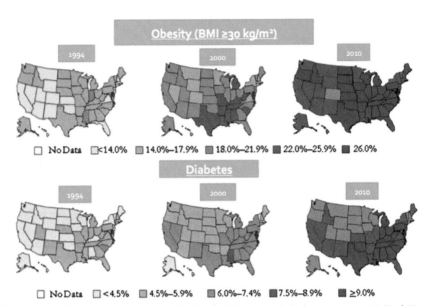

Fig. 3. Age-adjusted prevalence of obesity and diagnosed diabetes among United States adults aged 18 years and older. BMI, body mass index. (*From* Centers for Disease Control. Division of Diabetes Translation, National Diabetes Surveillance System. Available at http://www.cdc.gov/diabetes/statistics. Accessed March 3, 2013.)

on the planned procedure, a hematocrit assessment, and type and screen should be considered. If the patient is on hemodialysis, coordination with the dialysis schedule will be necessary. Optimally, surgery should be scheduled about 24 hours after dialysis to optimize fluid and electrolyte status.

EVALUATION OF SPECIFIC VASCULAR DISEASES

Patients with chronic vascular disease have many features in common, so all of these patients should be screened, then appropriately treated and risk stratified for these diseases. The following discussion focuses on specific therapy for each isolated vascular disease.

Cerebrovascular Disease

Epidemiology
The incidence of stroke in the United States is 700,000 per year, of which 500,000 are new strokes and 200,000 are recurrent strokes. The incidence of perioperative stroke

Table 3 Diabetes assessment levels	
	Goal
Blood pressure	<130/80 mm Hg
Low-density lipoprotein	<100 mg/dL if no coronary artery disease <70 mg/dL if coronary artery disease
Hemoglobin A_{1c}	<7%

Data from American Diabetes Association. Standards of medical care in diabetes—2012. Diabetes Care 2012;35(Suppl 1):S11–63.

in procedures other than cardiac, neurosurgical, and carotid artery surgery is between 0.05% and 7.4%. Mortality rates for perioperative stroke are extraordinarily high, with patients who have had a previous stroke having mortality rates as high as 87%.[18] Therefore, appropriately risk-stratifying this patient population and aggressive preoperative optimization is essential.

The epidemiology of patients who have strokes can help the perioperative physician screen for patients who are at higher risk of the disease (**Table 4**).[19]

Other risk factors for stroke include presence of carotid artery stenosis, higher total cholesterol and low-density lipoprotein levels, high fibrinogen levels, systolic hypertension, smoking, peripheral vascular disease, diabetes, known cerebrovascular disease, and history of atrial fibrillation.

Patients with a history of stroke should undergo careful evaluation to make sure they are well optimized before elective surgery, to decrease the risk of perioperative stroke and other perimorbid complications. In addition to the usual physical examination, one should perform a neurologic examination and document any preexisting deficits so that they can be compared with any new deficits that may develop in the perioperative period.

In patients with recent stroke, elective surgery should be delayed until the patient has had sufficient time to recover after the stroke. This delay must take place because after a stroke, cerebral autoregulation is impaired and the affected brain areas are dependent on systemic perfusion pressure such that episodes of hypotension, which frequently occur during anesthesia, can more readily lead to cerebral hypoperfusion (**Fig. 4**). Impaired autoregulation has been shown to begin within 8 hours after stroke, and lasts for between 2 and 6 months. Thus the exact amount of time to delay elective surgery after acute stroke is controversial, but 1 to 3 months seems reasonable.[20]

Given that patients with recent stroke often require anesthesia for urgent conditions including revascularization after stroke or hip/femur fractures, the perioperative physician may be asked to evaluate these patients in the immediate peristroke period. Of importance, both general anesthesia and a systolic blood pressure of less than 140 mm Hg were independent risk factors for worse neurologic outcomes in patients with acute ischemic stroke.[21] Whether this is because general anesthesia alone tends to decrease blood pressure, which then leads to brain hypoperfusion, or is due to an independent association with the stroke is unknown. Thus in evaluating these patients,

Table 4
Epidemiology of stroke

Population	Stroke Prevalence (%)
Native American	6.0
African American	4.0
Multiracial	4.6
Caucasian	2.3
Hispanic	2.6
Asian	1.6
Age >65 y	8.1
Male	2.7
Female	2.5
<12 y of formal education	4.4

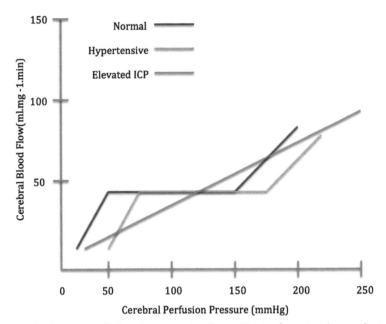

Fig. 4. Cerebral autoregulation in normotensive patients, hypertensive patients, and patients with elevated intracranial pressure (ICP).

considerable attention should be paid to the patient's blood pressure and antihypertensive medications. Permissive hypertension is often allowed immediately following stroke, so often these patients will be off their long-acting hypertensive agents. If they are on any long-acting agents, angiotensin-converting enzyme (ACE) inhibitors, angiotensin-II receptor blockers, and diuretics need to be discontinued at least on the morning of surgery if not for 24 hours beforehand, as they can lead to acute, refractory intraoperative hypotension.

Carotid Stenosis

Patients with carotid artery stenosis are at higher risk for stroke in general, and perioperative stroke in particular. Risk factors for carotid artery stenosis include male gender, age older than 65 years, smoking, hypertension, diabetes mellitus, and dyslipidemia.

As part of the perioperative examination, these patients should be questioned for the presence of known carotid stenosis, previous revascularization, and symptoms of carotid stenosis, and should also undergo auscultation of their carotid arteries to establish whether bruits are present.

In patients with known carotid stenosis, the perioperative physician should evaluate for recent symptoms of TIA/stroke, including ipsilateral transient visual changes, amaurosis fugax, contralateral weakness/numbness of an arm, leg, or the face, visual field defects, dysarthria, and aphasia. Symptoms of dizziness, generalized weakness, syncope/near syncope, floaters in the vision, and blurry vision are nonspecific and are not considered to be ischemic events.[22] Because symptomatic patients are at high risk for stroke, they may qualify for carotid revascularization and should be referred to a vascular surgeon before any elective surgical procedure.

In patients who are asymptomatic with known stenosis, one should ascertain the degree of stenosis, which can easily be done by obtaining their most recent vascular studies (carotid duplex scan/angiography, magnetic resonance imaging). Most asymptomatic patients do not qualify for revascularization; however, the degree of stenosis may alter the anesthetic management related to control of blood pressure, and thus is important information for the anesthesiologist.

Perioperative control of blood pressure is imperative, as TIA can be caused by hypoperfusion through poorly collateralized circulation. Uncontrolled hypertension will lead to a right shift of the patient's cerebral autoregulation curve (see **Fig. 4**), and the hemodynamic changes that occur under general anesthesia can thus put the patient at risk for hypoperfusion.

Patients who do not have known stenosis, but have risk factors, should be questioned for symptomatic stenosis. In the absence of symptoms, the value of screening patients for carotid stenosis is largely unknown. Studies have shown that the presence of carotid bruit is a poor predictor of carotid stenosis, although it does usually indicate the presence of generalized cerebrovascular and atherosclerotic disease. Evidence that supports these findings includes:

- The Framingham Heart Study, which showed that carotid bruits are associated with a double risk of stroke, but that most of these strokes occurred in vascular territories other than the bruit.[23]
- In patients with asymptomatic bruits, 1% to 3% annually have a stroke ipsilateral to the bruit.[23]
- The rate of myocardial infarction (MI) and cardiovascular death in patients with bruits is twice that in patients without bruits, and these patients are more likely to die from cardiovascular than cerebrovascular disease.[24]

Carotid artery stenosis: whom to revascularize

The decision on which patients require carotid revascularization and when this should occur will depend on patients' symptoms, degree of stenosis, risk factors, life expectancy, and type of elective surgery they are to undergo. Although the vascular surgeon will ultimately make this decision, it is important for the perioperative physician to know which patients might qualify, as this may lead to delay or cancellation of other surgical procedures that require coordination.

Patients with symptomatic stenosis require prompt evaluation by a vascular surgeon because the risk of ipsilateral stroke is highest within 90 days of initial symptoms. These patients almost always require revascularization unless the risk of the intervention is higher than the risk of the disease alone.

As regards revascularizing patients with asymptomatic stenosis, the evidence is less convincing. While certainly the risk of stroke and MI increases with increasing degrees of stenosis, because the surgical procedure itself carries a high risk of stroke, the risks and benefits must be carefully weighed. The degree of carotid stenosis increases the patient's risk of stroke; unselected patients have 0.1% risk of perioperative stroke, those with asymptomatic bruits 1%, and those with greater than 50% stenosis 3.6% risk of stroke.[19] Indications for carotid stenting or CEA in patients with asymptomatic carotid artery disease are summarized in **Table 5**.[22]

Abdominal Aortic Aneurysm

Given the high morbidity and mortality associated with abdominal aortic aneurysm (AAA) repair, they are not surgically repaired until they reach greater than 5.5 cm in diameter, as this is the size at which the yearly risk for rupture is equal to the risk of surgery.[25] Thus, many patients with unrepaired AAA will present for nonvascular surgery.

Table 5
Indications for carotid endarterectomy (CEA) in patients with asymptomatic carotid artery disease

For Patients with Surgical Risk <3% and Life Expectancy of at Least 5 y	
Proven indications	Ipsilateral CEA in stenotic lesions with >60% diameter reduction in distal outflow tract with or without ulceration and with or without antiplatelet therapy, irrespective of contralateral artery status
Acceptable indications	Unilateral CEA simultaneous with coronary artery bypass grafting (CABG) for lesions >60% with or without ulcerations with or without antiplatelet therapy, irrespective or contralateral artery status
Uncertain indications	Unilateral CEA for stenosis >50%
For Patients with Surgical Risk of 3%–5%	
Proven indications	None
Acceptable but not proven indications	Ipsilateral CEA for stenosis >75% with or without ulceration but in the presence of contralateral carotid artery stenosis of 75%–100%
Uncertain indications	Ipsilateral CEA for stenosis >75% irrespective of contralateral disease CABG required with bilateral asymptomatic stenosis >70%, unilateral CEA with CABG Unilateral carotid stenosis >70%, CABG required, ipsilateral CEA with CABG
For Patients with Surgical Risk of 5%–10%	
Proven indications	None
Acceptable but not proven indications	None
Uncertain indications	CABG required with bilateral asymptomatic stenosis >70%, unilateral CEA with CABG Unilateral stenosis >70% CABG required, ipsilateral CEA with CABG
Proven inappropriate indications	Ipsilateral CEA for stenosis >75% with or without ulceration, irrespective of contralateral carotid artery status

For patients with new abdominal bruits heard on preoperative physical examination, a computed tomography scan is warranted to evaluate for AAA before elective surgery so that the patient can be fully optimized.

AAA has an increasing prevalence with advancing age. Risk factors for AAA include advancing age, family history, male gender, and tobacco use. Noteworthy is that having a family history of AAA is a significant risk factor. First-degree male relatives of patients with AAA have 2 to 4 times the risk of normal, whereas females with first-degree relatives with AAA appear to have similar risk.[25] The perioperative physician should obtain a detailed family history and have a high index of suspicion for AAA in those with a family history of the disease.

Hypertension

Patients with AAA almost always present with contaminant hypertension. Given that hypertension and sudden increases in blood pressure are risks for aneurysm rupture, it is imperative for these patients to have good preoperative control of the hypertension. Because of the sympathetic surge that occurs during anesthesia and surgery, large swings in blood pressure can be seen, which is even more pronounced in patients with uncontrolled hypertension. Part of the preoperative evaluation should focus on determining the patient's actual resting blood pressure, and optimizing it before surgery with titration of current antihypertensives or addition of new ones. Furthermore, this patient population benefits from good heart-rate control, so titration of β-blockers might be appropriate.

If the patient is seen preoperatively and needs improved control of blood pressure, β-blockers, α-blockers, and ACE inhibitors are suitable agents, if the patient is not already taking them. Optimally these would be started at least several weeks before surgery and titrated to hemodynamic effect. In addition, retrospective studies show that β-blockade might reduce the risk of AAA expansion and rupture.[25]

Hereditary Risk Factors

Although the typical patient with AAA is an older man with a history of vascular disease, the perioperative physician should keep in mind that genetic connective tissue disorders such as Marfan syndrome predispose patients to aortic aneurysms. Thus, young patients with family history, associated comorbidities, and body habitus should be screened carefully for thoracic and aortic aneurysms.

Marfan Syndrome

Marfan syndrome is a connective tissue disease with an incidence of 1 in 3000 to 5000. It is characterized by patients with tall stature, long digits, scoliosis, pectus excavatum, ascending aortic dilation/dissection, valvular disorders, arrhythmias, and ocular disorders. The main issue in preoperative preparation of these patients is in dealing with their cardiac disorders, as the hemodynamic alterations of surgery and anesthesia could potentially lead to rupture of an undiagnosed aortic aneurysm.

Aortic root disease is the main cause of morbidity and mortality in this population, with 60% to 80% of adults with Marfan syndrome having dilation of the aortic root. The 2010 ACC/AHA/American Association for Thoracic Surgery (AATS) guidelines for thoracic aortic disease recommend that patients with Marfan syndrome have echocardiography to assess diameter of the aortic root at the time of diagnosis, and 6 months later and annually thereafter as long as the size of the aorta is stable and smaller than 45 mm. If rapid growth is noted or the size is greater than 45 mm, more frequent evaluation is recommended. The perioperative physician should make sure that these patients have had the appropriate cardiac imaging, as elective procedures should be canceled in favor of aortic root repair once the patient qualifies for such a procedure because the hemodynamic stress response of anesthesia and surgery can lead to aortic dissection. Although the exact diameter regarding which repair should be undertaken is controversial, the 2010 ACC/AHA/AATS guidelines recommend operation once the diameter is greater than 50 mm.[26]

Ensuring that these patients are on appropriate medical therapy in the perioperative period is also essential, as this can lower morbidity and mortality. β-Blockers are the standard of care in patients with Marfan syndrome; they have been shown to improve the elastic properties of the aorta as well as decrease myocardial contractility and pulse pressure. In the perioperative period, β-blockers decrease the sympathetic surge seen with anesthetic and surgical stimulation.

Patients who have had aortic valve replacement with a mechanical prosthetic valve will be on coumadin, and will need to be bridged with low molecular weight heparin

Table 6 Guidelines for patients requiring prophylaxis before endocarditis	
American Heart Association	**British Society for Antimicrobial Chemotherapy**
Prosthetic cardiac valves	Previous endocarditis
Previous endocarditis	Cardiac valve replacement surgery (mechanical or biological prosthetic valve)
Congenital heart disease Unrepaired cyanotic heart disease, including palliative shunts and conduits Completely repaired congenital heart defects with prosthetic material or device, whether placed by surgery or catheter intervention, during the first 6 mo after the procedure Repaired congenital heart disease with residual defects at the site or adjacent to the site of the prosthetic patch or prosthetic device Cardiac transplantation recipients who develop cardiac valvulopathy	Surgically constructed systemic or pulmonary shunt or conduit

in the perioperative period; they may also require prophylaxis for endocarditis (**Table 6**).[27]

Of note, endocarditis prophylaxis is only required in patients undergoing dental procedures, which are invasive to the gumline. Prophylaxis may also be considered in those undergoing procedures that involve incision or biopsy of the respiratory mucosa. In addition, if the procedure is being done to manage active infection, prophylaxis is recommended.

Finally, patients with Marfan syndrome have facial anomalies, which can cause retroagnathia and high arched palate, and lead to difficulty with intubation. If available, old anesthetic records should be obtained to look for prior difficulty with intubation, which would alert the anesthesiologist to the need for immediate availability of equipment for difficult airways.

Peripheral Vascular Disease

In evaluating the patient with peripheral vascular disease (PVD) for anesthesia, the focus should be on optimizing the patient's medical comorbidities. Patients with PVD are at very high risk for CAD, cerebrovascular disease, carotid artery stenosis, and diabetes mellitus (DM). In fact, 75% of patients with PVD have CAD.[28] Furthermore, because of claudication, their functional capacity may be limited and symptoms of CAD may be masked. For this reason, care must be taken in risk-stratifying these patients and determining whether a preoperative stress test is indicated.

SUMMARY

Patients with chronic vascular disease usually have multiple medical comorbidities including CAD, DM, cerebrovascular disease, CRI, smoking, and hypertension, which require careful attention from the perioperative physician for optimization before proceeding to the operating room for anesthesia. In addition, depending on the patient's underlying vascular disease, additional workup and screening may be necessary for adequate perioperative optimization.

REFERENCES

1. Klopfenstein C, Forster A, Van Gessel E. Anesthetic assessment in an outpatient consultation clinic reduces preoperative anxiety. Can J Anaesth 2000;47(6):511–5.
2. Wijeysundera D, Austin P, Beattie W, et al. A population-based study of anesthesia consultation before major noncardiac surgery. Arch Intern Med 2009;169(6):595–602.
3. Fleisher L, Beckman J, Brown K, et al. 2009 ACCF/AHA focused update on perioperative beta blockade incorporated into the ACC/AHA 2007 guidelines on perioperative cardiovascular evaluation and care for noncardiac surgery. J Am Coll Cardiol 2009;54(22):e13–118.
4. Apfelbaum J, Connis R, Nickinovich, et al. Practice advisory for preanesthesia evaluation: an updated report by the American Society of Anesthesiologists Task Force on Preanesthesia Evaluation. Anesthesiology 2012;116(3):522–38.
5. Reitze N, Lurati Buse G, Bollinger D, et al. The predictive ability of pre-operative B-type natriuretic peptide in vascular patients for major adverse cardiac events. An individual patient data meta-analysis. J Am Coll Cardiol 2011;58:522–9.
6. Devereaux P, Yang H, Yusuf S, et al. Effects of extended-release metoprolol succinate in patients undergoing non-cardiac surgery (POISE trial): a randomised controlled trial. Lancet 2008;371(9627):1839–47.
7. Douketis J, Berger P, Dunn A, et al. The perioperative management of antithrombotic therapy: American College of Chest Physicians evidence-based clinical practice guidelines, 8th edition. Chest 2008;133(Suppl 6):299S–339S.
8. Guyatt G, Akl E, Crowther M, et al. Executive summary: Antithrombotic therapy and prevention of thrombosis, 9th ed: American College of Chest Physicians evidence-based clinical practice guidelines. Chest 2012;141(Suppl 2):7S–47S.
9. Valgimigli M, Campo G, Monti M, et al. Short- versus long-term duration of dual-antiplatelet therapy after coronary stenting: a randomized multicenter trial. Circulation 2012;125(16):2015–26.
10. Ferreira-Gonzalez I, Marsal J, Ribera A, et al. Double antiplatelet therapy after drug-eluting stent implantation: risk associated with discontinuation with the first year. J Am Coll Cardiol 2012;60(15):1333–9.
11. McAlister F, Bertsch K, Bradley J, et al. Incidence of and risk factors for pulmonary complications after nonthoracic surgery. Am J Respir Crit Care Med 2005;171(5):514–7.
12. Arozullah A, Daley J, Henderson W, et al. Multifactorial risk index for predicting postoperative respiratory failure in men after major noncardiac surgery. The National Veterans Administration Surgical Quality Improvement Program. Ann Surg 2000;232(2):242–53.
13. Liu S, Wu C. Effect of postoperative analgesia on major postoperative complications: a systematic update of the evidence. Anesth Analg 2007;104(3):689–702.
14. Woehlck H, Connolly L, Cinquegrani M, et al. Acute smoking increases ST depression in humans during general anesthesia. Anesth Analg 1999;89(4):856–60.
15. Centers for Disease Control and Prevention. National diabetes fact sheet, 2011. Available at: http://www.cdc.gov/diabetes/pubs/pdf/ndfs_2011.pdf. Accessed March 3, 2013.
16. Finfer S, Chittock D, Su S, et al. Intensive versus conventional glucose control in critically ill patients. N Engl J Med 2009;360(13):1283–97.

17. American Diabetes Association. Standards of medical care in diabetes—2012. Diabetes Care 2012;35(Suppl 1):S11-63. Available at: http://care.diabetesjournals.org/content/35/Supplement_1/S11.full.pdf+html. Accessed March 3, 2013.

18. Blacker DJ, Flemming KD, Link MJ, et al. The preoperative cerebrovascular consultation: common cerebrovascular questions before general or cardiac surgery. Mayo Clin Proc 2004;79:223-9.

19. Norris E. Anesthesia for vascular surgery. In: Miller RD, Eriksson LI, Fleisher LA, et al, editors. Miller's anesthesia. 7th edition. Orlando (FL): Churchill-Livingstone; 2009. p. 1985-2044.

20. Donovan A, Flexman A, Gelb A. Blood pressure management in stroke. Curr Opin Anaesthesiol 2012;25:516-22.

21. Fischer SP, Bader AM, Sweitzer BJ. Preoperative evaluation. In: Miller RD, Eriksson LI, Fleisher LA, et al, editors. Miller's anesthesia. 7th edition. Orlando (FL): Churchill-Livingstone; 2009. p. 1001-66.

22. Mackey W. Cerebrovascular disease. In: Cronewell J, Johnston W, editors. Rutherford's vascular surgery. 7th edition. Philadelphia: Saunders Elsevier; 2010. p. 1386-99.

23. Lanzino G, Rabinstein A, Brown R. Treatment of carotid artery stenosis: medical therapy, surgery, or stenting? Mayo Clin Proc 2009;84:362-8.

24. Wolf PA, Kannel WB, Sorlie P, et al. Asymptomatic carotid bruit and risk of stroke. The Framingham study. JAMA 1981;245:1442-5.

25. Hirsch AT, Haska ZJ, Hertzer NR, et al. ACC/AHA 2005 practice guidelines for the management of patients with peripheral arterial disease (lower extremity, renal mesenteric, and abdominal aortic): a collaborative report from the American Association for Vascular Surgery/Society for Vascular Surgery, Society for Cardiovascular Angiography and Interventions, Society for Vascular Medicine and Biology, Society of Interventional Radiology and the ACC/AHA Task Force on Practice Guidelines (Writing Committee to Develop Guidelines for the Management of Patients with Peripheral Arterial Disease) endorsed by the American Association of Cardiovascular and Pulmonary Rehabilitation; National Heart, Lung, and Blood Institute; Society for Vascular Nursing, TransAtlantic Inter-Society Consensus; and Vascular Disease Foundation. Circulation 2006;113:1474-547.

26. Hiratzka LF, Bakris GL, Beckman JA, et al. 2010 ACCF/AHA/AATS/ACR/ASA/SCA/SCAI/SIR/STS/SVM guidelines for the diagnosis and management of patients with thoracic aortic disease: a report of the American College of Cardiology Foundation/American Heart Association Task Force on Practice Guidelines, American Association for Thoracic Surgery, American College of Radiology, American Stroke Association, Society of Cardiovascular Anesthesiologists, Society for Cardiovascular Angiography and Interventions, Society of Interventional Radiology, Society of Thoracic Surgeons, and Society for Vascular Medicine. Circulation 2010;121:e266-371.

27. Wilson W, Taubert KA, Gewitz M, et al, American Heart Association Rheumatic Fever, Endocarditis, and Kawasaki Disease Committee, American Heart Association Council on Cardiovascular Disease in the Young, American Heart Association Council on Clinical Cardiology, American Heart Association Council on Cardiovascular Surgery and Anesthesia, Quality of Care and Outcomes Research Interdisciplinary Working Group. Prevention of infective endocarditis: guidelines from the American Heart Association: a guideline from the American Heart Association Rheumatic Fever, Endocarditis, and Kawasaki Disease Committee, Council on Cardiovascular Disease in the Young, and the Council on Clinical Cardiology, Council on Cardiovascular Surgery and Anesthesia, and the Quality of Care

and Outcomes Research Interdisciplinary Working Group. Circulation 2007;116: 1736–54.

28. Biller J, Feinberg WM, Castaldo JE, et al. Guidelines for carotid endarterectomy: a statement for healthcare professionals from a Special Writing Group of the Stroke Council, American Heart Association. Circulation 1998;97:501–9.

Patients with Chronic Pulmonary Disease

Caron M. Hong, MD, MSc[a],*, Samuel M. Galvagno Jr, DO, PhD[b]

KEYWORDS

- Postoperative pulmonary complications • Preoperative preparation
- Chronic obstructive pulmonary disease • Anesthesia • Preoperative assessment
- Anesthesia and coexisting pulmonary disease • Asthma • Restrictive lung disease

KEY POINTS

- Preoperative evaluations are essential for individuals with chronic pulmonary disease to minimize postoperative pulmonary complications and perioperative morbidity and mortality.
- A detailed history and physical examination, including an assessment of functional status, is the most important means of predicting and preparing for postoperative pulmonary complications.
- Smoking is a risk factor for cancer, cardiovascular disease, and chronic respiratory disorders and a cessation goal should be 8 weeks before surgery.
- Chronic pulmonary disease, including chronic obstructive pulmonary disease, asthma, restrictive lung disease, obstructive sleep apnea, and obesity, has an associated risk of postoperative pulmonary complications and necessitates specific preoperative assessments to aid in risk reduction and appropriate surgical and anesthetic management.

PREOPERATIVE PATIENT ASSESSMENT

A meticulous preoperative evaluation of the patient with pulmonary disease is indicated because both regional and general anesthesia have the potential to precipitate numerous untoward physiologic effects.[1] These effects are caused by positive pressure ventilation, patient positioning, and the drugs used to induce and maintain general anesthesia.[2] Up to 90% of patients develop some degree of atelectasis during anesthesia.[3] Compression atelectasis results from patient positioning and loss of functional residual capacity (FRC). Hence, obesity and larger proportions of poorly

Disclosures: None.
[a] Department of Anesthesiology, University of Maryland School of Medicine, 22 South Greene Street, S11C0, Baltimore, MD 21201, USA; [b] Department of Anesthesiology, Shock Trauma Center, University of Maryland School of Medicine, 22 South Greene Street, T1R83, Baltimore, MD 21201, USA
* Corresponding author.
E-mail address: chong@anes.umm.edu

Med Clin N Am 97 (2013) 1095–1107
http://dx.doi.org/10.1016/j.mcna.2013.06.001   medical.theclinics.com
0025-7125/13/$ – see front matter Published by Elsevier Inc.

aerated lung areas predispose patients to ventilation-perfusion mismatching. Reabsorption atelectasis results when lower tidal volumes are used with a high Fio_2. Oxygen rapidly diffuses across the alveolar membrane, causing a pressure difference that leads to airway collapse.[2] FRC decreases significantly during general anesthesia; a decline of up to 50% of baseline may result because of a loss of inspiratory muscle tone and cephalad displacement of the diaphragm,[4,5] leading to increased shunting, dead space, and hypoxemia.[6] General anesthesia induces numerous other deleterious biologic effects on the respiratory system, including decreased alveolar macrophage activity, inhibition of mucociliary clearance, and decreased surfactant production.[5] All of these effects have the potential to cause precipitous changes in arterial oxygen concentration and postoperative pulmonary complications in patients with preexisting pulmonary disease.

Postoperative pulmonary complications (PPC) occur in approximately 10–30% of all patients who require general anesthesia.[5] PPC increase morbidity and mortality and are more costly than venous thromboembolic, cardiovascular, or infectious complications following surgery.[7] Fortunately, with a careful history and physical examination, many PPCs can be anticipated and potentially prevented.[6]

One of the most important preoperative assessments is a detailed description of the patient's quality of life.[7,8] An adequate activity level, as assessed by a validated questionnaire or simple questions about mobility, ability to climb 2 flights of stairs without dyspnea, and other markers of fitness has been independently associated with improved short-term mortality after major abdominal surgery.[9] Functional status is also assessed as a part of the Postoperative Pneumonia Risk Index.[6,10] This instrument incorporates type of surgery, age, functional status, and blood urea nitrogen level (BUN) to assess the risk of developing postoperative pneumonia (**Table 1**).

Any patient with dyspnea or cough must be evaluated carefully with a focused history and physical examination. A history of cardiac failure, American Society of Anesthesiologists (ASA) class ≥ 2 (**Table 2**), advanced age, chronic obstructive pulmonary disease (COPD), or a history of functional dependence have been shown to be significant risk factors for PPC.[6]

The risk for serious PPC, such as acute respiratory distress syndrome, is low (0.2%), but higher in patients with renal failure, COPD, emergency surgery, or in patients who have received numerous anesthetics.[11]

The "cough test" is performed by having the patient take a deep breath and cough once. A positive finding is defined as repeated coughing after the first cough.[6,12] This test has been shown to be a predictor of PPC.[12] Abnormal physical examination findings, such as adventitious lung sounds, have been shown to be highly associated with PPC (OR = 5.8); no individual spirometric variable has been as highly correlated with PPC.[13,14]

PREOPERATIVE TESTING

A general suggested approach to assessing the complaint of dyspnea is outlined in **Fig. 1**. Although the list of indications for pulmonary function tests (PFTs) is lengthy,[15] PFTs have a limited role in predicting PPC. In general, PFTs are recommended before surgery in patients undergoing lung resection or to classify the degree of lung impairment (ie, COPD) when there is uncertainty about the extent of disease.[5,13] PFTs may also be considered to determine the baseline lung function in patients with myasthenia gravis. PFTs alone do not reliably predict risk better than clinical evaluation alone, and the use of spirometry is fraught with limitations.[13,14,16] Although a postoperative forced expiratory volume in 1 second (FEV_1) greater than 40% has been shown to

Table 1 The postoperative pneumonia risk index	
Type of surgery	
Abdominal aortic aneurysm repair	15
Thoracic	14
Upper abdominal	10
Neck	8
Neurosurgery	8
Vascular	3
Age	
>80 y old	17
79–79 y old	13
60–60 y old	9
50–59 y old	4
Functional status	
Totally dependent	10
Partially dependent	6
Weight loss >10% in past 6 mo	7
History of COPD	5
General anesthesia	4
Impaired sensorium	4
History of stroke	4
BUN (mg/dL)	
<8	4
22–30	2
>30	3
Other factors	
Blood transfusion >4 U	3
Emergency surgery	3
Steroid use for chronic condition	3
Current smoker within 1 y	3
Alcohol intake >2 drinks/d	2

Scoring: 0–15 points, 0.24%; 16–25 points, 1.18%; 26–40 points, 4.6%; 41–55 points, 10.8%; >55 points, 15.9%.

Data from Canet J, Mazo V. Postoperative pulmonary complications. Minerva Anestesiol 2010;76:138–43; and Arouzullah A, Khuri S, Henderson W, et al. Development and validation of a multifactorial risk index for predicting postoperative pneumonia after major noncardiac surgery. Ann Intern Med 2001;135:847–57.

be associated with fewer PPC, the best assessment is a detailed description of the patient's quality of life.[8,17] In many cases, the FEV_1 alone may be inadequate. If PFTs are obtained, the FEV_1/Q (perfusion) ratio, combined with the FEV_1/Ht (height in centimeters), may be superior for determining functional status in young and old patients with severe lung disease.[16,18]

Laboratory testing is rarely helpful when evaluating patients with respiratory disease. Baseline arterial blood gas determinations have not been shown to help with risk stratification, but if available for a patient with advanced lung disease, may serve

Table 2
The ASA physical status classification system

ASA Physical Status 1	A normal healthy patient
ASA Physical Status 2	A patient with mild systemic disease (eg, mild intermittent asthma)
ASA Physical Status 3	A patient with severe systemic disease (eg, advanced COPD, congestive heart failure)
ASA Physical Status 4	A patient with severe systemic disease that is a constant threat to life (eg, active respiratory failure, stage IV COPD)
ASA Physical Status 5	A moribund patient who is not expected to survive without the operation (eg, a severe asthmatic requiring an exploratory laparotomy for necrotic bowel)
ASA Physical Status 6	A declared brain-dead patient whose organs are being removed for donor purposes

Data from American Society of Anesthesiologists. 2011 relative value guide package. Chicago: American Society of Anesthesiologists; 2011.

to establish baseline values for later comparison because therapy is adjusted in the intensive care unit.[5] Elevated levels of BUN (>30 mg/dL) and decreased levels of serum albumin (<3 g/dL) have been shown to predict PPC.[13,19]

Radiographic tests, such as chest computed tomography (CT) or chest radiography, are only useful when attempting to diagnose acute causes of dyspnea. Echocardiography should be considered for patients with heart failure as a cause (see **Fig. 1**).

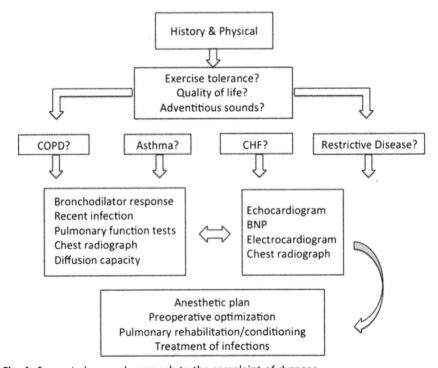

Fig. 1. Suggested general approach to the complaint of dyspnea.

SMOKING CESSATION

Smoking is a well-defined risk factor for PPC and a major independent risk factor for cancer, cardiovascular disease, and chronic respiratory disorders.[20–22] Smoking and comorbidities directly related to tobacco use have been shown to increase airway reactivity, decrease mucociliary clearance, and impede wound healing.[6] Although the cessation of smoking 48 hours before surgery decreases carboxyhemoglobin levels and cyanide levels, sputum production increases and symptoms of cough may worsen acutely.[22] In a recent systematic review that included 25 studies, the risk of PPC was similar in smokers who quit less than 2 or 2–4 weeks before surgery.[23] Ideally, to avoid PPCs, smokers should quit 8 weeks before surgery.[5,21] Smoking cessation has been shown to improve immune function and wound healing in addition to the salutary effects on pulmonary function and avoidance of PPC.[21]

CHRONIC OBSTRUCTIVE PULMONARY DISEASE

COPD is a leading cause of morbidity and mortality worldwide and is responsible for greater than 100,000 deaths per year in the United States.[24,25] COPD is defined by a pulmonary component that is characterized by "persistent airflow limitation" that is not fully reversible and "usually progressive and associated with an enhanced chronic inflammatory response."[24] The pathophysiological effects of COPD are summarized in **Fig. 2**.

Smoking is well-established as the leading risk factor for COPD, but other causes, such as occupational exposures, air pollution, lung development abnormalities, and genetic factors, may be responsible. A postbronchodilator FEV_1/forced vital capacity (FVC) ratio less than 0.70 confirms the presence of airflow limitation and is recommended for the diagnosis and assessment of the severity of COPD.[24] Both the FEV_1 and the FEV_1/FVC ratio are used to classify the stages of COPD according to the Global Initiative for Chronic Obstructive Lung Disease (GOLD-COPD), as listed in **Table 3**.[24] It is unlikely that PFTs will unmask high-stage patients with severe

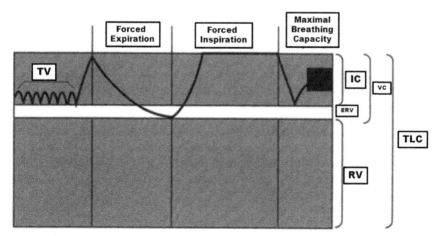

Fig. 2. Representative spirogram for a patient with COPD. ERV, expiratory reserve volume; IC, inspiratory capacity; RV, residual volume; TLC, total lung capacity; TV, tidal volume; VC, vital capacity. In advanced COPD, the inspiratory capacity and expiratory reserve volume are decreased, whereas the residual volume is greatly increased. (*From* Galvagno S. Emergency pathophysiology. Jackson (WY): Teton NewMedia; 2004; with permission.)

Table 3		
GOLD-COPD staging, based on severity of postbronchodilator airflow limitation		
Stage 1	Mild	$FEV_1 \geq 80\%$ predicted
Stage 2	Moderate	$50\% \leq FEV_1 < 80\%$ predicted
Stage 3	Severe	$30\% \leq FEV_1 < 50\%$ predicted
Stage 4	Very severe	$FEV_1 < 30\%$ predicted

Data from Vestbo J, Hurd SS, Agusti AG, et al. Global strategy for the diagnosis, management, and prevention of chronic obstructive pulmonary disease: GOLD executive summary. Am J Respir Crit Care Med 2013;187:347–65.

disability, and the level of physical tolerance (ie, stair climbing) has been shown to correlate well with PFT data.[14,26] Furthermore, PFTs do not reliably predict PPC in patients with COPD (see **Table 3**).[13,14]

In stages 1 to 2, the principles of management are centered around prevention, vaccination, pulmonary rehabilitation, and long-acting bronchodilators. In stage 3, inhaled glucocorticoids are added. In stage 4, patients require supplemental oxygen and are often severely physically debilitated.

In addition to a thorough history and physical examination, additional ancillary tests may be considered for high-stage COPD patients. Chest radiographs and chest CT studies are indicated only to rule out infection or other coexisting disease, such as carcinoma. An electrocardiograph (ECG) should be obtained in most COPD patients because signs of right heart strain (ie, right ventricular hypertrophy) may prompt the need for additional testing. Coexisting coronary artery disease is common in COPD patients,[26] and in stage 2 COPD or greater, an ECG or pharmacologic stress test is recommended if the patient reports poor exercise tolerance. Routine laboratory testing is not very helpful, although malnutrition is common in COPD patients, as potentially indicated by a low serum albumin level.

The major preoperative goal of management for patients with COPD involves the prevention of PPC, such as pneumonia, bronchospasm, respiratory failure with prolonged mechanical ventilation, or COPD exacerbation.[26] Smoking cessation is imperative for COPD patients and has been shown to decrease the incidence of PPC.[5,26] Bronchodilators should be continued up to the day of surgery, understanding that bronchodilators rarely improve FEV_1 more than 10% in patients with COPD.[26] Nevertheless, these agents should be continued before, during, and after surgery.[26] Prophylactic use of antibiotics is not recommended, but infections should be treated promptly when identified. Preoperative pulmonary conditioning may be helpful in some high-stage COPD patients, and in some studies this has been shown to decrease the incidence of PPC.

Recognition and treatment of a COPD exacerbation is a primary concern, because progression to surgery during an acute exacerbation will invariably increase the incidence of PPC as well as other systemic complications.[27] An exacerbation is defined as an acute event characterized by worsening of the patient's respiratory status, worse than usual daily variation.[24] One of the most common precipitating factors is a viral or bacterial upper respiratory tract infection. A thorough history will reveal changes in baseline dyspnea, worsening cough, or changes in sputum production beyond normal day-to-day variation.[24] COPD exacerbations are treated with short-acting inhaled β-agonists with or without anticholinergics (ie, ipratropium). Systemic corticosteroids and antibiotics have been shown to improve FEV_1, shorten recovery time, and reduce the length of hospital stay.[24] Similar effects with low-dose compared with high-dose steroids have been observed in at least one study, and preoperative use of corticosteroids has not been shown to increase the risk of wound healing or postoperative pneumonia.[26–28] Ideally, postponement of surgery during a COPD exacerbation is strongly advisable.

ASTHMA

Asthma is one of the most common diseases, affecting more than 300 million people worldwide,[29] in every sector of the population, without prejudice. It is attributed to 1 in 250 deaths, most preventable.[29] Therefore, asthma has been the topic of global public health intervention movements in the past few decades to implement practice guidelines to improve management and prevent morbidity and mortality.

Asthma occurs from acute airway obstruction secondary to inflammation and hyperresponsiveness. Oftentimes, COPD and asthma present simultaneously in adults and it is difficult to distinguish between the two entities. Specific preoperative preparations for COPD should be followed as mentioned above. It has been demonstrated for more than 50 years that surgical patients with asthma have an increased risk for perioperative complications and, when treated adequately before surgery, these patients have less postoperative complications.[30] Therefore, a thorough preoperative evaluation, including a physical examination, management of any electrolyte abnormalities secondary to medications such as B_2 agonists, an ECG to identify cardiac arrhythmias or abnormalities, continuation of asthma treatment, and treatment of other associated comorbidities, such as cor pulmonale, is essential. Identification of the usefulness of current medication, the number of medications needed, and precipitating factors are helpful to determine the severity of disease as well as managing avoidance of exposure during the perioperative period (ie, latex). The usefulness of spirometry and arterial blood gas analysis is questionable, as attacks are usually acute and resolve, and abnormalities may not be apparent. If, however, FEV_1 values during an exacerbation are less than 80% of the patient's personal best, corticosteroids should be prescribed.[31] Special attention should be given to these patients who receive steroids within 6 months of surgery, as they should receive systemic doses of steroids during the surgical period with a rapid wean within 24 hours postoperatively.[31]

Therapeutic considerations for optimization in the preoperative period include two categories: quick-acting and long-acting medications. The quick-acting medications for acute exacerbations include B_2 selective adrenergic agonists (metered-dose inhalers), such as albuterol, and an enantiomer, levalbuterol, with fewer side effects.[32] Corticosteroids can be used for more difficult to control attacks. Close monitoring of electrolytes with B_2 agonist treatment is essential. Long-acting medications include long-acting B_2 selective agonists, such as salmeterol, inhaled steroids, leukotriene modifier, inhaled anticholinergics, and IgE immunotherapy. To decrease the risk of postoperative complications, these patients should continue their medication regimen preoperatively and through the perioperative period.

RESTRICTIVE LUNG DISEASE

There are numerous pathophysiological states and disease processes that may be classified as restrictive lung disease. Causes are either pulmonary (parenchymal) or extrapulmonary (**Box 1**).

Restrictive pulmonary diseases are characterized by a reduction of lung volume and both total and vital capacity. Hence, patients with restrictive lung disease are at risk for exaggerated pulmonary dysfunction postoperatively.

Box 1
Restrictive lung disorders

Pulmonary causes

- Sarcoidosis
- Silicosis
- Tuberculosis
- Hypersensitivity pneumonitis
- Eosinophilic granulomatosis
- Pulmonary alveolar proteinosis
- Lung resection
- Atelectasis
- Acute respiratory distress syndrome
- Pulmonary edema

Extrapulmonary causes

- Obesity
- Skeletal/costovertebral deformities (eg, scoliosis)
- Sternal deformities (eg, pectus excavatum)
- Neuromuscular disorders
- Pneumothorax

The preoperative assessment of the patient with a restrictive lung disorder depends on the underlying cause. Exercise tolerance is important, and if impaired, the incidence of PPC may be increased. Chest radiographs are frequently obtained, but may only be helpful if comparison studies are available or if the study is being used to monitor the progression of the underlying disease. Similarly, CT studies are only indicated if tracheal compression or other associated pathologic condition is suspected. Preoperative arterial blood gases analysis may provide an estimate of baseline oxygenation and ventilation to be expected at the end of surgery.[33]

Unfortunately, there are very few evidence-based recommendations for the preoperative management of patients with restrictive lung disease. Some pulmonary conditions, such as hypersensitivity pneumonitis and sarcoidosis, may exhibit a degree of airway hyperreactivity and should be treated in a manner similar to COPD.[33] As with all pulmonary disease, preoperative management should be aimed at optimizing the patient's physiology with the goal of preventing PPC and additional morbidity and mortality.

OBSTRUCTIVE SLEEP APNEA

Obstructive sleep apnea (OSA) is an independent risk factor for mortality.[34,35] The prevalence of OSA in middle-aged men is 4% and 2% in women[35] and continues to increase. OSA is defined as multiple episodes of upper airway obstruction that occur during sleep, usually associated with oxygen desaturation.[36] It is secondary to anatomic features and pathologic abnormality resulting in decreased upper airway diameter and decreased patency during sleep. Risk factors are both anatomic and pathologic and OSA can present as acute, subacute, or chronic with severity of mild to severe (**Table 4**).

Table 4
Characterization and risk factors of OSA

	Characterization of OSA Severity	Risk Factors
Mild	Mild sleepiness	Male
	Mild insomnia	Obesity
	Minimal sleep disturbances	Nasopharyngeal abnormalities
	Mild oxygen desaturations	Hypertrophied tonsils and adenoids
	Benign cardiac arrhythmias	Severe upper respiratory tract
Moderate	Moderate sleepiness	infections
	Mild insomnia	Chronic allergic rhinitis
	Apneic episodes associated with	Craniofacial abnormalities
	moderate oxygen desaturation	
	Cardiac arrhythmias	
Severe	Severe sleepiness	
	Most sleep associated with respiratory	
	disturbances	
	Severe oxygen desaturations	
	Severe cardiac arrhythmias	
	Associated cardiopulmonary dysfunction	

Data from American Academy of Sleep Medicine. International classification of sleep disorders, revised: Diagnostic and coding manual. Chicago: American Academy of Sleep Medicine; 2001.

In addition to the increase of risk of mortality with OSA, there are associated multiorgan diseases, including hypertension, congestive heart failure, coronary artery disease, arrhythmias, stroke, deep vein thrombosis, and renal disease.[37] Individuals with OSA have a decreased lifespan of 20 years and are at increased risk for perioperative complications, including reintubation, hypoxia, hypercapnia, sudden respiratory arrest, hemodynamic alterations, and myocardial infarction.[13] Moreover, more than 80% are undiagnosed,[37] making the surgical preoperative assessment critical to optimize morbidity and mortality in these patients. There have been a few preoperative questionnaires developed to assess the risk of OSA that have lacked sensitivity, leaving the overnight polysomnography the "gold standard" for diagnosis. However, in the preoperative setting, there are many limitations to overnight polysomnography, including scheduling, facility availability, cost, and convenience. Chung and colleagues[38] demonstrated the "STOP-Bang" questionnaire with an increased sensitivity of greater than 80% and improved negative predicted value in patients with moderate to severe OSA. This questionnaire allows for a practitioner to assess quickly for those at risk for OSA preoperatively with minimal training (**Table 5**).

A thorough preoperative assessment that identifies OSA as a possible risk can lead to investigation of other organ system insufficiency that should be addressed before elective surgeries. Patients with OSA or high risk for OSA should have routine chemistry and cell count analysis in conjunction with an ECG. If the patient's OSA is moderate to severe, preoperative arterial blood gas analysis and chest radiograph should be considered to establish baseline levels. An extended evaluation is needed for those treated with continuous positive airway pressure, including treatment settings and compliance, to aid in the anesthetic plan and perioperative management. Preoperative patient optimization is imperative to decrease perioperative complications, including morbidity, unplanned intensive care unit transfers, hospital length of stay, and mortality associated with OSA.[13]

Table 5 Components of the "STOP-Bang" questionnaire and scoring system	
Components of the "STOP-Bang" Questionnaire	**Scoring System**
Snoring	High risk: >3 yes
Daytime *T*iredness	Low risk <3 yes
Observed apnea	
Hypertension (*Pressure*)	
BMI >35 kg/m²	
Age >50 y old	
Neck circumference >40 cm	
Male (Gender)	

Abbreviation: BMI, body mass index.
Data from Chung F, Yegneswaran B, Liao P, et al. STOP questionnaire: a tool to screen patients for obstructive sleep apnea. Anesthesiology 2008;108:812–21.

OBESITY

In 2010, about 35% of adults in the United States were obese, with obesity-related conditions leading the cause of preventable deaths.[39] This number has doubled since 1980 and continues to increase. Obesity is most often categorized by using the ratio of weight in kilograms to height in meters squared, otherwise known as body mass index (BMI). There are multiple associated comorbidities including coronary heart disease, hypertension, stroke, type 2 diabetes mellitus, cancer, and premature death, which are all beyond the scope of this article (**Table 6**). However, physiologic effects of

Table 6 Physiologic changes associated with obesity	
Respiratory mechanics	Restrictive lung disease and decreased compliance (resulting in decreased FRC, ERV, FEV_1, FVC, TLC, RV), increased work of breathing, and increased atelectasis
Risk for OSA	5% of obese population
Anatomic changes	Increased upper airway adipose/soft tissue
Cardiovascular changes	Increased oxygen consumption Increased cardiac work and CO_2 production Increased blood volume Pulmonary hypertension Left ventricular hypertrophy Increased risk for arrhythmia
GERD	Increased intra-abdominal pressures Increased gastric acidic contents Increased risk for aspiration
Alterations in pharmacokinetics and pharmacodynamics	Affects volume of distribution Affects peak plasma concentrations, clearance, and elimination
Other comorbidities	Hypertension, hyperlipidemia, non-insulin-dependent diabetes mellitus and functional dependence
DVT	Doubled risk for DVT

Abbreviations: DVT, deep vein thrombosis; GERD, gastroesophageal reflux disease; RV, residual volume; TLC, total lung capacity.
Data from Refs.[40–44]

obesity on the pulmonary system and the preoperative assessments that need to be addressed before surgery are important to mention.

Although studies, to date, have not demonstrated any increased risk for postoperative complications,[13] the physiologic effect and changes must be acknowledged and optimization and treatment initiated, when possible, before surgical procedure. There are modifications for every medical sector that occur when an obese patient undergoes surgery. It may be these modifications that aid in the undifferentiated morbidity and mortality in this group perioperatively. A physical examination that incorporates a detailed pulmonary examination, assessment of OSA risk (as mentioned above), airway management, and functional status is critical.

SUMMARY

PPC are costly and a serious complication following surgery. Because PPC occur in more than 25% of patients requiring general anesthesia, preoperative diligence is imperative to reducing morbidity and mortality. This diligence is especially critical in patients with chronic pulmonary disease, including smokers, and patients with COPD, asthma, restrictive lung disease, OSA, and obesity. With a detailed preoperative assessment and appropriate preoperative testing, the risk of PPC, and subsequent sequelae, can be minimized in these challenging patients.

REFERENCES

1. Manku K, Bacchetti P, Leung JM. Prognostic significance of postoperative in-hospital complications in elderly patients. I. Long-term survival. Anesth Analg 2003;96:583–9 [table of contents].
2. Bruells CS, Rossaint R. Physiology of gas exchange during anaesthesia. Eur J Anaesthesiol 2011;28:570–9.
3. Coussa M, Roietti S, Schnyder P, et al. Prevention of atelectasis formation during the induction of general anesthesia in morbidly obese patients. Anesth Analg 2004;98:1491–5.
4. Wahba R. Perioperative functional residual capacity. Can J Anaesth 1991;38: 384–400.
5. Rock P, Rich PB. Postoperative pulmonary complications. Curr Opin Anaesthesiol 2003;16:123–31.
6. Canet J, Mazo V. Postoperative pulmonary complications. Minerva Anestesiol 2010;76:138–43.
7. Sweitzer BJ, Smetana GW. Identification and evaluation of the patient with lung disease. Anesthesiol Clin 2009;27:673–86.
8. Kearney D, Lee T, Reilly J, et al. Assessment of operative risk in patients undergoing lung resection. Chest 1994;105:753–9.
9. Dronkers JJ, Chorus AM, van Meeteren NL, et al. The association of pre-operative physical fitness and physical activity with outcome after scheduled major abdominal surgery. Anaesthesia 2013;68:67–73.
10. Arouzullah A, Khuri S, Henderson W, et al. Development and validation of a multi-factorial risk index for predicting postoperative pneumonia after major noncardiac surgery. Ann Intern Med 2001;135:847–57.
11. Blum JM, Stentz MJ, Dechert R, et al. Preoperative and intraoperative predictors of postoperative acute respiratory distress syndrome in a general surgical population. Anesthesiology 2013;118:19–29.

12. McAlister F, Bertsch K, Man J, et al. Incidence of and risk factors for pulmonary complications after noncardiothoracic surgery. Am J Respir Crit Care Med 2005; 171:514–7.
13. Smetana GW. Preoperative pulmonary evaluation: identifying and reducing risks for pulmonary complications. Cleve Clin J Med 2006;73(Suppl 1):S36–41.
14. Lawrence V, Dhanda R, Hislebeck S, et al. Risk of pulmonary complications after elective abdominal surgery. Chest 1996;110:744–50.
15. Barreiro TJ, Perillo I. An approach to interpreting spirometry. Am Fam Physician 2004;69:1107–14.
16. Bernstein W. Pulmonary function testing. Curr Opin Anaesthesiol 2012;25:11–6.
17. Brunelli A, Varela G, Rocco G, et al. A model to predict the immediate postoperative FEV1 following major lung resections. Eur J Cardiothorac Surg 2007;32: 783–6.
18. Miller M, Pedersen O. New concepts for expressing forced expiratory volume in 1 s arising from survival analysis. Eur Respir J 2010;35:873–82.
19. Arozullah A, Daley J, Henderson W, et al. Multifactorial risk index for predicting postoperative respiratory failure in men after major noncardiac surgery. The National Veterans Administration Surgical Quality Improvement Program. Ann Surg 2000;232:242–53.
20. Thomsen T, Villebro N, Moller AM. Interventions for preoperative smoking cessation. Cochrane Database Syst Rev 2010;(7):CD002294.
21. Quraishi SA, Orkin FK, Roizen MF. The anesthesia preoperative assessment: an opportunity for smoking cessation intervention. J Clin Anesth 2006;18:635–40.
22. Warner DO. Helping surgical patients quit smoking: why, when, and how. Anesth Analg 2005;101:481–7 [table of contents].
23. Wong J, Lam DP, Abrishami A, et al. Short-term preoperative smoking cessation and postoperative complications: a systematic review and meta-analysis. Can J Anaesth 2012;59:268–79.
24. Vestbo J, Hurd SS, Agusti AG, et al. Global strategy for the diagnosis, management, and prevention of chronic obstructive pulmonary disease: GOLD executive summary. Am J Respir Crit Care Med 2013;187:347–65.
25. Edrich T, Sadovnikoff N. Anesthesia for patients with severe chronic obstructive pulmonary disease. Curr Opin Anaesthesiol 2010;23:18–24.
26. Mandra A, Simic D, Stevanovic V, et al. Preoperative considerations for patients with chronic obstructive pulmonary disease. Acta Chir Iugosl 2011;58:71–5.
27. Spieth PM, Guldner A, de Abreu MG. Chronic obstructive pulmonary disease. Curr Opin Anaesthesiol 2012;25:24–9.
28. Lindenauer P, Pekow P, Lahti M, et al. Association of corticosteroid dose and route of administration with risk of treatment failure in acute exacerbation of chronic obstructive pulmonary disease. JAMA 2010;303:2359–67.
29. Masoli M, Fabian D, Holt S, et al. The global burden of asthma: executive summary of the GINA Dissemination Committee report. Allergy 2004;59:469–78.
30. Shnider S, Papper E. Anesthesia for the asthmatic patient. Anesthesiology 1961; 22:886–92.
31. Yamakage M, Iwasaki S, Namiki A. Guideline-oriented perioperative management of patients with bronchial asthma and chronic obstructive pulmonary disease. J Anesth 2008;22:412–28.
32. Woods BD, Sladen RN. Perioperative considerations for the patient with asthma and bronchospasm. Br J Anaesth 2009;103(Suppl 1)):i57–65.
33. Groeben H. Strategies in the patient with compromised respiratory function. Best Pract Res Clin Anaesthesiol 2004;18:579–94.

34. Marshall NS, Wong KK, Liu PY, et al. Sleep apnea as an independent risk factor for all-cause mortality: the Busselton Health Study. Sleep 2008;31:1079–85.
35. Young T, Palta M, Dempsey J, et al. The occurrence of sleep-disordered breathing among middle-aged adults. N Engl J Med 1993;328:1230–5.
36. American Academy of Sleep Medicine. The international classification of sleep disorders, revised. Diagnostic and coding manual. 2001. Available at: http://www.esst.org/adds/ICSD.pdf.
37. Young T, Evans L, Finn L, et al. Estimation of the clinically diagnosed proportion of sleep apnea syndrome in middle-aged men and women. Sleep 1997;20:705–6.
38. Chung F, Yegneswaran B, Liao P, et al. STOP questionnaire: a tool to screen patients for obstructive sleep apnea. Anesthesiology 2008;108:812–21.
39. Ogden CL, Carroll MD, Kit BK, et al. Prevalence of obesity in the United States, 2009-2010. NCHS Data Brief 2012;(82):1–8.
40. Salome CM, King GG, Berend N. Physiology of obesity and effects on lung function. J Appl Physiol 2010;108:206–11.
41. Pedoto A. Lung physiology and obesity: anesthetic implications for thoracic procedures. Anesthesiol Res Pract 2012;2012:154208.
42. Koenig SM. Pulmonary complications of obesity. Am J Med Sci 2001;321:249–79.
43. Catenacci VA, Hill JO, Wyatt HR. The obesity epidemic. Clin Chest Med 2009;30:415–44, vii.
44. Allman-Farinelli M. Obesity and venous thrombosis: a review. Semin Thromb Hemost 2011;37:903–7.

Patients with Chronic Kidney Disease

Alicia Gruber Kalamas, MD[a],*, Claus U. Niemann, MD[a,b]

KEYWORDS

- Chronic kidney disease (CKD) • Acute kidney injury (AKI) • Preoperative assessment
- Preoperative management • Preoperative evaluation

KEY POINTS

- Patients with chronic kidney disease (CKD) are particularly susceptible to further renal impairment during hospitalizations or surgical intervention.
- Preoperative efforts should focus on identifying patients with risk factors for CKD in order to risk stratify them based on the degree of impairment and the nature of the proposed procedure.
- Maintenance of an adequate renal perfusion pressure with fluids and inotropic agents, the mainstays of hemodynamic optimization, may protect against acute kidney injury.
- None of the pharmacological interventions that have been used to prevent acute kidney injury have convincingly demonstrated a benefit during the perioperative period.
- Nephrotoxic drugs, such as nonsteroidal antiinflammatory drugs and aminoglycoside antibiotics should be used with caution or avoided during the perioperative period.

INTRODUCTION

Chronic kidney disease (CKD) is increasingly recognized as a major public health problem worldwide. In the US alone, roughly 1 in 10 adult Americans has CKD with the highest incidence and prevalence amongst patients > 65 years old. These patients are at significant risk for excessive morbidity and mortality during the perioperative period even when adjusted for other variables such as hypertension and diabetes. Given the tremendous health and cost burden of end-stage renal disease (ESRD), preventing or avoiding progression of CKD to ESRD is critical. Therefore, identifying patient and procedural related risk factors and implementing risk mitigation strategies to prevent further deterioration of renal function during the perioperative period is of

[a] Department of Anesthesia and Perioperative Care, University of California, San Francisco, 521 Parnassus Avenue, PO Box 0648, San Francisco, CA 94143-0648, USA; [b] Department of Surgery, Division of Transplantation, University of California, San Francisco, 521 Parnassus Avenue, PO Box 0648, San Francisco, CA 94143-0648, USA
* Corresponding author.
E-mail address: grubera@anesthesia.ucsf.edu

Med Clin N Am 97 (2013) 1109–1122
http://dx.doi.org/10.1016/j.mcna.2013.07.002
0025-7125/13/$ – see front matter © 2013 Elsevier Inc. All rights reserved.

paramount importance. In this chapter we will review patient risk stratification; preoperative evaluation and management; and perioperative interventions aimed at renal protection.

DEFINITION AND CAUSES OF CHRONIC KIDNEY DISEASE

Chronic kidney disease (CKD) is defined according to the presence or absence of kidney damage and level of kidney function, irrespective of the type of kidney disease, and is often diagnosed and staged using the 2002 National Kidney Foundation Kidney Disease Outcomes Quality Initiative (NKF KDOQI) guidelines. These guidelines include a 5 stage classification system based on glomerular filtration rate (GFR) and evidence of kidney damage (e.g. proteinuria, glomerular hematuria, abnormal imaging, abnormal renal biopsy)[1] (Table 1). All individuals with a GFR <60 mL/min/1.73 m^2 or evidence of kidney damage for 3 months are classified as having CKD. Conversely, individuals with a GFR 60 to 89 mL/min/1.73 m^2 without kidney damage are classified as "decreased GFR". Decreased GFR without recognized markers of kidney damage (e.g. proteinuria) is common in older adults, and is usually considered "normal for age". The consequences of age-related decline in GFR without kidney damage are not known. Conversely, 'moderate' or clinically significant CKD refers to CKD stages 3 (GFR 30–59 ml/min) and 4 (GFR 15–29 ml/min), with <60 ml/min chosen as a cutoff because it represents loss of about 50% of normal renal function. A recent meta-analysis of eight cohorts of 845,125 general and high-risk people confirms the marked and graded increased risk for ESRD in those with a GFR less than 60 ml/min (stage 3 CKD).[2] Patients with a GRF of < 25 ml/min are considered to be candidates for kidney transplantation and stage 5 CKD is ESRD and is identified by a GFR less than 15 ml/min or the need for renal replacement therapy (RRT) (e.g. hemodialysis, peritoneal dialysis).

In the United States, diabetes mellitus, hypertension, and glomerulonephritis cause approximately 75% of all adult cases of CKD (www.usrds.org, accessed 3/26/2013). Arterial hypertension can either be a cause or consequence of CKD and is associated with its progression. Under normal conditions, renal blood flow (RBF) is autoregulated over a broad range of systemic mean arterial pressure (MAP) (80–160 mm Hg). Chronic hypertension, diabetes, and high protein intake disturb the autoregulatory mechanisms and increase the pressure load to the renal vasculature, resulting in glomerulosclerosis.[3] Proteinuria can further accelerate injury to the tubulointerstitium, and is an independent promoter of the progression of renal disease.[4]

THE IMPACT OF CKD DURING HOSPITALIZATION AND THE PERIOPERATIVE PERIOD

Although the perioperative challenges and management of patients with ESRD are well appreciated, patients with CKD are particularly susceptible to further renal

Table 1
National Kidney Foundation K/DOQI: stages of chronic kidney disease (CKD)

Stage of CKD	Description	GFR (mL/min/1.73 m^2)
I	Kidney damage with normal or increased GFR (eg, early diabetic nephropathy)	≥90 mL/min
II	Kidney damage with mildly reduced GFR	60–89
III	Moderately reduced GFR	30–59
IV	Severely reduced GFR	15–29
V	End-stage renal disease	<15 or need for dialysis

impairment during hospitalizations or surgical intervention.[5] This patient population fits the commonly used second-hit injury paradigm with some stable chronic baseline organ dysfunction that is disproportionately aggravated when exposed to acute physiologic stresses such as hypotension, hypovolemia, or drug toxicity.

Acute Kidney Injury

Acute kidney injury (AKI), often graded by the RIFLE (Risk, Injury, Failure, Loss, ESRD; as proposed by the Acute Dialysis Quality Initiative) or AKIN (Acute Kidney Injury Network) criteria, is generally defined by an increase in serum creatinine by 50%, a corresponding decline of 50% or more in the GFR, or the need for renal replacement therapy (RRT; eg, dialysis, hemofiltration, renal transplantation). It is a serious condition that not only affects kidney structure and function acutely but also in the long term. AKI is observed in 5% to 7% of acute care hospitalizations but accounts for up to 20% of admissions to intensive care units (ICU).[6–8] Even modest changes in serum creatinine, as small as 0.3 mg/dL, are associated with increased risk-adjusted morbidity, length of hospital stay, and mortality. Increases in serum creatinine of greater than 0.5 mg/dL have been associated with an adjusted 6.5-fold increase in the odds of death and increased hospital length of stay (LOS).[9]

Survivors of AKI incur long-term risks for developing CKD and ESRD compared with those without AKI, with even mild, reversible AKI conveying risk of persistent tissue damage.[10] Over a 4-month period in 1996, Nash and colleagues[7] prospectively followed 4622 medical and surgical admissions and identified 332 patients (7.2% of admissions) who developed AKI. The most common causes of AKI were decreased renal perfusion (39%), nephrotoxin administration (16%), contrast administration (11%), and major surgery (9%). Only 38.6% experienced complete recovery of renal function, whereas almost 20% were discharged with an increased creatinine or on chronic dialysis. The in-hospital mortality of 19.4% is similar to that seen in other cohorts of hospitalized patients.[6–8] In patients hospitalized in the intensive care unit, the mortality of patients with AKI has been reported as high as 50% to 60%.[9,11,12]

Prediction of Risk: Patient-related and Procedure-related Risk Factors

AKI after any surgical procedure is usually the result of a combination of factors, including comorbid conditions, the nature and extent of the surgical procedure (eg, cardiopulmonary bypass, liver transplantation), and complications during the perioperative period (eg, low perfusion states). However, preoperative renal insufficiency, as measured by GFR, is the most important risk factor for developing AKI after a surgical procedure. Patients with GFR greater than 60 mL/min without additional risk factors (e.g. intraoperative hypotension) are unlikely to develop serious postoperative complications. In a cohort of patients with normal renal function undergoing noncardiac surgery, there was a low risk of postoperative AKI (0.8%) and an even lower risk of requiring RRT (0.1%).[13]

In contrast, preexisting CKD not only increases a patient's risk for AKI but is an independent risk factor for postoperative death and cardiovascular events, with even mild preoperative renal dysfunction identified as a powerful predictor of perioperative morbidity and mortality.[14–19]

Several studies in patients undergoing major aortic or lower extremity vascular procedures have noted increased perioperative risk in patients with an estimated GFR less than 60 mL/min.[20,21] In a large cohort of patients requiring infrainguinal vascular surgery, preoperative renal insufficiency was independently associated with postoperative myocardial infarction, cardiac arrest, reintubation, and death.[22] Analysis of operative outcomes in patients undergoing thoracoabdominal aneurysm surgery with cross clamping identified advanced age and preoperative CKD as risk factors for post-operative dialysis.[21] Although postoperative renal dysfunction and perioperative mortality seem to be less frequent in patients undergoing endovascular abdominal aortic aneurysm (AAA) repair, other studies have found no benefit in long-term survival between the two approaches.[23–26]

Although high-risk vascular procedures such as thoracic aneurysm repair or AAA repair are associated with a high risk of renal dysfunction, there is emerging evidence that even common surgeries such as laparoscopic procedures may be implicated in transient renal dysfunction.[27] In a single-center study that examined more than 300 gastric bypass surgeries, the incidence of postoperative AKI was 8.5%. Factors associated with increased risk included higher body mass index (BMI), hyperlipidemia, and preoperative use of angiotensin-converting enzyme (ACE) inhibitors/angiotensin receptor blocker (ARB) agents.[28]

In a study of more than 10,000 patients who underwent radical prostatectomy at the Mayo Clinic from 1990 to 2004, GFR was strongly associated with all-cause mortality and nonprostate cancer death. On multivariate analysis, after controlling for age, BMI, prostate-specific antigen doubling time, Gleason score, and clinical stage, GFR remained a statistically significant predictor of all-cause mortality.[29]

Of all surgical procedures, AKI in the cardiac surgery patient is associated with the highest rates of morbidity and mortality. Lassnigg and colleagues[19] showed a 2-fold increase in the risk for death for patients who experienced no change or a small increase (0.5 mg/dL) in serum creatinine 48 hours after cardiothoracic surgery compared with patients who experienced a small decline in serum creatinine during the same time frame. In a similar population, Loef and colleagues[30] showed an association between a 25% increase in serum creatinine during the first postoperative week and short-term and long-term (8 years) mortality. In a more recent trial, patients on dialysis undergoing coronary artery bypass surgery carried a 6-fold increase in operative mortality and 3-fold increase in the frequency of stroke, septicemia, prolonged ventilation, and hospital LOS compared with patients with a normal GFR.[15] It is unclear at this time whether recent advances in surgical technique resulting in a higher percentage of off-pump cases will have a beneficial effect on the incidence of perioperative renal dysfunction, and various studies have reported conflicting results.[31–34]

Contrast-induced Nephropathy

There are a growing number of imaging and interventional procedures that depend on iodinated contrast media and consequently pose the risk of contrast-induced AKI. Contrast-induced nephropathy (CIN) is the third leading cause of hospital-acquired AKI and accounts for up to 10% of AKI cases in hospitalized patients.[35] Although the incidence of contrast-induced AKI is low (1%–2%) in the general population, the incidence of CIN may be as high as 50% in some high-risk patient subgroups, such as those with diabetes mellitus and preexisting renal impairment. Patients who develop CIN sustain an increase in both short-term and long-term mortality whether or not CKD was present before contrast exposure.[36,37]

Risk Indices

Several studies have attempted to produce risk indices to predict postoperative AKI and need for RRT after cardiac surgery. Chertow and colleagues[38] were among the first to develop a preoperative renal risk stratification algorithm based on a large population database from the Veterans Affairs Coronary Artery Surgery Study (>40,000 patients from 42 centers). To improve on the clinical usefulness of the risk index, Thakar and colleagues[39] developed a clinical score based on a large cohort of patients

(>30,000) from a single center (Cleveland Clinic Foundation). In contrast with the work of Chertow and colleagues,[38] in that study, all surgical procedures were well represented and only recipients of a renal transplant and patients who were on preoperative dialysis were excluded. By incorporating a graded severity of multiple risk factors, Thakar and colleagues[39] developed and internally validated a clinical risk assessment tool with improved predictive accuracy compared with prior indices (**Table 2**). More recently, Wijeysundera and colleagues[40] developed and validated a simplified renal index (SRI) based on patients who underwent cardiac surgery under cardiopulmonary bypass (CPB) at 2 Canadian centers (**Table 3**). In 2008, Candela-Toha and colleagues[41] externally validated and compared the performance of the 2 clinical scores published by Thakar and colleagues[39] and Wijeysundera and colleagues.[40] Both models were useful for discriminating between patients who will and will not develop AKI after cardiac surgery, with values for the areas under the receiving operator characteristics curves of 0.86 (95% confidence interval, 0.81–0.9) and 0.82 (95% confidence interval, 0.76–0.87), respectively.

For noncardiac surgery, Kheterpal and colleagues[42] developed and validated a risk index to predict AKI for patients undergoing general surgery using data acquired from a large national data set. The investigators identified 11 independent preoperative predictors: age 56 years or older, male sex, emergency surgery, intraperitoneal surgery, diabetes mellitus necessitating oral or insulin therapy, active congestive heart failure, ascites, hypertension, mild or moderate preoperative renal insufficiency, and preoperative serum creatinine greater than 1.2 mg/dL. The incidence of AKI increased with risk

Table 2	
Risk index to predict AKI requiring dialysis after cardiac surgery	
Risk Factor	**Points**
Female	1
CHF LVEF<35%	1
Preoperative IABP	2
COPD	1
IDDM	1
Prior surgery	1
Emergency surgery	2
Surgery type: Valve only	1
CABG + valve	2
Other	2
Preoperative Cr: 1.2 to <2.1 mg/dL	2
2.1 mg/dL or greater	5
Score	**Risk (%)**
0–2	0.4
3–5	2
6–8	8
9–13	21

Abbreviations: CABG, coronary artery bypass graft; CHF, congestive heart failure; COPD, chronic obstructive pulmonary disease; IABP, intra-aortic balloon pump, IDDM, insulin-dependent diabetes mellitus; LVEF, left ventricular ejection fraction.

Table 3
Risk index to predict AKI requiring dialysis after cardiac surgery

Risk Factor	Points
eGFR≤30 ml/min	2
eGFR 31–60 ml/min	1
DM	1
LVEF≤40%	1
Previous cardiac surgery	1
Surgery other than CABG/ASD repair	1
Urgent/emergent procedure	1
Preoperative IABP	1

Score/Risk Class	
Low risk <1% (0–1 points)	<1%
Intermediate risk 2%–5% (2–3 points)	2-5%
High risk 10% (≥4 points)	10%

Abbreviations: ASD, atrial septal defect; DM, diabetes mellitus; eGFR, estimated GFR.

class and was consistent across the derivation and validation cohorts (**Table 4**). Of 152,244 operations reviewed, 762 (1.0%) were complicated by AKI. Class V patients (6 or more risk factors) had a 9% incidence of AKI. Overall, patients experiencing AKI had an 8-fold increase in 30-day mortality.

PREOPERATIVE EVALUATION

Preoperative efforts should focus on identifying patients with risk factors for CKD in order to risk stratify them based on the degree of impairment and the nature of the proposed procedure. Furthermore, the possibility of slowing the decline of renal function and preoperative optimization of renal function should be assessed.

However, lack of physician awareness of CKD and the associated risks is still widespread.[43] Because most patients are asymptomatic, CKD is underdiagnosed and, if acknowledged during acute hospital care or surgery, often not included in the clinical decision making. Therefore, the first step in risk assessment is identification of common diseases associated with CKD through a careful history and physical examination and basic laboratory tests. Because it is not possible to directly

Table 4
Risk index for general surgery patients

Preoperative Risk Class	AKI Incidence (%) Derivation Cohort	AKI Incidence (%) Validation Cohort
Class 1 (0–2 risk factors)	0.2	0.2
Class 2 (3–4 risk factors)	0.8	0.8
Class 3 (4 risk factors)	1.8	2.0
Class 4 (5 risk factors)	3.3	3.6
Class 5 (≥6 risk factors)	8.9	9.5

Risk factors: age 56 years or older, male sex, emergency surgery, intraperitoneal surgery, diabetes mellitus necessitating oral or insulin therapy, congestive heart failure, ascites, hypertension, mild or moderate preoperative renal insufficiency; preoperative serum creatinine > 1.2 mg/dL.

measure kidney function or the GFR, a surrogate is needed. The endogenous marker most commonly used to measure kidney function is creatinine. Creatinine is a breakdown product of creatine phosphate in muscle and a surrogate marker of muscle mass. Therefore any condition that affects muscle mass or muscle metabolism decreases the reliability of creatinine to assess kidney function. For example, people who are frail, elderly or critically ill and have serum creatinine levels within the normal range may have a substantial reduction in kidney function. GFR is usually estimated from a single blood level of creatinine using the Cockcroft-Gault or Modification of Diet in Renal Disease (MDRD) equations. Estimating equations like the MDRD are derived from large populations of patients and provide the best estimate of mean GFR for a group of people of a certain age, race, gender, and serum creatinine value. Thus, the reported estimated GFR (eGFR) is the best estimate of a patient's GFR; it is not the patient's actual GFR.

CKD is associated with pathophysiologic changes in many organ systems. Accelerated atherosclerosis, vascular calcification, valvular heart disease, conduction abnormalities, and left ventricular hypertrophy are features of CKD and multiple studies show a strong independent association between CKD and cardiovascular disease.[44,45] Although cardiovascular complications are the leading cause of mortality in patients with ESRD, the excess cardiovascular risk is demonstrable in patients with early CKD, with the highest relative risk of mortality in the youngest patients.[46] Therefore, careful cardiac risk assessment is required for all patients undergoing intermediate-risk and high-risk surgery per American College of Cardiology/ American Heart Association guidelines.[47]

Autonomic neuropathy with reduced baroreceptor sensitivity, sympathetic hyperactivity, and parasympathetic dysfunction may have significant effects on arterial pressure and predispose to the development of arrhythmias during surgery.[48] The development of clinically relevant peripheral neuropathy (in the absence of diabetic neuropathy), conversely tends to be a late complication that is typically limited to patients with end-stage kidney disease (stage 5 CKD). Gastroparesis occurs in as many as 12% of patients with long-standing diabetes and an estimated 50% of people on dialysis.[49] The main symptoms include early satiety, nausea, vomiting, and bloating, and are associated with aspiration pneumonia.[50]

Decreased renal function interferes with the kidneys' ability to maintain fluid and electrolyte homeostasis. The ability to concentrate urine declines early and is followed by decreases in ability to excrete phosphate, acid, and potassium. When CKD is advanced, the ability to dilute urine is lost, and urinary volume does not respond readily to variations in water intake. Maximum sodium excretion is a function of GFR and the impaired ability to excrete a sodium load predisposes these patients to volume overload, especially when large volumes of saline solutions are administered.

Anemia develops in the course of CKD and is caused by several factors, the most common of which is abnormally low erythropoietin levels. The severity of anemia in CKD is related to the duration and extent of kidney failure, with the lowest hemoglobin levels found in anephric patients and those who commence dialysis at severely decreased levels of kidney function.[51,52]

CKD is associated with a variety of disorders of calcium and phosphorus metabolism. Decreased kidney function leads to reduced phosphorus excretion and consequent phosphorus retention; reduced kidney mass leads to decreased calcitriol production; and decreased calcitriol production with consequent reduced calcium absorption from the gastrointestinal tract contributes to hypocalcemia. Hypocalcemia, reduced calcitriol synthesis, and increased serum phosphorus levels stimulate the production of parathyroid hormone, resulting in secondary hyperparathyroidism, and patients may have signs or symptoms of renal osteodystrophy (bone mineralization deficiency).[53]

Patients at various clinical stages of CKD display a wide range of derangements in all aspects of hemostasis and therefore experience a broad spectrum of clinical manifestations that lead to considerable morbidity and mortality. The early stages of CKD are dominated by hemostatic abnormalities that suggest impaired fibrinolysis and enhanced prothrombosis. As CKD advances, the procoagulant abnormalities persist but, in addition, patients start to have platelet dysfunction that typically manifests with an increased risk of cutaneous, mucosal, or serosal bleeding.[54]

PREOPERATIVE OPTIMIZATION

Patients who have unexplained CKD identified at the time of preoperative evaluation should have elective surgery postponed pending further work-up to determine the cause and to identify and treat reversible causes of renal disease. There are several medications that can either cause spurious increases in creatinine or true reductions in the GFR. Under certain conditions, the serum creatinine level can increase without reflecting a change in the GFR. For example, an increase in serum creatinine can result from increased intake of protein and creatine supplements. The antibiotic trimethoprim-sulfamethoxazole, cimetidine, and other H2-blockers (eg, famotidine and ranitidine) can similarly cause an increase in the measured serum creatinine from their effects on the secretion of creatinine in the tubules. This increase can result in a self-limited and reversible increase in the serum creatinine level of as much as 0.4 to 0.5 mg/dL (depending on baseline serum creatinine level) without having any measurable effects on the GFR.

In contrast, use of ACE inhibitors and ARBs can lead to decreases in GFR and hyperkalemia. These classes of drugs are used not only to optimize blood pressure control but can be prescribed to prevent progression of proteinuric CKD. Patients who begin taking or have a dose increase in ACE inhibitors or ARBs may experience an increase in the serum creatinine level reflecting a decrease in GFR. Although an increase in serum creatinine of 20% to 30% is acceptable, it is important to confirm that the serum creatinine level stabilized after initiation of therapy. In patients with an increase in creatinine level of more than 20% to 30% or in those with uncontrollable hyperkalemia, the ACE inhibitor or ARB may need to be discontinued or titrated to a lower dose before surgery.[55] Nephrotoxic drugs, such as nonsteroidal antiinflammatory drugs and aminoglycoside antibiotics should be used with caution or avoided during the perioperative period.

PERIOPERATIVE INTERVENTIONS FOR RENAL PROTECTION FOR PATIENTS WITH CKD

Although adequate control of hypertension in the perioperative setting is important to maintain renal function as well as to avoid other perioperative complications, overzealous correction of blood pressure may result in relative renal hypoperfusion and worsening renal function. The most common cause of perioperative acute tubular necrosis is hypovolemia and hypotension leading to hypoxic injury in the medullary region.[56]

In a study of non-critically ill patients with multiple co-morbidities, a decrease in systolic blood pressure relative to a pre-morbid value (so-called relative systolic hypotension) was a significant independent predictor of the development of AKI. Therefore, targets for blood pressure in the perioperative period should probably focus on correction of relative hypotension rather than on absolute blood pressure (defined as a systolic blood pressure <90 mm Hg).[57]

Although few studies have been published that address CKD and its perioperative management, including possible prevention by therapeutic interventions, maintenance of renal perfusion remains the most important prophylactic measure to protect renal function. Renal perfusion may be preserved by pursuing adequate volume and cardiac output by means of fluids and inotropic drugs, which are the mainstays of so-called hemodynamic optimization or goal-directed therapy. In a meta-analysis that included 20 studies and more than 4220 participants, postoperative acute renal injury was significantly reduced by perioperative hemodynamic optimization compared with a control group.[58]

Further evidence for the renal protective effects of hydration in the setting of CKD exists for patients undergoing radiographic studies requiring intravenous contrast agents. Solomon and colleagues[59] showed that hydration with 0.45% saline reduced the incidence of nephropathy as measured by serum creatinine compared with saline in combination with furosemide or mannitol. Although subsequent studies in patients undergoing procedures involving intravenous contrast have shown a better protection from 0.9% saline than from 0.45%, presumably because of more effective volume expansion,[60] hyperchloremic acidosis may develop after administration of the 0.9% normal saline and may adversely affect renal function.[61]

PHARMACOLOGIC INTERVENTIONS

There is no reliable evidence suggesting any benefit of specific pharmacologic interventions in preventing postoperative renal injury.[62] Although a small or renal-dose dopamine infusion may have a benefit in volume management by increasing renal blood flow and urine output, there is increasing evidence that it does not have any renal protective effect.[63,64] Furthermore, dopamine even at low doses can induce tachyarrhythmias, myocardial ischemia, and extravasation into a vein can cause severe necrosis. Therefore, routine administration of dopamine to prevent AKI is not recommended.

Fenoldopam is a highly selective type 1 dopamine agonist that preferentially dilates the renal and splanchnic vasculature. A systematic review of 13 studies in patients undergoing cardiovascular surgery showed that fenoldopam significantly reduced the need for RRT and in-hospital death.[65] While additional studies are warranted, fenoldopam may be a likely candidate for the prevention of AKI, particularly in critically ill patients, if the positive results obtained in some recent trials are confirmed.

Although loop diuretics such as furosemide are frequently used to preserve intraoperative urine output, there is no evidence to support their use in the prevention of AKI. Loop diuretics may, however, convert an oliguric into a non-oliguric form of AKI that may allow for easier fluid management. Two recent meta-analyses concluded that loop diuretics were neither associated with improved survival benefit in AKI nor with better recovery of renal function despite a reduction in the oliguric period.[66,67] The osmotic diuretic mannitol is routinely used during kidney transplantation.[68] It is an intravascular volume expander and may function as a free-radical scavenger as well as an osmotic diuretic. Administration of mannitol immediately before vessel clamp removal reduces the incidence of AKI, as indicated by a lower requirement of post-transplant dialysis.[69,70] Several small RCTs, however, found no reduction in the incidence of AKI with mannitol plus intravenous fluids compared with intravenous fluids alone in a variety of settings, including: CABG, traumatic rhabdomyolysis, vascular, and biliary tract surgery.[71,72]

There is evidence that increased renal free-radical production may in part be responsible for the renal injury in both ischemic and nephrotoxic AKI. N-acetylcysteine

(NAC) is very effective in neutralizing certain free radicals in vitro and several clinical trials have evaluated the efficacy of NAC, mainly in the prevention of CIN and post-cardiac surgery AKI. Many, but not all, studies have shown NAC to have a protective effect on CIN when administered before the onset of renal insult.[73] Conversely, recent meta-analyses and several randomized controlled trials (RCTs) investigating the effectiveness of prophylactic administration of NAC in the prevention of AKI following cardiac surgery have failed to demonstrate a benefit.[74]

Several studies have focused on the prevention of CIN, which has a high incidence in patients with CKD. A single randomized clinical trial has suggested that hydration with sodium bicarbonate may be superior to sodium chloride; it has been hypothesized that alkalinization of the urine reduces free radical tubular injury.[75] However, follow-up studies have suggested limited benefit from bicarbonate therapy and additional research is warranted.

SUMMARY

The presence of CKD is associated with increased perioperative mortality even when adjusted for other variables such hypertension or diabetes. However, lack of physician awareness of CKD and the associated risks is still widespread.[43] CKD is frequently underdiagnosed and, if acknowledged during acute hospital care or surgery, often not included in the clinical decision making. Asking whether the patient is hyperkalemic or symptomatic is no longer sufficient to determine whether a patient with CKD is optimized for surgery.

At present, the best available evidence indicates that successful identification, risk stratification, and intervention should take place in the preoperative evaluation phase. Universal acceptance of preoperative GFR calculations and new markers of CKD such as cystatin C will help identify and risk stratify patients. Nephrotoxic drugs should be identified and, if possible, discontinued before surgery. Maintenance of renal perfusion pressure should be pursued by ensuring normovolemia and adequate cardiac output. During the immediate perioperative phase, pharmacological interventions seem to be of limited value. With the possible exception of NAC for CIN, most interventional studies have been inconclusive or nonbeneficial. Prospective randomized studies are needed that specifically enroll patients with established CKD undergoing surgery.

REFERENCES

1. National Kidney Foundation. K/DOQI clinical practice guidelines for chronic kidney disease: evaluation, classification, and stratification. Am J Kidney Dis 2002; 39(2 Suppl 1):S1–266.
2. Astor BC, Matsushita K, Gansevoort RT, et al. Lower estimated glomerular filtration rate and higher albuminuria are associated with mortality and end-stage renal disease. A collaborative meta-analysis of kidney disease population cohorts. Kidney Int 2011;79(12):1331–40.
3. Ravera M, Re M, Deferrari L, et al. Importance of blood pressure control in chronic kidney disease. J Am Soc Nephrol 2006;17(4 Suppl 2):S98–103.
4. Peterson JC, Adler S, Burkart JM, et al. Blood pressure control, proteinuria, and the progression of renal disease. The Modification of Diet in Renal Disease Study. Ann Intern Med 1995;123(10):754–62.
5. Palevsky PM. Perioperative management of patients with chronic kidney disease or ESRD. Best Pract Res Clin Anaesthesiol 2004;18(1):129–44.

6. Kellerman PS. Perioperative care of the renal patient. Arch Intern Med 1994; 154(15):1674–88.

7. Nash K, Hafeez A, Hou S. Hospital-acquired renal insufficiency. Am J Kidney Dis 2002;39(5):930–6.

8. Thakar CV, Christianson A, Freyberg R, et al. Incidence and outcomes of acute kidney injury in intensive care units: a Veterans Administration study. Crit Care Med 2009;37(9):2552–8.

9. Chertow GM, Burdick E, Honour M, et al. Acute kidney injury, mortality, length of stay, and costs in hospitalized patients. J Am Soc Nephrol 2005;16(11): 3365–70.

10. Murugan R, Kellum JA. Acute kidney injury: what's the prognosis? Nat Rev Nephrol 2011;7(4):209–17.

11. Metnitz PG, Krenn CG, Steltzer H, et al. Effect of acute renal failure requiring renal replacement therapy on outcome in critically ill patients. Crit Care Med 2002;30(9):2051–8.

12. Uchino S, Kellum JA, Bellomo R, et al. Acute renal failure in critically ill patients: a multinational, multicenter study. JAMA 2005;294(7):813–8.

13. Kheterpal S, Tremper KK, Englesbe MJ, et al. Predictors of postoperative acute renal failure after noncardiac surgery in patients with previously normal renal function. Anesthesiology 2007;107(6):892–902.

14. Mathew A, Devereaux PJ, O'Hare A, et al. Chronic kidney disease and postoperative mortality: a systematic review and meta-analysis. Kidney Int 2008;73(9): 1069–81.

15. Cooper WA, O'Brien SM, Thourani VH, et al. Impact of renal dysfunction on outcomes of coronary artery bypass surgery: results from the Society of Thoracic Surgeons National Adult Cardiac Database. Circulation 2006;113(8):1063–70.

16. Devbhandari MP, Duncan AJ, Grayson AD, et al. Effect of risk-adjusted, non-dialysis-dependent renal dysfunction on mortality and morbidity following coronary artery bypass surgery: a multi-centre study. Eur J Cardiothorac Surg 2006; 29(6):964–70.

17. Hillis GS, Croal BL, Buchan KG, et al. Renal function and outcome from coronary artery bypass grafting: impact on mortality after a 2.3-year follow-u. Circulation 2006;113(8):1056–62.

18. Ix JH, Mercado N, Shlipak MG, et al. Association of chronic kidney disease with clinical outcomes after coronary revascularization: the Arterial Revascularization Therapies Study (ARTS). Am Heart J 2005;149(3):512–9.

19. Lassnigg A, Schmidlin D, Mouhieddine M, et al. Minimal changes of serum creatinine predict prognosis in patients after cardiothoracic surgery: a prospective cohort study. J Am Soc Nephrol 2004;15(6):1597–605.

20. Baele HR, Piotrowski JJ, Yuhas J, et al. Infrainguinal bypass in patients with end-stage renal disease. Surgery 1995;117(3):319–24.

21. Schepens MA, Defauw JJ, Hamerlijnck RP, et al. Surgical treatment of thoracoabdominal aortic aneurysms by simple crossclamping. Risk factors and late results. J Thorac Cardiovasc Surg 1994;107(1):134–42.

22. O'Hare AM, Feinglass J, Sidawy AN, et al. Impact of renal insufficiency on short-term morbidity and mortality after lower extremity revascularization: data from the Department of Veterans Affairs' National Surgical Quality Improvement Program. J Am Soc Nephrol 2003;14(5):1287–95.

23. Blankensteijn JD, de Jong SE, Prinssen M, et al. Two-year outcomes after conventional or endovascular repair of abdominal aortic aneurysms. N Engl J Med 2005;352(23):2398–405.

24. Johnson ML, Bush RL, Collins TC, et al. Propensity score analysis in observational studies: outcomes after abdominal aortic aneurysm repair. Am J Surg 2006;192(3):336–43.

25. Park B, Danes S, Drezner AD, et al. Endovascular abdominal aortic aneurysm repair at Hartford Hospital: a six year experience. Conn Med 2006;70(6):357–62.

26. Wald R, Waikar SS, Liangos O, et al. Acute renal failure after endovascular vs open repair of abdominal aortic aneurysm. J Vasc Surg 2006;43(3):460–6 [discussion: 466].

27. Perez J, Taura P, Rueda J, et al. Role of dopamine in renal dysfunction during laparoscopic surgery. Surg Endosc 2002;16(9):1297–301.

28. Thakar CV, Kharat V, Blanck S, et al. Acute kidney injury after gastric bypass surgery. Clin J Am Soc Nephrol 2007;2(3):426–30.

29. Tollefson MK, Boorjian SA, Gettman MT, et al. Preoperative estimated glomerular filtration rate predicts overall mortality in patients undergoing radical prostatectomy. Urol Oncol 2012. [Epub ahead of print].

30. Loef BG, Epema AH, Smilde TD, et al. Immediate postoperative renal function deterioration in cardiac surgical patients predicts in-hospital mortality and long-term survival. J Am Soc Nephrol 2005;16(1):195–200.

31. Cheng DC, Bainbridge D, Martin JE, et al. Does off-pump coronary artery bypass reduce mortality, morbidity, and resource utilization when compared with conventional coronary artery bypass? A meta-analysis of randomized trials. Anesthesiology 2005;102(1):188–203.

32. Chukwuemeka A, Weisel A, Maganti M, et al. Renal dysfunction in high-risk patients after on-pump and off-pump coronary artery bypass surgery: a propensity score analysis. Ann Thorac Surg 2005;80(6):2148–53.

33. Weerasinghe A, Athanasiou T, Al-Ruzzeh S, et al. Functional renal outcome in on-pump and off-pump coronary revascularization: a propensity-based analysis. Ann Thorac Surg 2005;79(5):1577–83.

34. Moller CH, Penninga L, Wetterslev J, et al. Off-pump versus on-pump coronary artery bypass grafting for ischaemic heart disease. Cochrane Database Syst Rev 2012;(3):CD007224.

35. McCullough PA. Contrast-induced acute kidney injury. J Am Coll Cardiol 2008; 51(15):1419–28.

36. McCullough PA, Adam A, Becker CR, et al. Risk prediction of contrast-induced nephropathy. Am J Cardiol 2006;98(6A):27K–36K.

37. Nikolsky E, Aymong ED, Dangas G, et al. Radiocontrast nephropathy: identifying the high-risk patient and the implications of exacerbating renal function. Rev Cardiovasc Med 2003;4(Suppl 1):S7–14.

38. Chertow GM, Lazarus JM, Christiansen CL, et al. Preoperative renal risk stratification. Circulation 1997;95(4):878–84.

39. Thakar CV, Arrigain S, Worley S, et al. A clinical score to predict acute renal failure after cardiac surgery. J Am Soc Nephrol 2005;16(1):162–8.

40. Wijeysundera DN, Karkouti K, Dupuis JY, et al. Derivation and validation of a simplified predictive index for renal replacement therapy after cardiac surgery. JAMA 2007;297(16):1801–9.

41. Candela-Toha A, Elias-Martin E, Abraira V, et al. Predicting acute renal failure after cardiac surgery: external validation of two new clinical scores. Clin J Am Soc Nephrol 2008;3(5):1260–5.

42. Kheterpal S, Tremper KK, Heung M, et al. Development and validation of an acute kidney injury risk index for patients undergoing general surgery: results from a national data set. Anesthesiology 2009;110(3):505–15.

43. Perazella MA, Khan S. Increased mortality in chronic kidney disease: a call to action. Am J Med Sci 2006;331(3):150–3.
44. Go AS, Chertow GM, Fan D, et al. Chronic kidney disease and the risks of death, cardiovascular events, and hospitalization. N Engl J Med 2004;351(13): 1296–305.
45. Schiffrin EL, Lipman ML, Mann JF. Chronic kidney disease: effects on the cardiovascular system. Circulation 2007;116(1):85–97.
46. London GM. Cardiovascular disease in chronic renal failure: pathophysiologic aspects. Semin Dial 2003;16(2):85–94.
47. Fleisher LA, Beckman JA, Brown KA, et al. ACC/AHA 2007 guidelines on perioperative cardiovascular evaluation and care for noncardiac surgery: a report of the American College of Cardiology/American Heart Association Task Force on Practice Guidelines (Writing Committee to Revise the 2002 Guidelines on Perioperative Cardiovascular Evaluation for Noncardiac Surgery): developed in collaboration with the American Society of Echocardiography, American Society of Nuclear Cardiology, Heart Rhythm Society, Society of Cardiovascular Anesthesiologists, Society for Cardiovascular Angiography and Interventions, Society for Vascular Medicine and Biology, and Society for Vascular Surgery. Circulation 2007;116(17):e418–99.
48. Savica V, Musolino R, Di Leo R, et al. Autonomic dysfunction in uremia. Am J Kidney Dis 2001;38(4 Suppl 1):S118–21.
49. Camilleri M. Clinical practice. Diabetic gastroparesis. N Engl J Med 2007; 356(8):820–9.
50. Tao Y, Yan Z, Sha J, et al. Severe gastroparesis causing postoperative respiratory complications in a heart-lung recipient. J Thorac Dis 2010;2(2):121–3.
51. Fisher JW. Mechanism of the anemia of chronic renal failure. Nephron 1980; 25(3):106–11.
52. McGonigle RJ, Wallin JD, Shadduck RK, et al. Erythropoietin deficiency and inhibition of erythropoiesis in renal insufficiency. Kidney Int 1984;25(2):437–44.
53. Sherrard DJ, Hercz G, Pei Y, et al. The spectrum of bone disease in end-stage renal failure–an evolving disorder. Kidney Int 1993;43(2):436–42.
54. Jalal DI, Chonchol M, Targher G. Disorders of hemostasis associated with chronic kidney disease. Semin Thromb Hemost 2010;36(1):34–40.
55. Bakris GL, Weir MR. Angiotensin-converting enzyme inhibitor-associated elevations in serum creatinine: is this a cause for concern? Arch Intern Med 2000; 160(5):685–93.
56. Sear JW. Kidney dysfunction in the postoperative period. Br J Anaesth 2005; 95(1):20–32.
57. Liu YL, Prowle J, Licari E, et al. Changes in blood pressure before the development of nosocomial acute kidney injury. Nephrol Dial Transplant 2009;24(2): 504–11.
58. Brienza N, Giglio MT, Marucci M, et al. Does perioperative hemodynamic optimization protect renal function in surgical patients? A meta-analytic study. Crit Care Med 2009;37(6):2079–90.
59. Solomon R, Werner C, Mann D, et al. Effects of saline, mannitol, and furosemide to prevent acute decreases in renal function induced by radiocontrast agents. N Engl J Med 1994;331(21):1416–20.
60. Mueller C, Buerkle G, Buettner HJ, et al. Prevention of contrast media-associated nephropathy: randomized comparison of 2 hydration regimens in 1620 patients undergoing coronary angioplasty. Arch Intern Med 2002;162(3): 329–36.

61. Reid F, Lobo DN, Williams RN, et al. (Ab)normal saline and physiological Hartmann's solution: a randomized double-blind crossover study. Clin Sci (Lond) 2003;104(1):17–24.
62. Zacharias M, Conlon NP, Herbison GP, et al. Interventions for protecting renal function in the perioperative period. Cochrane Database Syst Rev 2008;(4):CD003590.
63. Schenarts PJ, et al. Low-dose dopamine: a physiologically based review. Curr Surg 2006;63(3):219–25.
64. Carcoana OV, Mathew JP, Davis E, et al. Mannitol and dopamine in patients undergoing cardiopulmonary bypass: a randomized clinical trial. Anesth Analg 2003;97(5):1222–9.
65. Landoni G, Biondi-Zoccai GG, Marino G, et al. Fenoldopam reduces the need for renal replacement therapy and in-hospital death in cardiovascular surgery: a meta-analysis. J Cardiothorac Vasc Anesth 2008;22:27–33.
66. Sampath S, Moran JL, Graham PL, et al. The efficacy of loop diuretics in acute renal failure: Assessment using Bayesian evidence synthesis techniques. Crit Care Med 2007;35(11):2516–24.
67. Bagshaw SM, Delaney A, Haase M, et al. Loop diuretics in the management of acute renal failure: a systematic review and metaanalysis. Crit Care Resusc 2007;9:60–8.
68. Schnuelle P, Johannes van der Woude F. Perioperative fluid management in renal transplantation: a narrative review of the literature. Transpl Int 2006; 19(12):947–59.
69. Weimar W, Geerlings W, Bijnen AB. A controlled study on the effect of mannitol on immediate renal function after cadaver donor kidney transplantation. Transplantation 1983;35:99.
70. Tiggeler RG, Berden JH, Hoitsma AJ, et al. Prevention of acute tubular necrosis in cadaveric kidney transplantation by the combined use of mannitol and moderate hydration. Ann Surg 1985;201:246.
71. Schetz M. Should we use diuretics in acute renal failure? Best Pract Res Clin Anaesthesiol 2004;18:75–89.
72. Yallop KG, Sheppard SV, Smith DC. The effect of mannitol on renal function following cardio-pulmonary bypass in patients with normal pre-operative creatinine. Anaesthesia 2008;63:576–82.
73. McCullough PA. Contrast-induced acute kidney injury. J Am Coll Cardiol 2008; 51:1419–28.
74. Ashworth A, Webb ST. Does the prophylactic administration of N-acetylcysteine prevent acute kidney injury following cardiac surgery? Interact Cardiovasc Thorac Surg 2010;11(3):303–8.
75. Merten GJ, Burgess WP, Gray LV, et al. Prevention of contrast-induced nephropathy with sodium bicarbonate: a randomized controlled trial. JAMA 2004;291: 2328–34.

Patients with Chronic Endocrine Disease

Mary Josephine Njoku, MD

KEYWORDS

- Diabetes mellitus • Adrenal insufficiency • Hyperthyroidism • Hypothyroidism
- Acromegaly • Pheochromocytoma • Carcinoid

KEY POINTS

- The goal of preoperative management of chronic endocrine disease is to minimize the impact of the associated comorbidities on the perioperative course by maintaining physiologic and metabolic homeostasis.
- There are few evidence-based guidelines for preoperative management of chronic endocrine disease; hence this review is based on recent subspecialty society consensus guidelines and professional society clinical practice recommendations.
- This review summarizes the key features and clinical considerations related to preoperative management and planning for the care of patients of common endocrine disorders (diabetes mellitus, adrenal insufficiency, thyroid disease), a less common disorder but one that has significant perioperative implications (acromegaly), and 2 disorders for which preoperative management is essential to good postoperative outcomes (pheochromocytoma and carcinoid syndrome).

INTRODUCTION

The American Society of Anesthesiologists Committee on Standards and Practice Parameters recently published the updated practice advisory for the preparation of patients for surgery.[1] Although the standards are designed to assist in basic decision making by the anesthesiologist, one aspect of these guidelines should be highlighted: the importance of the integration of pertinent information for the appropriate assessment of the severity of the patient's medical condition in advance of the procedure. In addition to perioperative management, the practitioner who cares for the patient with endocrine disease is important in the coordination of patient care, including providing information related to risk stratification, assessment of the extent of disease control, defining the current state of hormonal-metabolic balance, and providing guidance

Department of Anesthesiology, University of Maryland School of Medicine, University of Maryland Hospital, 22 South Greene Street, S11C, Baltimore, MD 21201, USA
E-mail address: mnjoku@anes.umm.edu

Med Clin N Am 97 (2013) 1123–1137
http://dx.doi.org/10.1016/j.mcna.2013.07.001   medical.theclinics.com
0025-7125/13/$ – see front matter © 2013 Elsevier Inc. All rights reserved.

for perioperative pharmacologic and medical management. For perioperative testing, the cost of repeating endocrine assays for the sole purpose of preprocedure documentation may be prohibitive. Selective tests may be repeated when the information may assist in optimizing perioperative care or if the course of care will be altered by the additional information.

There are few randomized controlled trials and evidence-based guidelines related to preoperative management of patients with endocrine disease. The majority of recommendations are adapted from meta-analyses, professional society consensus statements, and current literature reviews. Some endocrinopathies may not result in chronic disease because the medical and/or surgical therapy to control or eradicate the disease (eg, pheochromocytoma) is sufficient. Other endocrinopathies (eg, diabetes, acromegaly, recurrent carcinoid) may result in chronic disease because of the range of comorbidities that occur with or without treatment.

DIABETES MELLITUS

Since 2001, the literature related to glycemic control has been extensive, probably influenced by the increasing number of diagnosed and undiagnosed diabetics presenting for medical care, and the recognition of the relationship between blood glucose variability and adverse outcomes.[2–4] The proponents of tight glycemic control (blood glucose target 80–110 mg/dL) recognized the relationship between the severity of hyperglycemia and the extent of a myocardial infarction[5]; the association between fasting glucose and the risk of cardiovascular events in patients with and without diabetes[6]; reduced morbidity and mortality among critically ill patients with a stay in the intensive care unit (ICU) of longer than 3 days; and reduced morbidity, including the prevention of newly acquired kidney injury, accelerated weaning from mechanical ventilation, and decreased length of stay in the ICU and hospital.[3] As a result, tight glycemic control and intensive insulin therapy were incorporated into the standards of care in many centers, and glycemic control has been used as a hospital performance measure by the National Hospital Inpatient Quality Measure (NHIQM), the Surgical Care Improvement Project (SCIP), and the Joint Commission (JC), and is a component of Pay for Performance (P4P). Since 2009 intensive glucose control has been reevaluated, recognizing that tight glycemic control targets increase the risk of severe hypoglycemia (blood glucose 40 mg/dL) in some patients, may increase mortality risk, and may only benefit specific patient populations (eg, the critically ill and brittle diabetics).[7,8]

In 2009, the American Association of Clinical Endocrinologists (AACE) and the American Diabetes Association (ADA) updated the Consensus Statement on inpatient glycemic management, providing less stringent glycemic targets for critically ill and non–critically ill patients, and recommendations for treatment options and monitoring.[9] The recommendations (**Box 1**) include the administration of insulin to critically ill patients for persistent serum glucose level of 180 mg/dL and higher to achieve a target of 140 to 180 mg/dL. The glucose target for non–critically ill patients receiving insulin is less than 140 mg/dL when fasting and less than 180 mg/dL for random measurements. Scheduled, subcutaneous insulin with basal nutritional and correction components are recommended for achieving and maintaining control in the noncritical population. In addition, noninsulin agents are not suitable for most hospitalized patients who require treatment of hyperglycemia because of their pharmacokinetics and variable half-lives, making the agents less amenable to rapid titration.

Because the AACE-ADA recommendations did not specifically address patients undergoing ambulatory surgical procedures, the Society for Ambulatory Anesthesia

> **Box 1**
> **Summary of AACE-ADA consensus on inpatient glycemic control**
>
> *Critically Ill Patients: Treat with Intravenous Insulin*
> - Initiate insulin infusion, for persistent hyperglycemia 180 mg/dL or greater
> - Use validated protocols
> - Glucose target 140 to 180 mg/dL
>
> *Non–Critically Ill Patients*
> - If treated with subcutaneous insulin
>   - Premeal blood glucose less than 140 mg/dL
>   - Random blood glucose less than 180 mg/dL
>   - Scheduled subcutaneous insulin with basal, nutritional, correction components
> - Reassess insulin regimen if blood glucose levels less than 100 mg/dL
>
> *Noninsulin Agents*
> - Not recommended for hyperglycemia treatment of hospitalized patients
> - May be appropriate in selected patients
>
> *Data from* Moghissi E, Korytkowski M, DiNardo M, et al. American Association of Clinical Endocrinologists and American Diabetes Association consensus statement on inpatient glycemic control. Endocr Pract 2009;15(4):1–17.

(SAMBA) developed a consensus statement on blood glucose management in diabetic patients.[10] The recommendations, a result of a systematic review of the literature from January 1980 to November 2009, are based on general principles of blood glucose control in diabetics, drug pharmacology, data gathered from inpatient surgical populations, review articles, clinical experience, and judgment. These guidelines are summarized in **Box 2**. The SAMBA recommendations for preoperative management include an assessment of the level of glycemic control with measurement of glycosylated hemoglobin, documentation of the types and doses of antidiabetic agents, assessment of the frequency and symptoms of hypoglycemia, and an assessment of the patient's level of understanding and participation in self-management.

For patients who are treated with oral hypogycemic and noninsulin injectable agents, the SAMBA recommendation is to withhold the medicine on the day of surgery until normal oral intake resumes. For patients treated with insulin, the recommendation is to continue basal insulin unless there is a history of hypoglycemia. For the patient who is fasting before surgery, insulin regimens are summarized as follows: (1) no change required for continuous subcutaneous insulin pump but may reduce to sleep basal rates; (2) decrease morning dose of intermediate-acting and fixed combination insulin doses by 50% to 75%; (3) hold short-acting and rapid-acting insulin on the morning of surgery. The goals of perioperative ambulatory management are to minimize fluctuations in the glycemic management regimen, avoid hypoglycemia, and resume oral intake, when appropriate, soon after surgery.

In 2013, the ADA revised the standards of medical care in diabetes, based on new evidence published since 2011. The ADA guidelines are intended for use in conjunction with clinical judgment by patients and clinicians who manage diabetes.[11] Although the guidelines do not specifically address preoperative management of the patient with diabetes, the recommendations related to chronic management are relevant. The content related to the assessment of glycemic control, pharmacologic

Box 2
SAMBA consensus statement on blood glucose management in diabetic patients for ambulatory surgery

Preoperative Information Related to Glycemic Control

- Hemoglobin A_{1c}
- Type and dose of antidiabetic therapy
- Hypoglycemia: occurrence, frequency, manifestations, blood glucose at which symptoms occur
- Hospitalizations related to glycemic control
- Assess patient's ability to reliably test glucose and manage diabetes

Management of Preoperative Oral Antidiabetic and Noninsulin Injectable Therapy

- Hold on the day of surgery until normal food intake is resumed

Management of Preoperative Insulin Therapy

- Day before surgery
  - No change in basal insulin regimen, unless history of hypoglycemia
- Day of surgery
  - Insulin pump: no change
  - Long-acting insulin: 75% to 100% of morning dose
  - Intermediate-acting insulin and fixed-combination insulin: 50% to 75% of morning dose
  - Short-acting, rapid-acting, and noninsulin injectables: hold morning dose

Optimal Intraoperative Blood Glucose Level

- Well-controlled diabetes: less than 180 mg/dL
- Poorly controlled diabetes: maintain preoperative baseline values
  - Hypoglycemic symptoms may occur at normal blood glucose levels

Regimen to Maintain Optimal Blood Glucose Level

- Subcutaneous rapid-acting insulin analogues
- Dosing schedule based on time to peak effect

Optimal Perioperative Blood Glucose Monitoring

- Measure blood glucose level before surgery and before discharge home
- Intraoperative blood glucose monitoring every 1 to 2 hours, depending on duration and type of insulin

Hypoglycemia Management

- Diagnosis
  - Glucose less than 70 mg/dL or
  - Based on symptoms: sweating, palpitations, weakness, fatigue, confusion, behavioral changes, seizure, altered level of consciousness
- Treatment
  - Glucose 10 to 25 g, oral or intravenous
  - Glucagon 1 mg subcutaneously, if unable to ingest or if no intravenous access

Other Considerations:

- Preoperative hydration
- Nausea and vomiting prophylaxis

Data from Joshi GP, Chung F, Vann MA, et al. SAMBA consensus statement on perioperative blood glucose management in diabetic patients undergoing ambulatory surgery. Anesthesiology 2010;111(6):1378–87.

treatment, intercurrent illness and hypoglycemia, and discharge planning are applicable to the care of the patient preparing for surgery (**Box 3**).

Based on the 2012 American College of Physicians Clinical Practice Guidelines, there are more than 11 unique classes of oral pharmacologic agents used for the treatment of type 2 diabetes (**Box 4**). Metformin is first-line monotherapy, when not contraindicated. When monotherapy is inadequate because of failure to reach glycemic targets, the addition of a second agent (combination therapy) is recommended, and at times insulin therapy may be required. Hypoglycemia is more common with sulfonamides and with metformin-sulfonurea combination therapy. The thiazolidinediones are associated with an increased risk of heart failure, and may be contraindicated in patients with preexisting serious heart failure.[12] Metformin has been associated with lactic acidosis, but it is not clear if the lactic acidosis is due to the accumulation of metformin in patients with renal dysfunction (creatinine >1.4) or if this occurs in patients who are predisposed to lactic acidosis or renal insufficiency, independent of metformin therapy (eg, hypoxemia, shock, acute myocardial infarction, acute congestive heart failure, liver dysfunction, surgery, intravenous contrast administration). Because

---

Box 3
American Diabetes Association standards of medical care in diabetes

Glycemic Recommendations for Nonpregnant Adults with Diabetes

- Hemoglobin A_{1c} less than 7%
- Peak preprandial (before meals and snacks) capillary plasma glucose 70 to 130 mg/dL
- Peak postprandial capillary plasma glucose less than 180 mg/dL

Individual Goals Based On:

- Duration of diabetes
- Age/life expectancy
- Comorbid conditions
- Cardiovascular or microvascular complications
- Hypoglycemia unawareness

Pharmacologic Management

Type 1 diabetes

- Three to 4 injections of basal and postprandial insulin or subcutaneous insulin infusion

Type 2 diabetes

- Metformin, preferred initial agent
- Add second oral agent or insulin, if first-line therapy at maximal tolerated dose or hemoglobin A_{1c} greater than target

Hypoglycemia (Glucose<70 mg/dL)

- Assess for symptomatic and asymptomatic hypoglycemia
- Treatment
  - Glucose 15 to 20 g (intravenous or oral)
  - Glucagon 0.5 to 1 IU (subcutaneous, intravenous, intramuscular)
  - Reassess glycemic targets

Data from American Diabetes Association. Standards of medical care in diabetes—2013. Diabetes Care 2013;36(Suppl 1):S11–66.

Box 4
Pharmacologic treatment options for diabetes

Oral Antidiabetic Agents	Noninsulin Injectables	Insulin
Metformin	Exenatide	Short to rapid acting:
Chlorpropamide	Pramlintide	Regular
Tolbutamide		
Glimepiride		Lispro
Glipizide		Aspart
Glyburide		
Repaglinide		Glulisine
Nateglinide		Intermediate acting:
Rosiglitazone		
Pioglitazone		NPH insulin
Acarbose		Zinc insulin
Miglitol		
Sitagliptin		Long acting:
Saxagliptin		Glargine
		Detemir
		Mixed insulins

Data from Joshi GP, Chung F, Vann MA, et al. SAMBA consensus statement on perioperative blood glucose management in diabetic patients undergoing ambulatory surgery. Anesthesiology 2010;111(6):1378–87.

---

of the benefits (lower all-cause mortality, decreased cardiovascular mortality, fewer hypoglycemic episodes) in the management of type 2 diabetes in conjunction with lifestyle modification, metformin continues to be first-line therapy; and unless there is a contraindication to its use, metformin should be continued in the perioperative period.[12]

Hyperglycemic crises, diabetic ketoacidosis (DKA), and hyperosmolar hyperglycemic state (HHS) are associated with high mortality. Surgery for patients who present with a hyperglycemic crisis should be postponed for treatment and for the identification and management of the precipitating cause. The diagnostic criteria for DKA and HHS, as summarized by Kitabchi and colleagues,[13] are outlined in **Table 1**. For the

Table 1
Diagnostic criteria for DKA and HHS

	DKA			HHS
	Mild	**Moderate**	**Severe**	**HHS**
Plasma glucose (mg/dL)	>250	>250	>250	>600
Arterial pH	7.25–7.3	7.00 to <7.24	<7.00	>7.30
Serum HCO_3^- (mEq/L)	15–18	10 to <15	<10	>18
Urine or serum ketone	+	+	+	Small
Effective serum osmolality	Variable	Variable	Variable	>320 mOsm/kg
Anion gap	>10	>12	>12	Variable
Mental status	Alert	Alert/drowsy	Stupor/coma	Stupor/coma

Data from Moghissi E, Korytkowski M, DiNardo M, et al. American Association of Clinical Endocrinologists and American Diabetes Association consensus statement on inpatient glycemic control. Endocr Pract 2009;15(4):1–17.

patient who presents on the day of surgery with hyperglycemia (glucose $\geq$250 mg/dL), the suggested approach is to determine whether there has been an intercurrent illness, a change in medication management, or another precipitating cause. The initial laboratory assessment should include plasma glucose, serum electrolytes, bicarbonate, blood urea nitrogen (BUN), creatinine, serum osmolality, serum or urine ketones, and the calculation of anion gap. If there is no identified precipitating cause, if the serum bicarbonate, osmolarity, and anion gap are normal, and ketones are not present, then it is reasonable to proceed with the procedure, provided that the glucose decreases with hydration and insulin. If the response to treatment is considered inadequate or if in the clinician's judgment the risk outweighs the benefit, elective surgery should be postponed until the hyperglycemia, DKA, or HHS are resolved, until the patient has returned to the regimen that preceded the hyperglycemia, or until the glycemic treatment regimen is less variable and the glucose is stable.

Continuous glucose monitoring (CGM), together with intensive insulin therapy with subcutaneous insulin infusion delivered by pump, is being used increasingly for patients with type 1 diabetes. CGM devices can be continued during surgery as long as the device does not interfere with the surgical field.[14] The CGM glucose value should be confirmed with a serum measurement. When the patient is not receiving oral intake, the insulin delivery device should be reset to the patient's usual fasting dose.

ADRENAL INSUFFICIENCY

Adrenal insufficiency (AI) is classified based on the site of hypothalamic-pituitary-adrenal (HPA) axis dysfunction. Primary AI is the result of failure of the adrenal gland. The most common causes of primary AI are autoimmune adrenalitis, infection, postsurgical adrenalectomy, and sepsis. Secondary AI is the result of inadequate corticotropin for stimulation of the adrenal cortex, which may be due to atrophy of the adrenal cortex or exogenous glucocorticoid suppression of pituitary corticotropin. Common conditions associated with secondary AI include the therapeutic use of steroids to treat autoimmune disease, inflammatory disease, chronic lung disease, or asthma, or when steroids are used for organ transplantation. Tertiary AI is caused by impaired ability of the hypothalamus to secrete corticotropin-releasing hormone (CRH). In patients receiving a chronic replacement dose of steroids, the incidence of perioperative AI is probably low, and most reports of suspected AI are not based on biochemical confirmation. In practice, many patients receive perioperative steroid replacement, often in supraphysiologic doses. This practice is probably based on a 1994 recommendation for steroid replacement related to the degree of surgical stress.[15,16] In 2008, Marik and Varon[17] reviewed the literature from the period 1966 to 2007 related to perioperative stress-dose steroids for patients' undergoing surgical procedures. Their findings and recommendations recognize the differences in stress responses for patients receiving therapeutic doses of corticosteroids (eg, immunosuppression regimen after transplantation), but with an intact, though suppressed, HPA axis and stress response in patients with primary dysfunction of the HPA axis (eg, primary or secondary adrenal failure, Addison disease, congenital adrenal hyperplasia, hypopituitarism) requiring physiologic replacement. The recommendations based on their review are summarized in **Box 5**. The recommended doses of hydrocortisone are based on the physiologic responses to the stress of the surgical procedure as described by Salem and colleagues.[16]

For the practitioner managing the patient with chronic AI, the preoperative management and preparation should include the medical history, including the etiology of AI,

---

Box 5
Perioperative stress doses of corticosteroids

Patients Receiving Therapeutic Doses of Corticosteroids (eg, organ transplant)

- Continue usual daily dose
- No stress dose required
- No need to test adrenal function
- Consider stress dose in patients with volume refractory hypotension
  - Hydrocortisone 100 mg intravenously then 50 mg every 6 hours, until symptom resolution

Patients Receiving Physiologic Replacement Doses of Corticosteroids (eg, primary AI)

- Hydrocortisone 50 mg intravenously (one dose), for minor surgery
- Hydrocortisone 50 mg intravenously every 8 hours, for 48 to 72 hours, for major surgery

---

the history of previous adrenal crises and the precipitating cause(s), the chronic medication replacement regimen including dose and frequency, and the history of any medical or physiologic changes that may predispose to acute adrenal dysfunction. Laboratory evaluation should include electrolytes, BUN, creatinine, and glucose. The decision to administer steroids should be based on: the normal diurnal cortisol secretion in the absence of HPA dysfunction; chronic steroid dose; duration of treatment; anticipated recovery from HPA suppression after cessation of treatment; and the route of chronic steroid administration (topical, inhaled, oral, or intravenous).

Replacement is usually required for patients taking steroid doses that exceed a daily dose of 5 mg prednisone, 25 mg hydrocortisone, 4 mg triamcinolone, or 0.75 mg dexamethasone. The recommended replacement is a single dose of 50 mg hydrocortisone for minor surgery, and for major surgery 50 mg, 3 times a day, for 48 to 72 hours. For those patients receiving therapeutic doses of corticosteroids, the recommendation is to continue the usual daily dose prior to and including the day of surgery. Additional stress-dose steroids are usually not required.

The utility of repeating preoperative adrenal function tests is limited. If a patient develops hypotension during a procedure that is refractory to administration of intravenous fluids, the recommendation is to administer an initial dose of 100 mg hydrocortisone, followed by 200 mg/d (eg, 50 mg every 6 hours). Hydrocortisone is then continued until the stress resolves and when the patient is able to resume the preoperative steroid regimen. Mineralocorticoid replacement (fludrocortisone or equivalent) is usually not required unless it is a component of the chronic replacement regimen for primary AI. Moreover, hydrocortisone has mineralocorticoid activity in doses that exceed 100 mg/d and in the absence of primary adrenal failure. Most patients with AI do not show signs of aldosterone deficiency because mineralocorticoid secretion is primarily modulated by the renin-angiotensin system.

THYROID DISEASE

The goal of perioperative management of the patient with thyroid disease is to maintain the euthyroid state. In 2012, the AACE together with the American Thyroid Association published clinical practice guidelines for the management of hypothyroidism in adults.[18] Similarly, in 2011, evidence-, expert-, and consensus-based guidelines were developed for the management of hyperthyroidism.[19] Both these sets of recommendations refer to the management of the ambulatory patient with previously established hypothyroidism or hyperthyroidism.

The symptoms of hypothyroidism can be subclinical or overt. Dry skin, cold sensitivity, fatigue, muscle cramps, voice changes, and constipation are common symptoms. Hypothyroidism may be associated with a prolonged ankle-jerk relaxation time, carpal tunnel syndrome, bradycardia, and sleep apnea. A low serum thyrotropin level is the primary marker of the disease. L-Thyroxine is the primary treatment. Therapeutic end points for the management of hypothyroidism are related to resolution of symptoms, return to a normal resting heart rate, and normalization of cholesterol, anxiety, sleep pattern, menstrual cycle, creatinine kinase, hepatic transaminases, and thyrotropin levels.

Hyperthyroidism, a subset of thyrotoxicosis, is due to increased synthesis and secretion of thyroid hormone by the thyroid gland. Thyroid hormone excess increases basal metabolic rate and thermogenesis, reduces systemic vascular resistance, and may result in weight loss, tachycardia, atrial fibrillation, heart failure, neuropsychiatric dysfunction, anxiety, emotional lability, irritability, and muscle weakness and tremor. The primary treatment is β-blockade (propranolol, atenolol, metoprolol, nadolol, esmolol) for control of a heart rate in excess of 90 beats/min or for patients with concomitant cardiovascular disease. Oral calcium-channel blockers (verapamil, diltiazem) may be effective alternative agents for control of heart rate in patients with β-blocker intolerance.

The management of the patient with chronic thyroid dysfunction requires an assessment of symptoms, documentation of the medication regimen, and a detailed assessment of cardiovascular symptoms to elicit the presence of arrhythmias, heart failure, or ischemic heart disease. The primary purpose of the preoperative and preprocedure management is to establish and maintain the euthyroid state. For patients with a history of hypothyroidism, oral thyroid hormone replacement therapy should continue through the day of surgery and afterward. For patients with a history of hyperthyroidism, β-adrenergic blockade and the usual doses of antithyroid medications (propylthiouracil, methimazole, potassium iodide) should continue perioperatively. Propylthiouracil is associated with agranulocytosis, and methimazole and propylthiouracil are associated with hepatotoxicity. In some patients, hyperthyroidism may be associated with elevated liver enzymes. Patients receiving antithyroid agents may require baseline preoperative laboratory screening, including white blood cell count and differential and liver enzymes.

Changes in thyroid size, position, shape, and nodularity may influence the management of the airway. The physician responsible for the chronic care of the patient may be the first to elicit the symptoms associated with airway compromise and the potentially challenging perioperative airway. Findings that may be associated with airway changes are neck discomfort, stridor, swelling, dysphagia, hoarseness, changes in voice, and positional symptoms. The physical examination should include the position of the trachea and an assessment for positional dyspnea or dysphagia. Preprocedure imaging (chest radiograph, computed tomography scan) can help in evaluating the degree of tracheal compression or displacement. In some cases, flexible fiberoptic examination of the larynx may be needed to document the ease of access to the glottis as well as the preprocedure or preintubation position and function of the vocal cords.

Thyroid storm, or life-threatening thyrotoxicosis, may occur preoperatively, and is related to the abrupt cessation of antithyroid drugs, unrecognized or inadequately treated thyrotoxicosis, or exposure to exogenous iodine. The diagnosis requires a high index of suspicion in the presence of symptoms of thermoregulatory dysfunction, hemodynamic lability, gastrointestinal symptoms, and central nervous system disturbance.[19] The treatment of thyroid storm targets each step in thyroid hormone synthesis, release, and site of action. Conversion of triiodothyronine to thyroxine is blocked by β-adrenergic blockade, Propylthiouracil, and corticosteroids. Synthesis of new thyroid hormone is blocked by methimazole and inorganic iodide. Moreover, inorganic iodide blocks the release of thyroid hormone. Symptomatic treatment also includes acetaminophen, cooling, and volume replacement. If the symptoms of thyrotoxicosis are recognized in advance, surgery should be postponed until the patient is rendered euthyroid. Consultation with an endocrinologist is indicated for the management of thyrotoxicosis, and for the management of hyperthyroidism in children, pregnant women, patients with concomitant cardiac disease, or if present with another complicated endocrine disease (AI) or when there is difficulty achieving a euthyroid state.

ACROMEGALY

Excess of growth hormone (GH) is associated with multisystem comorbidities, and the presenting features depend on the timing of GH hypersecretion. If GH excess occurs before the closure of the epiphyseal plates, the result is accelerated vertical growth and, sometimes, gigantism. If GH excess occurs after epiphyseal closure, the result is acromegaly. Acromegaly is characterized, on physical examination, by enlargement of the skull, hands, and face; large tongue; protrusion of the brow and jaw; swelling of vocal cords; and a deep voice. In 2009, the Acromegaly Consensus Group published consensus guidelines for disease management.[20] In 2011, the AACE published updated guidelines for the diagnosis and treatment of acromegaly.[21] Although the guidelines do not specifically address the patient with GH excess who is presenting for nonpituitary surgery or other procedures, they do provide a comprehensive framework for assessing and managing the patient. The 2011 recommendations of the AACE are summarized in **Box 6**.

Acromegaly is associated with several comorbidities that may affect or confound perioperative management, including somatic enlargement, jaw overgrowth, joint pain, and carpal tunnel syndrome. Osteoarthropathy may affect the access to the operative site and positioning of the patient for surgery. Jaw overgrowth may influence the ability to achieve adequate mask fit and maintain airway patency, and may adversely affect the ability to achieve bag-mask ventilation. Central sleep apnea, which results in altered respiratory control, and obstructive sleep apnea as a result of craniofacial and soft-tissue changes, are associated with acromegaly. Patients with acromegaly and sleep apnea warrant more intense postprocedural monitoring and vigilance because of the increased sensitivity of the central nervous system (CNS) to the respiratory depressant effects of narcotics and sedatives, the associated risk of airway obstruction (macroglossia, epiglottis hypertrophy), and an attenuated hypoxic respiratory drive. GH-associated CNS changes (headaches, visual changes), may confound the postoperative assessment of a neurologic change. Complete documentation of the patient's baseline may save the cost of repeating tests and may facilitate timely assessment of new findings in the perioperative period.

Therapeutic options for acromegaly are medical, surgical, and radiation. Medical therapy is based on 3 types of agents: dopamine antagonists, somatostatin analogues, and GH receptor antagonists. The dopamine antagonists cabergoline and bromocriptine may cause nausea, vomiting, orthostatic hypotension, headache, and nasal congestion. Cabergoline has been associated with echocardiographic valvular abnormalities in patients who also have Parkinson's disease. The somatostatin analogues octreotide and lanreotide may cause nausea, poor glycemic control, and bradycardia. The GH receptor antagonist pegvisomant may cause enlargement of pituitary tumor, flu-like symptoms, allergic reactions, and increased liver enzymes.

Box 6
Acromegaly: comorbidities influencing perioperative management

Acral	Cardiovascular	Pulmonary	Endocrine	Neurologic	Other
Somatic enlargement	Cardiomyopathy, left ventricular hypertrophy, impaired systolic and diastolic function, arrhythmias, conduction abnormalities	Sleep apnea	Diabetes mellitus	Headache	Fatigue
Jaw overgrowth			Menstrual irregularities	Visual field loss	Generalized weakness
Arthralgias			Hyper- and Hypoprolactinemia	Diplopia	Diaphoresis
Osteoarthropathy			Primary hyperparathyroidism associated with multiple endocrine neoplasia (MEN)-1		
	Hypertension		Post-therapy hypopituitarism		

Data from Katznelson L, Atkinson JL, Cook DM, et al, American Association of Clinical Endocrinologists. American Association of Clinical Endocrinologists medical guidelines for clinical practice for the diagnosis and treatment of acromegaly—2011 update. Endocr Pract 2011;17(Suppl 4):1–44.

For the preparation of the patient with GH excess for nonpituitary surgery, the following points should be considered:

- Perform a comprehensive history, documentation of physical findings, and medication regimen including side effects.
- Obtain laboratory evaluation including electrolytes, glucose, BUN, creatinine, and liver function tests when indicated. Once the diagnosis of GH excess is established, repeat assays for GH, insulin-like growth factor I, oral glucose tolerance test, or prolactin are usually not needed preoperatively.
- Assess cardiovascular risk with testing based on risk profile, and signs and symptoms.
- Anticipate additional perioperative monitoring and the use of continuous positive airway pressure (if used preoperatively) if the patient has sleep apnea.
- If pituitary surgery has been performed previously, consider additional screening for symptoms of pituitary failure, hypothyroidism, adrenal dysfunction, syndrome of inappropriate antidiuretic hormone secretion, and diabetes insipidus; and plan for hormone supplementation when indicated.

NEUROENDOCRINE TUMORS

Functional and nonfunctional neuroendocrine tumors originate from several tissue sites. The diseases may occur sporadically or as part of a familial genetic syndrome. Because the diseases are numerous, this review focuses on the preoperative preparation of patients with pheochromocytoma and carcinoid syndrome.

Pheochromocytomas are neuroendocrine tumors that present with symptoms of adrenergic excess as result of the production, storage, and secretion of catecholamines and their metabolites. The most common presenting signs are hypertension, palpitations, headache, diaphoresis, and pallor. Less common findings are fatigue, nausea, weight loss, constipation, flushing, and fever. The signs and symptoms are similar to other disease presentations and are not specific to pheochromocytoma, so the initial diagnosis may be missed in the absence of biochemical confirmation. Morbidity is due to the effects of catechol excess on end organs, including the cardiovascular system. The North American Neuroendocrine Tumor Society Consensus Guidelines were developed in 2010 to provide a standardized framework for the diagnosis, management of symptoms, selection of medical therapy, indications for surgery for focal disease, and options for management of advanced disease, which may include radiotherapy and systemic chemotherapy.[22,23] Although the primary goal of surgery is curative, some patients develop advanced, multifocal disease that is not amenable to surgical resection.

The goals for preoperative management for endocrine and nonendocrine surgery for the patient with pheochromocytoma are similar (**Box 7**). The preprocedure preparation includes an assessment of the current symptoms and signs of the disease, the current medical therapy, medication doses and frequency, and screening for and management of concomitant end-organ dysfunction (cardiovascular, neurologic, renal, endocrine). It may be helpful to know the specific catecholamine secreted by the tumor (epinephrine, norepinephrine, dopamine). The degree of biochemical control is based on control of blood pressure and other symptoms (tachycardia, flushing) with α-blockade. Phenoxybenzamine, 10 to 20 mg/d, is the primary agent for outpatient control. Shorter-acting α-adrenergic agents (prazosin, terazosin, doxazosin) may be used for long-term control of symptoms for patients with metastatic disease. α-methyltyrosine may be added if symptom control is inadequate with α-blockade alone. If β-blockade is a component of the medical regimen, it is important to know the

---

Box 7
Pheochromocytoma: presurgical preparation and optimization

Diagnosis

- Consider association with other hereditary syndromes:
  ○ MEN-2
  ○ Neurofibromatosis type 1
  ○ Von Hippel–Lindau syndrome
  ○ Osler-Weber-Rendu syndrome
  ○ Familial paraganglioma

Preoperative Medical Management: Begin 10 to 14 Days Before Surgery

- α-Blockade: administer with or without elevated catecholamines
  ○ Phenoxybenzamine (by mouth) 10 to 20 mg/d or
  ○ Phentolamine (intravenous) 2.5 to 5 mg bolus titrated to effect
- Alternative agents
  ○ Calcium-channel blockers or
  ○ Short-acting selective α1-blocking agents
    ■ Prazosin
    ■ Terazosin
    ■ Doxazosin
- Tyrosine hydroxylase blockers
  ○ α-Methyltryrosine
- β-Blockade (only after α-blockade)
  ○ Use for control of tachyarrhythmias or angina
- Intravascular volume expansion

---

indications (angina, arrhythmia, coronary artery disease). It is recommended that β-blockade not be instituted until adequate α-blockade has been achieved to avoid unopposed α activity. Medications should be continued before surgery, during surgery, and immediately after surgery. Parenteral agents (phentolamine, 2.5–5 mg every 1–2 hours) may be substituted if the oral α-blocking agents are not feasible.

Evaluation for the presence or absence of cardiac disease or cardiac dysfunction is essential, because cardiomyopathy may result from the effect of chronic catechol excess, and coronary artery disease may be an unrelated comorbidity. The resting electrocardiogram and echocardiogram may be helpful in guiding perioperative management. Additional cardiac workup should be based on symptoms, signs, and risk factors. Intravascular volume deficits should be assessed and replaced up to 7 days before the scheduled endocrine or nonendocrine surgery in the patient with pheochromocytoma. Hyperglycemia may be related to catechol excess, and warrants close monitoring and management.

Carcinoids tumors originate from neuroendocrine tissues located in the lungs, thymus, or gastrointestinal tract. Carcinoids that originate in the lung are associated with corticotropin secretion and Cushing syndrome; those that originate in the gastrointestinal tract are associated with carcinoid syndrome with the secretion of serotonin, histamine, or tachykinins. Common carcinoid syndrome symptoms are flushing and diarrhea. Right-sided cardiac valvular abnormalities (tricuspid regurgitation and pulmonic stenosis) are associated with the disease.[23] Flushing mimics an allergic response; hence an understanding of the patient's symptoms and presentation are essential to management, because the approach to treatment will differ based on the diagnosis. Once the diagnosis of carcinoid is established, repeated assays of 5-hydroxyindoleacetic acid are not required for surveillance before nonendocrine surgery. Octreotide (short-acting octretotide: subcutaneous 150–250 µg 3 times a day; long-acting, slow-release octreotide: intramuscular 20–30 mg once a month) is prescribed for chronic management and symptom control. If the disease is progressive or metastatic, interferon-α may be used for its antitumor effect. Side effects of octreotide that may affect preoperative management include hyperglycemia or hypoglycemia and bradycardia, and inhibitory effects on other pituitary thyrotropin and GH secretion. The preprocedural optimization of the patient with carcinoid syndrome requires the control of symptoms with octreotide, and the monitoring and management of its side effects.

SUMMARY

Treatment options that reduce disease burden have allowed several endocrinopathies to be managed as chronic diseases. The current professional society consensus statements and guidelines were developed using specialist experts, current practice, consensus panels, and reviews of the existing literature. Most of these guidelines do not specifically address the care of the patient who is undergoing nonendocrine surgery. However, the principles for management are applicable to preoperative preparation of the patient presenting for surgery or other procedures. Because endocrine disorders have multisystem effects, preoperative optimization requires the recognition of the comorbidities associated with the endocrine disorder that are related to the disease itself and to its treatment. Preoperative preparation should include assessment of the course of the disease, and documentation of the therapy's medication regimen and side effects. For the practitioner managing the patient before surgery, communication and documentation of the premorbid condition and the coordination of care with those who will care for the patient during and after surgery (anesthesiologists, surgeons, hospitalists, and other internists) is essential.

REFERENCES

1. Committee on Standards and Practice Parameters, Apfelbaum JL, Connis RT. Practice advisory for preanesthesia evaluation—an updated report by the American Society of Anesthesiologists Task Force on Preanesthesia Evaluation. Anesthesiology 2012;116(3):522–38.
2. Van Den Berghe G, Wouters P, Weekers F, et al. Intensive insulin therapy in critically ill patients. N Engl J Med 2001;345(19):1359–67.
3. Van den Berghe G, Wilmer A, Hermans G, et al. Intensive insulin therapy in the medical ICU. N Engl J Med 2006;354(5):449–61.
4. International Surviving Sepsis Campaign Guidelines Committee. Surviving sepsis campaign. International guidelines for management of severe sepsis and septic shock: 2008. Crit Care Med 2008;36(1):296–327.
5. Gu W, Pagel PS, Warltier DC, et al. Modifying cardiovascular risk in diabetes mellitus. Anesthesiology 2003;98(3):774–9.

6. Suleiman M, Hammerman H, Boulos M, et al. Fasting glucose is an important in-dependent risk factor for 30-day mortality in patients with acute myocardial infarction: a prospective study. Circulation 2005;111(6):754–60.
7. NICE-SUGAR Study Investigators. Intensive versus conventional glucose control in critically ill patients. N Engl J Med 2009;360(13):1283–97.
8. Lipshutz AK, Gropper MA. Perioperative glycemic control: an evidence based re-view. Anesthesiology 2009;110(2):408–21.
9. Moghissi E, Korytkowski M, DiNardo M, et al. American Association of Clinical En-docrinologists and American Diabetes Association consensus statement on inpa-tient glycemic control. Endocr Pract 2009;15(4):1–17.
10. Joshi GP, Chung F, Vann MA, et al. SAMBA consensus statement on perioperative blood glucose management in diabetic patients undergoing ambulatory surgery. Anesthesiology 2010;111(6):1378–87.
11. American Diabetes Association. Standards of medical care in diabetes—2013. Diabetes Care 2013;36(Suppl 1):S11–66.
12. Qaseem A, Humphrey L, Sweet D, et al. Oral pharmacologic treatment of type 2 diabetes mellitus: a clinical practice guideline from the American College of Phy-sicians. Ann Intern Med 2012;156:218–31.
13. Kitabchi A, Umpierrez GE, Miles JM, et al. Consensus statement: hyperglycemic crises in adult patient with diabetes. Diabetes Care 2009;32(7):1335–43.
14. Rice MJ, Coursin DB. Continuous measurement of glucose: facts and challenges. Anesthesiology 2012;116(1):199–204.
15. Axelrod L. Perioperative management of patients treated with glucocorticoids. Endocrinol Metab Clin North Am 2003;32(2):367–83.
16. Salem M, Tainsh RE, Bromberg J, et al. Perioperative glucocorticoid coverage. A reassessment 42 years after emergence of a problem. Ann Surg 1994;219:416–25.
17. Marik PE, Varon J. Requirement of perioperative stress doses of corticosteroids. Arch Surg 2008;143(12):1222–6.
18. Garber JR, Cobin RH, Gharib H, et al. Clinical practice guidelines for hypothyroid-ism in adults: cosponsored by the American Association of Clinical Endocrinolo-gists and the American Thyroid Association. Endocr Pract 2012;18(6):989–1028.
19. Bahn RS, Burch HB, Cooper DS, et al. Hyperthyroidism and other causes of thyro-toxicosis: management guidelines of the American Thyroid Association and Amer-ican Association of Clinical Endocrinologists. Endocr Pract 2011;17(3):456–520.
20. Melmed S, Colao A, Barkan M, et al. Guidelines for acromegaly management: an: update. J Clin Endocrinol Metab 2009;94(5):1509–17.
21. Katznelson L, Atkinson JL, Cook DM, et al. American Association of Clinical En-docrinologists. American Association of Clinical Endocrinologists medical guide-lines for clinical practice for the diagnosis and treatment of acromegaly—2011 update. Endocr Pract 2011;17(Suppl 4):1–44.
22. Chen H, Sippel R, O'Dorisio MS, et al. The North American Neuroendocrine Tu-mor Society consensus guideline for the diagnosis and management of neuroen-docrine tumors. Pancreas 2010;39(6):775–8.
23. National Comprehensive Cancer Network Guidelines. Version 1. 2012. Neuroen-docrine Tumors Copyright 2013, National Comprehensive Cancer Network, Inc. All Rights Reserved..

Patients with Immunodeficiency

Michael J. Hannaman, MD*, Melissa J. Ertl, MD

KEYWORDS

- Immunocompromised • Preoperative • Human immunodeficiency virus • Cancer
- Transplant

KEY POINTS

- Immunosuppressed individuals with human immunodeficiency virus, cancer, and in the period surrounding organ transplantation should be evaluated in a broad, though targeted, systems-based manner for dysfunction relating to both their underlying disease state and medical treatment.
- Communication during this time among the many specialists managing these patients is essential in facilitating thorough evaluations while minimizing redundancy.
- As insight is gained into the immune response in the perioperative period, the future holds potential for individualizing our medical therapy based on more sophisticated immunologic profiling. Until such a time, clinicians must continue to rely on sound judgment and evidence-based practice guidelines to optimize outcomes within this growing and challenging population.

HUMAN IMMUNODEFICIENCY VIRUS

The human immunodeficiency virus (HIV) remains an important contributor to our population of immunosuppressed patients both in the United States and worldwide, despite remarkable strides in recent years. The acquired immunodeficiency syndrome (AIDS), first described more than 30 years ago,[1,2] has led to more than 640,000 deaths in the United States since the beginnings of the epidemic, with more than 20,000 of these occurring in 2009 alone.[3] It is estimated that in the United States more than 50,000 new infections occur annually, with current figures placing the number of people living with HIV/AIDS at 1.1 million. These numbers are more staggering when viewed globally, with current worldwide estimates at 34 million people living with HIV, and 2.5 million new infections taking place annually, or more than 7000 daily.[4–7] Among those with HIV in the United States, it is estimated that some 18% are unaware of it, and even among those who carry a known diagnosis of being

Disclosures: None.
Department of Anesthesiology, University of Wisconsin School of Medicine and Public Health, B6/319 Clinical Science Center, 600 Highland Avenue, Madison, WI 53792-3272, USA
* Corresponding author.
E-mail address: hannaman@wisc.edu

Med Clin N Am 97 (2013) 1139–1159
http://dx.doi.org/10.1016/j.mcna.2013.06.002
0025-7125/13/$ – see front matter © 2013 Elsevier Inc. All rights reserved.

HIV positive, 50% are not receiving regular care.[8-11] Routine HIV testing is now recommended for all persons ages 13 to 64 years but, yet again, some 18% of those infected do not realize it,[9] thus about one-third of patients with HIV are diagnosed late in their illness.[8]

Steady progress has led to numerous successes in our treatment of this disease, with highly active retroviral therapy (HAART) having an extremely profound impact. Indeed, HIV mortality rates, which rose steadily through the 1980s and peaked in 1995, have declined significantly, with the age-adjusted HIV death rate dropping 80% since that time,[12] mostly attributable to HAART. As of 2008, HIV was the sixth leading cause of death in those ages 25 to 44, down from first in 1995.[13] Progression to AIDS, quality of life, and survival are dramatically improved for those with adequate access to health care resources.[14,15]

It is estimated that roughly 20% to 25% of those infected with HIV will require surgery at some point in their illness.[16] As survival with this disease improves, as well as our comfort level in working with HIV-positive individuals, more will need to undergo surgical and anesthetic interventions. It is important that practitioners understand the risks and benefits involved when evaluating the health of these patients perioperatively. The aim of this article is to educate and update perioperative clinicians on several of these considerations.

Perioperative HAART

A key concept in understanding of the pathophysiologic impact of HIV/AIDS is its multiorgan system involvement. The infection itself, plus opportunistic infections, neoplastic sequelae, and the medications necessary to manage these issues can contribute to the overall pathologic state.[17] A more complete discussion on HAART medication initiation and management is covered elsewhere,[18] but HAART generally involves the use of antiretroviral agents (ARVs) from 5 different classes, combined to achieve more effective treatment while keeping the overall toxicity and risk of resistance low. These 5 classes are categorized by their mechanism of viral inhibition (**Table 1**), and are listed chronologically in the order in which they were developed.[19]

As with any medication, the common adverse effects and drug interactions these patients may manifest in the perioperative period are important to understand.[20] In broad terms these side effects, listed in **Table 2**, generally include mitochondrial dysfunction, metabolic abnormalities, bone marrow suppression, allergic reactions,[17,21] and the immune recovery syndrome.

Table 1
Antiretroviral medications by mechanism of action

Mechanism of Antiretroviral Action	Examples
Nucleoside/nucleotide reverse transcriptase inhibitors (NRTI/NtRTI)	Zidovudine (AZT), didanosine, zalcitabine, stavudine, lamivudine, abacavir
Nonnucleoside reverse transcriptase inhibitors (NNRTI)	Nevirapine, delavirdine, efivirenz
Protease inhibitors (PI)	Amprenavir, fosamprenavir, atazanavir, saquinavir, ritonavir, indinavir, nelfinavir
Fusion inhibitors	Enfuvirtide
Integrase inhibitors	Raltegravir

Data from Littlewood K. The immunocompromised adult patient and surgery. Best Pract Res Clin Anaesthesiol 2008;21(3):588.

Table 2
Side effects of antiretroviral medication

Adverse Effects	Resultant Side Effects
Mitochondrial dysfunction	Lactic acidosis, hepatic toxicity, pancreatitis, peripheral neuropathy, cardiomyopathy, pancreatitis, hepatic steatosis, lipoatrophy, proximal myopathy, polymyositis
Metabolic abnormalities	Fat maldistribution (lipodystrophy) and body habitus changes, dyslipidemia, hyperglycemia, glucose intolerance, insulin resistance, osteopenia, osteoporosis, osteonecrosis, arthritis
Bone marrow suppression	Anemia, neutropenia, thrombocytopenia
Allergic reactions	Rashes, hypersensitivity responses
Immune recovery syndrome	*Mycobacterium avium* abscesses, *Mycobacterium leprae* lesions, sarcoidosis, Graves disease, PML, SLE, antiphospholipid syndrome, vasculitis, primary biliary cirrhosis, hepatitis, polymyositis, uveitis, ITP

Abbreviations: ITP, idiopathic thrombocytopenic purpura; PML, progressive multifocal leukoencephalopathy; SLE, systemic lupus erythematosus.
Data from Leelanukrom R. Anesthetic considerations of the HIV-infected patients. Curr Opin Anaesthesiol 2009;22:412–8; and Hoffman RM, Currier JS. Management of antiretroviral treatment-related complications. Infect Dis Clin North Am 2007;21:103–32.

Mitochondrial enzyme synthesis is known to be significantly disrupted by HAART.[22] One consequence is a state of lactic acidosis, which can range from mild to severe,[23] and be variable in terms of both its incidence and presentation.[24,25] The perioperative physician should be aware of potential interactions between ARVs and anesthetic agents so as to accurately assess their impact on the patient's ability to successfully undergo surgery. Anesthetic agents can induce pharmacodynamic changes that may affect the efficacy and toxicity of ARVs, while at the same time ARVs may affect the absorption, distribution, metabolism, and elimination of anesthetic drugs. Giving anesthetic agents that may result in renal and hepatic dysfunction specifically should be avoided if possible in patients on ARVs. In addition, there is some evidence to support avoiding prolonged propofol infusions in these patients because of mitochondrial toxicity and lactic acidosis.[26]

Other consequences of the mitochondrial toxicity of HAART include cardiomyopathy,[22,27,28] pancreatitis, hepatosteatosis, proximal myopathy, osteopenia,[29] peripheral neuropathy,[30] and lipoatrophy.[31] Lipodystrophy, another side effect of HAART that may be important in intraoperative airway management, refers to a pattern of peripheral lipoatrophy and central fat accumulation over the dorsocervical spine as well as the abdomen and breasts[32]; as with any alteration in normal airway anatomy, this can potentially make intubation challenging. Insulin resistance, glucose intolerance, and dyslipidemia can also potentially have a clinical impact,[33] but their cause and implications in the patient on HAART are only beginning to be fully understood.

Regarding hematologic issues while on HAART, myelosuppression and anemia are well characterized, and their extent and severity may have prognostic implications.[34] Hypersensitivity reactions should be recognized quickly in these patients, as they can range from mild rashes to life-threatening entities such as Stevens-Johnson syndrome.[35] The immune recovery syndrome is the consequence of a rapid and acute increase in CD4+ lymphocytes after the initiation of HAART, which may occur in some and be associated with significant clinical deterioration. The syndrome is manifested by a marked local and systemic inflammatory response, thought to be the result of progressive reconstitution of the immune system. Its consequences may be infectious, inflammatory, and otherwise. These disorders should be recognized and treated appropriately before undergoing elective surgery.

Preoperative Evaluation and Perioperative Considerations

Patients with HIV may present in any number of ways, and their disease severity may range from asymptomatic to severe (**Table 3**).[36] Their evaluation should follow accepted perioperative guidelines, with additional studies ordered depending on the severity of disease manifestations (**Table 4**). Laboratory studies should include complete blood count and coagulation values, and serum chemistries to evaluate electrolyte imbalances as well as liver and renal function. A chest radiograph should be ordered to screen for tuberculosis and other opportunistic infections. Cardiac studies including electrocardiogram (ECG) and echocardiogram can aid in assessing cardiomyopathy, if present.

If at all possible, ARVs should be continued perioperatively, as long as there are not surgical restrictions on gastrointestinal function and intake, although formal recommendations for this are lacking. Although no study has evaluated continuing versus withholding ARVs during surgery, the risks and benefits of holding them should strongly be considered before doing so. Only 2 ARVs, zidovudine and enfuvirtide, are available in parenteral form at present, and should be restricted to patients currently taking them who cannot take oral formulations.

A preoperative dialogue should be established between the preoperative practitioner managing a patient with HIV and the anesthesiologist to communicate concerns on both sides, as well as to exchange important information to be relayed to the patient. When deciding which anesthetic technique is best in patients with HIV, none has been proved to be safer than another. This decision should be made in context with how advanced the disease is at the time of surgery, and what other pathologic variables they may be manifesting. Regional anesthesia may be considered

Table 3 Clinical staging of HIV infection	
Stage 1 (asymptomatic)	No symptoms, persistent generalized lymphadenopathy
Stage 2 (mild symptoms)	Moderate weight loss (less than 10% of body weight), recurrent upper respiratory tract infection, oral and skin lesions
Stage 3 (advanced symptoms)	Severe weight loss (more than 10% of body weight), chronic diarrhea, persistent fever, oral lesion or candidiasis, pulmonary tuberculosis, severe bacterial infections, anemia, thrombocytopenia, neutropenia
Stage 4 (severe symptoms)	Wasting syndrome (more than 10% of body weight, or body mass index <18.5 kg/m^2), chronic diarrhea, persistent fever, recurrent bacterial infections, opportunistic infections, encephalopathy, nephropathy, cardiomyopathy, malignancy

Data from World Health Organization. WHO case definitions of HIV for surveillance and revised clinical staging and immunologic classification of HIV related disease in adult and children. World Health Organization. Geneva (Switzerland): WHO Press; 2007. Available at: http://www.who.int/hiv/pub/guidelines/HIVstaging150307.pdf.

Table 4	
Preoperative evaluation of the HIV-positive patient	
History and physical	Focusing on disease progression and organ dysfunction related to infection and drug therapy
Laboratory studies	CBC, INR, PT, PTT, serum electrolytes, LFTs, renal function tests
Imaging	Chest radiograph
Studies	ECG, echocardiogram

Abbreviations: CBC, complete blood count; ECG, electrocardiogram; INR, international normalized ratio; LFTs, liver function tests; PT, prothrombin time; PTT, partial thromboplastin time.

cautiously, depending on the extent of any central nervous system comorbidity and the extent of their immunosuppression and infectious risk. Neuraxial analgesia and epidural blood patches have been shown to be safe in obstetric patients with HIV[37] provided they lack neurologic symptomatology, but the full extent of any neurologic risk afterward is unclear. Blood transfusion in this population has been studied,[17] and is currently thought to lead to elevated HIV viral load in patients with advanced disease. Thus, it would seem prudent to avoid transfusions in these patients if the patient can tolerate them being withheld safely.

Finally, an emphasis should be placed on maintaining strict aseptic technique and taking infectious precautions when working with a patient with HIV. Heightened awareness of sterile technique, hand washing, and universal precautions for handling sharps are essential. Although there has yet to be a reported case of HIV transmission during anesthesia, it is important to have an institutional protocol in place to handle inadvertent exposures, as postexposure prophylaxis should be started as soon as possible.[38]

CANCER

It is estimated that in the year 2013, more than 580,000 Americans will die of cancer, almost 1600 people per day. More than 1.6 million new cancer diagnoses are projected in 2013 alone. It is the second most common cause of death after heart disease in the United States and the developed world, and accounts for nearly 1 in every 4 deaths.[39] At the same time, 5-year survival is up to 68% for the years 2002 to 2008, compared with 49% for 1975 to 1977.[40] More than 70% of these patients will develop symptoms related to primary or metastatic disease,[40] and many of these will require surgical intervention, either for primary tumor resection or emergently for complications of the disease.

The pathologic derangements of cancer require careful evaluation before proceeding with surgery. In addition to the disease state, the various treatment modalities, including chemotherapy and radiation, may have important perioperative implications. Severe derangements in nutrition, end-organ function, metabolism, and anatomic distortion may present to varying degrees depending on the type of cancer. Assessing the fitness of these patients for surgery can be challenging, as often the risks of undergoing the procedure are weighed against those of not proceeding with or delaying treatment.[41,42] Indeed, although clinicians always seek to optimize coexisting medical conditions before undergoing surgery and anesthesia, many cancer-related operations are often undertaken in a less than optimal state so as to avoid further metastasis.

Preoperative Evaluation and Perioperative Considerations

The physical presentation of these patients can vary from someone who is reasonably functional and able to carry on daily activities, to extreme physical debilitation, with poor nutrition, considerable pain, and other significant comorbidities. Along with a thorough history and physical examination, further laboratory evaluations and tests may be warranted (**Table 5**); these may include, but are not limited to, a complete blood count, serum electrolytes, liver function tests, and coagulation studies. Depending on the degree of cardiac involvement and type of surgery planned, a 12-lead ECG, echocardiogram, cardiac stress test, or coronary angiography may be advisable.[41] A chest radiograph should be considered if there is known or suspected primary or metastatic intrathoracic disease, pleural effusions, or other pulmonary disease processes that may have perioperative consequences. Consideration should be given to draining pleural effusions if there is any degree of pulmonary compromise; however, overly aggressive or repeated drainage should be discouraged owing to the risks of expansion pulmonary edema, as well as volume and protein depletion.

Immune compromise in oncologic patients results in several important considerations. Optimizing nutrition via appropriately timed perioperative feeding has also been shown to reduce infections, protein catabolism, and inflammatory markers.[43] The immunosuppressive effects of chemotherapeutic agents, specifically bone marrow suppression, can open the door to opportunistic infections. Replacing individual blood elements via transfusion or bone marrow stem cell stimulation, as well as maintaining coagulation homeostasis, may have a positive impact on patient survival.[41] These patients require strict adherence to aseptic principles, including hand hygiene, the use of barrier precautions, and timely perioperative antibiotic administration.

Although a comprehensive discussion of the specific effects of commonly used chemotherapeutic agents is beyond the scope of this article, it is important to have a general understanding of their physiologic impact. Examples within each class and their adverse effects are listed in **Table 6**. Such effects broadly include myelosuppression, central nervous system toxicity, nausea and vomiting, gastrointestinal upset, nephrotoxicity, cardiotoxicity, pulmonary toxicity, dermatotoxicity, and coagulopathy. At present, most investigations of the interactions of chemotherapy agents with anesthetic agents have been in vitro studies, with clinical relevance still open to debate.[44–48] Although all of these drugs may affect a patient's operative course, certain individual agents are highlighted here because of their higher degree of organ toxicity and overall greater potential impact on perioperative management.

Cardiac Toxicity

Chemotherapeutic drugs from several different classes, specifically from the anthracyclines, antimetabolites, and alkylating agent classes, are known to have cardiotoxic effects in addition to their chemotherapeutic benefits. The most studied and reported

Table 5 Preoperative evaluation of the patient with cancer	
History and physical	Focusing on disease progression and organ dysfunction related to tumor spread and drug therapy
Laboratory studies	CBC, INR, PT, PTT, serum electrolytes, LFTs, renal function tests
Imaging	Chest radiograph
Studies	ECG, echocardiogram, cardiac stress testing, coronary angiography, pulmonary function testing

Table 6
Classification of antineoplastic agents with common and/or important agents and effects

Antineoplastic Class and Subclass	Examples of Agents	Common and/or Important Effects (All Effects May Not Apply to All Agents in Class)
Alkylating agents	Cyclophosphamide Ifosfamide Melphalan Chlorambucil Busulfan Cisplatin Carboplatin Carmustine	Myelosuppression Neurotoxicity (including seizures and mental status changes) Gastrointestinal mucosal ulceration and denudation Hepatic veno-occlusion Nephrotoxicity Leukemogenesis Nausea and vomiting
Antimetabolites	Methotrexate Mercaptopurine Fluorouracil Gemcitabine Cytarabine	Myelosuppression Hepatic fibrosis in patients with preexistent autoimmune disease Elevation of hepatic transaminases Gastrointestinal mucosal ulceration and denudation Anorexia and nausea Cardiotoxicity with ischemic changes on ECG Noncardiogenic pulmonary edema Interstitial pneumonitis
Natural products		
Vinca alkaloids	Vinblastine Vincristine	Myelosuppression Nausea, vomiting, and anorexia SIADH Peripheral neuropathy Vocal cord paresis Fever
Epipodophyllotoxins	Etoposide Teniposide	Leukopenia Nausea and vomiting Fever Hepatic toxicity
Taxanes	Paclitaxel Docetaxel	Myelosuppression Myalgias "Stocking glove" neuropathy Hypersensitivity reactions Peripheral and pulmonary edema Pleural effusion
Antibiotics	Daunorubicin Dactinomycin Doxorubicin Mitomycin Mitoxantrone Bleomycin Mitomycin C	Myelosuppression Gastrointestinal mucosal ulceration and denudation Cardiotoxicity Pulmonary toxicity, including fibrosis Fever Raynaud's Coronary artery spasm Myelosuppression Hemolytic uremic syndrome Interstitial pulmonary fibrosis

(*continued on next page*)

Table 6
(continued)

Antineoplastic Class and Subclass	Examples of Agents	Common and/or Important Effects (All Effects May Not Apply to All Agents in Class)
Enzymes	L-Asparaginase	Hypersensitivity Hyperglycemia Spontaneous thrombosis (deficient factor S, factor C, or AT-III) Coagulopathy
Hormones and antagonists		
Adrenocortical suppressants	Mitotane Aminoglutethimide	Nausea and vomiting Dermatitis Adrenocorticoid suppression Hypothyroidism
Adrenocorticosteroids	Prednisone and equivalents	Adrenocortical insufficiency Glucose intolerance Fluid retention Hypernatremia Hypokalemia
Progestins and estrogens	Hydroxyprogesterone caproate Medroxyprogesterone acetate Megestrol acetate Diethylstilbestrol	Metabolic alkalosis Anorexia Elevated hepatic transaminases Venous thrombosis
Antiestrogens	Ethinyl estradiol Tamoxifen	Venous thrombosis
Aromatase inhibitors	Toremifene Anastrozole Letrozole	Retinal deposits and cataracts Elevated hepatic transaminases Venous thrombosis
Androgens	Exemestane Testosterone propionate	Arthralgia Sleep apnea Cholestatic jaundice
Antiandrogen	Fluoxymesterone Flutamide	Hypercalcemia Hepatic necrosis Cholestasis
Gonadotropin-releasing hormone analogue	Leuprolide	Methemoglobinemia Anaphylactoid reactions Dyspnea Leukopenia Osteoporosis Pulmonary embolism Vertigo
Miscellaneous Agents		
Substituted urea	Hydroxyurea	Myelosuppression Desquamative pneumonitis
Differentiating agents	Tretinoin Arsenic trioxide	Pulmonary infiltrates Pericardial effusion Elevated hepatic transaminases Hyperglycemia Lengthened QT interval
Protein tyrosine kinase inhibitors	Imatinib Gefitinib Erlotinib	Nausea and vomiting Pleural effusion Ascites Interstitial lung disease

(continued on next page)

Table 6 (continued)		
Antineoplastic Class and Subclass	**Examples of Agents**	**Common and/or Important Effects (All Effects May Not Apply to All Agents in Class)**
Proteasome inhibitors	Bortexomib	Elevated hepatic transaminases Myelosuppression Peripheral neuropathy
Biological response modifiers	Interferon-α Interleukin-2	Capillary leak syndrome Increased infection risk Cardiomyopathy Confusion
Antibodies	Rituximab Alemtuzumab Daclizumab Gemtuzumab Trastuzumab Cetuximab Bevacizumab	Bronchiolitis obliterans Fever Gastrointestinal obstruction Cardiomyopathy Supraventricular tachycardia Ventricular fibrillation Hepatic failure Oliguria Stevens-Johnson syndrome Myelosuppression

Abbreviation: SIADH, syndrome of inappropriate antidiuretic hormone secretion.

Adapted from Littlewood KE. The immunocompromised adult patient and surgery. Best Pract Res Clin Anaesthesiol 2008;22(3):585–609, with permission; and Chabner BA, Amertein PC, Druker BJ, et al. Antineoplastic agents. In: Brunton LL, Lazo JS, Perker KL, editors. Goodman and Gilman's The pharmacologic basis of therapeutics. New York: McGraw-Hill, Inc; 2006. Chapter 51; with permission.

agents include doxorubicin, daunorubicin, and epirubicin, and patients being treated with these agents should be carefully evaluated for cardiac dysfunction when considering surgery. Toxicity may occur in more than 20% of patients on these drugs,[49] with variable onset.

Other drugs with well-described cardiotoxic effects include cyclophosphamide, cisplatin, and mitomycin. Early changes can manifest as nonspecific T-wave changes, whereas late cardiotoxicity can result in congestive heart failure from left ventricular dysfunction. Cisplatin, for example, has a bimodal cardiovascular complication pattern: in early stages of treatment, patients may experience dysrhythmias, chest pain, and elevation of myocardial enzymes consistent with myocardial injury,[50] whereas complications such as left ventricular hypertrophy, ischemic cardiomyopathy, and hypertension may take as long as 2 decades to manifest themselves.[51] 5-Fluorouracil, of the antimetabolic agent class, may also cause dose-dependent cardiac ischemia.[52] Trastuzumab therapy has led to an increased incidence of congestive heart failure,[53,54] interleukin-2 has been shown at high doses to be associated with irreversible ischemic cardiac injury,[55] and arsenic trioxide may cause QT prolongation with inhalational anesthetics.[56] Known or suspected cardiac dysfunction in patients on any of these medications warrants evaluation via ECG, echocardiogram, stress testing, and coronary angiography, according to severity of disease and surgical risk.[41]

Pulmonary Toxicity

Like cardiac effects, pulmonary toxicity resulting from chemotherapy is variable in its presentation, and may be either early or late in onset. In general, early-onset symptoms include inflammatory interstitial pneumonitis, noncardiogenic pulmonary edema, and, less commonly, pleural effusions or bronchospasm. Late-onset toxicity most commonly manifests in the development of pulmonary fibrosis.

Also similarly to cardiac toxicity, pulmonary effects may appear from early to late in the treatment course. The more common early issues can include interstitial pneumonitis, noncardiogenic pulmonary edema, with pleural effusions and bronchospasm less common. The most studied of the agents causing these early effects is bleomycin, but inflammatory pneumonitis has been described in multiple other agents. Of the late effects, the most important is pulmonary fibrosis, and again bleomycin is the most noteworthy, although late-onset disease has also been described with busulfan, carmustine, and mitomycin.[57] Pulmonary toxicity may develop in 2% to 40% of patients on bleomycin therapy,[58] and up to 25% of patients previously treated with bleomycin undergoing surgery may develop postoperative respiratory insufficiency requiring prolonged intubation.[40] Receiving excessive intraoperative fluids, transfusions, lengthy surgery, and decreased vital capacity may make postoperative respiratory insufficiency more likely in these patients. Using a lower fraction of inspired oxygen intraoperatively may be beneficial in this patient subset, as lung injury may be exacerbated by oxidant pathways[59]; however, this approach may have negative consequences with regard to wound healing[60] and remains an area of controversy.

The impact of radiation therapy on pulmonary function should also be recognized, as the lungs are particularly sensitive to its deleterious effects, and this may have relevance perioperatively. Radiation pneumonitis develops in up to 15% of individuals undergoing high-dose radiation for lung cancer, as well as in a significant percentage of patients receiving radiation therapy for breast cancer.[57] Early symptoms include dyspnea or cough, which resolves in some patients but will progress in others. Pulmonary fibrosis develops in the progressive state, which may lead to respiratory failure and right heart failure over 12 to 24 months, after which the condition usually stabilizes.[61] Whether progression occurs or not seems to be determined by the amount of lung tissue injured, total radiation dose, and concomitant administration of chemotherapeutic agents with pulmonary toxicity.[62] Although advanced age or preexisting chronic lung disease do not appear to be major risk factors for developing radiation pneumonitis, they do worsen its overall impact.

Kidney, Liver, and Nerve Toxicity

Several antineoplastic drugs may have nephrotoxic effects, ranging from nonoliguric renal insufficiency to renal failure. Included among these are cisplatin, carboplatin, paclitaxel, methotrexate, and cyclophosphamide. These toxic effects may be exacerbated by other renal comorbidities such as diabetes and hyperglycemia, as well as high urate levels from tumor lysis. Nonsteroidal anti-inflammatory drugs are best avoided in these patients, thus affecting postoperative pain management options.

Liver enzyme elevation is commonly associated with many of the chemotherapy agents. Though this is generally transient, it may progress to more severe damage, and liver failure has been described.[63,64]

Neurotoxicity is a well-described issue in several of these agents. In the perioperative period, this may have unexpected consequences for the anesthesia provider. Vincristine, for instance, has been implicated in several case reports of vocal cord paralysis via recurrent laryngeal nerve injury.[65,66] This situation should be understood to place the patient at higher risk of nerve injury when undergoing procedures whereby there is already some risk of postoperative laryngeal dysfunction. Other drugs with neurotoxic effects include cisplatin, busulfan, and paclitaxel. Of note, a postoperative brachial plexopathy has been reported in a patient receiving cisplatin after an interscalene nerve block,[67] so regional anesthesia in patients on these medications should be performed only after very careful consideration of the risks and benefits. Special effort should also be given in proper positioning during surgery so as to avoid exacerbation of subclinical neurotoxicity during lengthy procedures.

TRANSPLANT

Another cohort of immunocompromised patients is those who have received organ transplants. The first ultimately successful transplant in 1954 was a kidney transplant between identical twin brothers. Since then, advances in surgical technique and immunosuppression have allowed thousands of patients to benefit from organ transplantation. The number of transplants performed yearly has increased over the last decade, as has patient survival. In 2011 alone more than 25,000 organs were transplanted in the United States,[68] and with 5-year patient survival rates as high as 91% among living-donor kidney transplant recipients,[69] more than 280,000 patients are living with functioning transplants in the United States today (**Tables 7** and **8**).[68] As the number of transplants performed increases and patient outcomes continue to improve, it becomes increasingly likely that physicians who do not work at transplant centers will care for transplant recipients presenting for nontransplant surgery and procedures.

Pretransplant Immune Dysfunction

Most organs contribute to the body's defense system in some way, and individuals awaiting organ transplant are often immunocompromised because of a combination of chronic disease and organ dysfunction. For example, the mucociliary action of the lungs is among the first lines of defense against inhaled particles, impairment of which predisposes a patient to airborne pathogens.[70] Liver disease is associated with spontaneous bacterial peritonitis and a higher risk of septicemia, in part attributable to shunting of portal blood, decreased ability of Kupffer cells to clear opsonized particles, neutrophil impairment, and decreased complement levels.[71] Similarly, decreased neutrophil function and complement deficiency can occur in patients with hyperglycemia from diabetes mellitus, illustrating the importance of pancreatic function in immunocompetence.[71]

Arguably the most complex but best described example of immune dysfunction related to organ failure occurs in renal disease. On one hand, renal failure is associated with a proinflammatory state characterized by hypercytokinemia. Hemodialysis has been widely implicated in contributing to this immunoactivation via interactions

Table 7 Organs transplanted in the United States, 2011[68]: adult transplant recipients	
Organ	**Number of Transplants**
Heart	1949
Lung	1804
Liver	4593
Kidney	16,055
Pancreas	1051
Intestine	129

Exceptions include lungs, which are reported as recipients 12 years old and older, and intestine, which are reported as pediatric and adult recipients combined.

Table 8
Patient survival after organ transplantation

Organ	Patient Survival (%)		
	1 y	5 y	10 y
Heart	88.3	74.9	56.0
Lung	83.3	54.4	28.6
Liver: deceased donor	88.4	73.8	60.0
Liver: living donor	91.0	79.0	69.9
Kidney: deceased donor	95.6	81.9	61.2
Kidney: living donor	98.5	91.0	77.1
Pancreas	97.8	88.7	76.1
Intestine	89.3	57.9	46.4
Heart-lung	80.6	44.9	29.0
Heart-kidney	95.8	77.6	58.8
Liver-kidney	87.4	71.4	58.9
Liver-intestine	63.3	58.0	39.0
Kidney-pancreas	95.7	87.2	71.4
Pancreas after kidney	97.0	84.5	67.5

Data from 2009 Annual Report of the US Organ Procurement and Transplantation Network and the Scientific Registry of Transplant Recipients: Transplant Data 1999-2008. Rockville (MD): US Department of Health and Human Services, Health Resources and Services Administration, Healthcare Systems Bureau, Division of Transplantation.

between the patient's blood and the dialyzing membrane, the presence of endotoxin in dialysate, and chronic vascular access.[72] However, it seems that there is also an accumulation of cytokines from decreased renal elimination and/or increased generation owing to uremia in renal failure, independent of dialysis.[72,73] This state of chronic immunoactivation and inflammation may contribute to the 50% mortality from cardiovascular disease seen in end-stage renal disease.[73] Conversely, renal failure is also associated with immunosuppression. Some of the impairments seen in the immune systems of patients with end-stage renal disease include hyporeactive monocytes, neutrophils with decreased bactericidal abilities, impaired T lymphocytes, and decreased numbers of B lymphocytes.[73] Vaccines against several pathogens, including hepatitis B, influenza, tetanus, and diphtheria, may be less effective in patients with end-stage renal disease, perhaps because of impaired T-lymphocyte function.[73] These defects contribute to the 20% mortality from infection seen in these patients,[73] and their propensity for infection and cardiovascular disease should be kept in mind during preoperative evaluation.

Posttransplant Immune Dysfunction

After patients with organ failure receive a transplant, the immune dysfunction related to their underlying condition may improve with improved organ function; however, they inevitably become immunocompromised for a different reason: the immunosuppressive medications necessary to prevent rejection of their transplanted organ. In general, patients require stronger immunosuppression in the immediate posttransplant period, termed induction immunosuppression, as well as during bouts of suspected rejection. Doses are eventually titrated down to maintenance levels. There are 4 major classes of commonly used immunosuppressants: corticosteroids, antibodies, antiproliferative/antimetabolic drugs, and calcineurin inhibitors. These agents are used in various combinations to lower the dose and associated side effects of any one in particular.

Corticosteroids, including hydrocortisone, prednisone, methylprednisolone, and dexamethasone, are commonly used in high doses for induction immunosuppression and treatment of acute rejection, as well as in lower doses for maintenance immuno-suppression. Although their actions on the immune system are broad, they are thought to primarily inhibit the production of T-cell cytokines, thereby impairing lymphocyte and macrophage function. Corticosteroids also suppress antibody and complement binding.[74] The side effects of corticosteroid treatment are many, and include fluid retention and hypertension, hyperlipidemia, glucose intolerance, potential adrenal suppression, osteoporosis and myopathy, glaucoma, poor wound healing, and increased risk of infections.[74]

Antibodies, such as antithymocyte globulin and basiliximab, are often used in the induction phase of immunosuppression. These drugs consist of monoclonal or poly-clonal antibodies that bind to specific antigens on B and T cells. These cells are then depleted from the circulation, via internalization of receptors, opsonization, lysis, or apoptosis.[74] Side effects include hypotension, tachycardia, bronchospasm, and fever during administration, owing to release of cytokines from lymphocytes.[74]

Antiproliferative and antimetabolic drugs include sirolimus, mycophenolate, and azathioprine. These drugs are primarily used as maintenance immunosuppressants, and inhibit the proliferation of B and T cells by interfering with various stages in their replication process.[74] As a class, their primary side effect is myelosuppression.[19] In addition, sirolimus may cause hyperlipidemia.[74]

Calcineurin inhibitors are also frequently used as maintenance immunosuppres-sants, and include cyclosporine and tacrolimus. These drugs block calcineurin phos-phatase activity, thereby impairing cytokine expression.[19] The most problematic side effect of this class is renal impairment, occasionally severe enough to necessitate dialysis and/or kidney transplantation, although they are also associated with hyper-tension, hyperlipidemia, neurotoxicity, and diabetes.[19,74] During preoperative evalua-tion, the side effects of these immunosuppressive agents should be understood so that their sequelae may be optimized before elective surgery.

Preoperative Evaluation and Perioperative Considerations

When a transplant recipient presents for nontransplant surgery, careful preoperative optimization, intraoperative management, and postoperative care are vital in achieving the best possible outcomes. Transplant patients are relatively medically complex and often have several significant medical comorbidities, whether preexist-ing or as a result of their immunosuppression. Cardiovascular disease, hypertension, hyperlipidemia, diabetes mellitus, renal insufficiency, and malignancy are all more common in this patient population.[75] In fact, metabolic syndrome is at least twice as prevalent in posttransplant patients as it is in the general population.[76]

Before any planned surgical procedure, a patient who has previously received an organ transplant should undergo a thorough preoperative evaluation, which should include a comprehensive history and physical examination, with particular attention to a review of systems and functional capacity. A decline in a transplant patient's func-tional capacity, and/or the presence of vague constitutional symptoms such as fatigue, malaise, lethargy, or anorexia, should raise concern for the presence of possible rejection, infection, or other acute process. Of course, more specific com-plaints should also be thoroughly investigated. It is important to remember that because of their immunosuppressed state and the altered physiology of their transplanted organs, transplant recipients may not display classic signs of infection such as fever and leukocytosis, and signs of rejection may be subtle. It is essential to maintain a high level of suspicion during the preoperative assessment, as morbidity is increased in transplant patients undergoing elective surgery during periods of acute rejection or infection.[75,77]

Most transplant patients have undergone a comprehensive cardiac evaluation before their transplant, and these records are often obtainable from the transplant center. Further preoperative workup may be indicated on an individual basis, however, given that these patients are generally at increased risk for cardiovascular disease owing to their comorbidities. If a significant amount of time has elapsed since the patient's last evaluation, or if, since that time, they have experienced a decline in their functional capacity or symptoms suggestive of cardiovascular disease, a chest radiograph, ECG, echocardiogram, or stress test may be warranted. Of importance, many of these patients may not experience classic anginal symptoms despite significant cardiac ischemia. For example, diabetic patients notoriously experience silent cardiac ischemia, as do heart transplant recipients because of the denervated nature of the transplanted heart.[75] Decreased exercise tolerance, cough, dyspnea, orthopnea, and peripheral edema should all raise suspicion and prompt further investigation.

In addition to appropriate cardiac evaluation and testing, other tests may be indicated preoperatively in transplant recipients. Because of the potential for myelosuppression in patients taking immunosuppressants, obtaining a complete blood count before surgery is reasonable. In addition, if neuraxial anesthesia is planned or if the potential for significant surgical blood loss is anticipated, preoperative evaluation of coagulation studies should be considered. As renal insufficiency from both calcineurin-inhibitor use and comorbidities is common in this population, determination of creatinine, blood urea nitrogen, and glomerular filtration rate preoperatively is advisable. As many transplant recipients have either diabetes mellitus or glucose intolerance, testing blood glucose and obtaining glycemic control before elective surgery is also desirable. Finally, evaluation of the patient's graft function preoperatively is essential, with the potentially indicated tests varying depending on which organ has been transplanted (**Table 9**). Each patient should be considered individually in the context of their overall clinical picture, focusing on their comorbidities, functional status, review of systems, and physical examination.

One of the most vital steps in the preoperative process should be communication with the patient's transplant center. The transplant center is often able to provide records that may minimize the need for redundant testing, as well as surgical operative notes that may be helpful for surgical planning. In addition, any unexpectedly abnormal examination findings, test results, or deviation from the patient's baseline functional capacity should be discussed with the transplant center during the preoperative workup. Communication with the transplant center about the patient's immunosuppression regimen is vital. Transplant recipients should generally be continued on their immunosuppressive medications with as little interruption as possible, and communication with the transplant center as well as with pharmacy can help formulate an appropriate plan for the perioperative period, when nil-by-mouth restrictions might otherwise interrupt the patient's normal medication schedule.

Intraoperative and Postoperative Management

When preoperatively counseling transplant recipients presenting for nontransplant surgery, it is important to understand that no single best intraoperative strategy has been demonstrated. Depending on the individual patient's medical condition and current surgical problem, the surgical team may elect to perform either an open or

Table 9
Organ-specific preoperative tests to consider in transplant recipients

Organ Transplanted	Preoperative Tests to Consider	Notes
Heart	Chest radiograph ECG Echocardiogram Stress testing Angiography	Biphasic and double P waves, and RBBB are common and of no clinical significance. New dysrhythmias, especially supraventricular, may indicate rejection.[8] 10%–20% have CAD at 1 y posttransplant, 50% at 5 y posttransplant.[8] Ischemia is often silent
Lung	Chest radiograph PFTs ABG	Infection and rejection may be difficult to distinguish, with infiltrates on chest radiograph, worsening PFTs, and decreased Pao_2 present in both[8]
Liver	Transaminases GGT Alkaline phosphatase Bilirubin Albumin INR/PTT Platelet count	Platelet function usually normalizes, but platelet count may remain decreased posttransplant[75]
Kidney	Creatinine Blood urea nitrogen Electrolytes Urinalysis	Creatinine may be normal or near-normal, but GFR is often diminished[75]
Pancreas	Blood glucose Amylase, lipase Electrolytes Acid-base status	Potential metabolic acidosis in patients with bladder drainage of the exocrine pancreas[75]
Intestine	Electrolytes Acid-base status Prealbumin Liver function tests	To assess nutritional status Coexisting liver dysfunction is common[75]

Abbreviations: ABG, arterial blood gas; CAD, coronary artery disease; ECG, electrocardiogram; GFR, glomerular filtration rate; GGT, γ-glutamyl transpeptidase; INR, international normalized ratio; PFTs, pulmonary function tests; PTT, partial thromboplastin time; RBBB, right bundle branch block.

minimally invasive procedure, and general, neuraxial, regional, local, and monitored anesthetics have all been safely preformed in appropriately selected posttransplant patients. Outpatient procedures are not strictly contraindicated, provided follow-up is adequate. A few salient points are covered here briefly.

As all transplant recipients are immunocompromised, avoidance of perioperative infections is of paramount concern. Invasive monitors and lines should be placed using a strict aseptic technique, and left in place only for as long as necessary. Arterial catheters and central lines placed in the groin should be avoided, when possible, because of the increased risk of infection.[75] Early postoperative extubation is desirable when possible, and oral endotracheal intubation is preferred over nasal, because of the increased risk of infection from the nasal route.[75] These guidelines apply to posttransplant patients in any setting, not just in the operating room.

In general, the standard guidelines for surgical antibiotic prophylaxis used for all patients should also be applied to transplant recipients.[19,75,78] Despite their immunocompromised state, there is no evidence that the bacteriology of their surgical-site infections differs from that of the general public, and empiric expansion of antimicrobial coverage to include atypical and opportunistic organisms is not indicated.[75,78] Prophylactic antibiotic administration for transplant recipients undergoing "clean" procedures that would not otherwise require prophylaxis has been advocated, albeit with limited supporting evidence.[19] Transplant recipients on chronic antibiotic prophylaxis should have this coverage continued perioperatively.[19]

The need for perioperative stress dose steroids in patients who take chronic exogenous glucocorticoids has been a subject of much debate. These patients may have blunting of the hypothalamic-pituitary-adrenal axis response to surgical stress. Despite this fact, clinically relevant hypotension during the perioperative period secondary to adrenal insufficiency is uncommon in these patients, and tends to respond to steroids given as "rescue" treatment.[79] Additional supplemental steroids are likely unnecessary in patients continued on their usual preoperative glucocorticoid regimen. Physiologic doses of supplemental steroids should be considered perioperatively in patients who have recently been withdrawn from glucocorticoid therapy, steroid-dependent patients with refractory hypotension, or critically ill steroid-dependent patients requiring vasopressors.[79]

There are no specifically contraindicated medications in this patient population in the perioperative period, although some considerations must be kept in mind. If a transplant recipient has residual hepatic or renal insufficiency, medications metabolized via a different route should be chosen, or doses should be adjusted accordingly and titrated to effect. Drugs with hepatotoxicity and renal toxicity should be avoided if possible. In addition, it is important to remember that heart transplant recipients, because of the denervated nature of the transplanted heart, will not respond normally to drugs with action via the autonomic nervous system (indirect-acting drugs), such as atropine.[75] Direct-acting drugs, such as epinephrine, should be used instead.

There are not many clinically relevant interactions between immunosuppressants and commonly used anesthetic drugs, though a few do deserve mention. Azathioprine and cyclosporine have been shown to decrease and increase the duration of action of muscle relaxants, respectively, and muscle-relaxant dosage should be titrated to effect accordingly.[75] In addition, there are several medications that may alter cyclosporine and tacrolimus blood levels, some of which are occasionally used in the perioperative setting (**Table 10**).

The patient's usual immunosuppressant regimen should be restarted as soon as possible after surgery. Immunosuppressant drug levels should be monitored postoperatively,[80,81] and communication with the transplant center and pharmacy should help guide any necessary adjustments.[75] Finally, graft function should be monitored

Table 10	
Perioperative drugs that affect cyclosporine and tacrolimus blood levels	
Increase Blood Levels	**Decrease Blood Levels**
Cimetidine	Carbamazepine
Diltiazem	Octreotide
Erythromycin	Phenobarbital
Fluconazole	Phenytoin
Metoclopramide	Rifampicin
Nicardipine	
Verapamil	

Data from Kostopanagiotou G, Smyrniotis V, Arkadopoulos N, et al. Anesthetic and perioperative management of adult transplant recipients in nontransplant surgery. Anesth Analg 1999;89:613–22.

to ensure that the transplanted organ has not been compromised during the perioperative period.

SUMMARY

Immunosuppressed individuals with HIV, cancer, and in the period surrounding organ transplantation each have unique considerations to be addressed during preoperative evaluation. These patients should be evaluated in a broad, though targeted, systems-based manner for dysfunction relating to both their underlying disease state and medical treatment. Communication during this time among the many specialists managing these patients is essential in facilitating thorough evaluations while minimizing redundancy. As insight is gained into the immune response in the perioperative period, the future holds potential for individualizing our medical therapy based on more sophisticated immunologic profiling. Until such a time, clinicians must continue to rely on sound judgment and evidence-based practice guidelines to optimize outcomes within this growing and challenging population.

REFERENCES

1. Gottlieb MS, Schroff R, Schanker HM, et al. *Pneumocystis carinii* pneumonia and mucosal candidiasis in previously healthy homosexual men: evidence of a new acquired cellular immunodeficiency. N Engl J Med 1981;305: 1425–31.
2. Centers for Disease Control and Prevention. Unexplained immunodeficiency and opportunistic infections in infants: New York, New Jersey, California. MMWR Morb Mortal Wkly Rep 1982;31:665–7.
3. Prejean J, Song R, Hernandez A, et al. Estimated HIV incidence in the United States, 2006-2009. PLoS One 2011;6(8):e17502.
4. UNAIDS. Report on the global AIDS epidemic; 2012. Available at: http://www.unaids.org/en/media/unaids/contentassets/documents/epidemiology/2012/gr2012/20121120_UNAIDS_Global_Report_2012_en.pdf.
5. UNAIDS. Together we will end AIDS; 2012. Available at: http://www.unaids.org/en/media/unaids/contentassets/documents/epidemiology/2012/jc2296_unaids_togetherreport_2012_en.pdf.
6. UNAIDS. World AIDS day report: results; 2012. Available at: http://www.unaids.org/en/media/unaids/contentassets/documents/epidemiology/2012/gr2012/JC2434_WorldAIDSday_results_en.pdf.
7. UNAIDS. Core slides: global summary of the AIDS epidemic; 2012. Available at: http://www.unaids.org/en/media/unaids/contentassets/documents/epidemiology/2012/201207_epi_core_en.pdf.
8. CDC. HIV surveillance report. vol. 22. 2012. Available at: http://www.cdc.gov/hiv/library/reports/surveillance/2010/surveillance_Report_vol_22.html.
9. CDC. HIV supplemental report 2012. vol. 17, No. 3 (Part A); 2012. Available at: http://www.cdc.gov/hiv/library/reports/surveillance/2010/surveillance_Report_vol_17_no_3.html.
10. CDC. Fact sheet: HIV in the United States: an overview; 2011. Available at: http://www.cdc.gov/hiv/library/factsheets/index.html.
11. CDC. Vital Signs: HIV Prevention Through Care and Treatment — United States. MMWR Morbid Mortal Wkly Rep 2011;60(47):1618–23.
12. NCHS. Health, United States, 2011; 2012. Available at: http://www.cdc.gov/nchs/data/series/sr_10/sr10_256.pdf.

13. CDC. Slide set: HIV mortality (through 2008). Available at: http://www.cdc.gov/hiv/pdf/statistics_surveillance_HIV_mortality.pdf.

14. Nieuwkerk PT, Hillebrand-Haverkort ME, Vriesendorp R, et al. Quality of life after starting highly active antiretroviral therapy for chronic HIV-1 infection at different CD4 cell counts. J Acquir Immune Defic Syndr 2007;45(5):600–1.

15. Van Sigham AI, van de Wiel MA, Chani AC, et al. Mortality and progression to AIDS after starting highly active antiretroviral therapy [see comment]. AIDS 2003;17(15):2227–36.

16. Eichler A, Eiden U, Kessler P. Aids and anesthesia. Anaesthesist 2000;49:1006–17 [in German].

17. Leelanukrom R. Anaesthetic considerations of the HIV-infected patients. Curr Opin Anaesthesiol 2009;22:412–8.

18. Tapper ML, Daar ES, Piliero PJ, et al. Strategies for initiating combination antiretroviral therapy. AIDS Patient Care STDS 2005;19(4):224–38.

19. Littlewood K. The immunocompromised adult patient and surgery. Best Pract Res Clin Anaesthesiol 2008;22(3):585–609.

20. Hofman P, Nelson AM. The pathology induced by highly active antiretroviral therapy against human immunodeficiency virus: an update. Curr Med Chem 2006;13(26):3121–32.

21. Hoffman RM, Currier JS. Management of antiretroviral treatment-related complications. Infect Dis Clin North Am 2007;21:103–32.

22. Carr A. Toxicity of antiretroviral therapy and implications for drug development. Nat Rev Drug Discov 2003;2(8):624–34.

23. Shambelan M, Benson CA, Carr A, et al. Management of metabolic complications associated with antiretroviral therapy for HIV-1 infection: recommendations of an International AIDS Society-USA panel. J Acquir Immune Defic Syndr 2002;31(3):257–75.

24. Geddes R, Knight S, Moosa MY, et al. A high incidence of nucleoside reverse transcriptase inhibitor (NRTI)-induced lactic acidosis in HIV-infected patients in a South African context. S Afr Med J 2006;9(8):722–4.

25. Wester CW, Okezie OA, Thomas AM, et al. Higher-than-expected rates of lactic acidosis among highly active antiretroviral therapy-treated women in Botswana: preliminary results from a large randomized clinical trial. J Acquir Immune Defic Syndr 2007;46(3):318–22.

26. Wolf A, Weir P, Segar P, et al. Impaired fatty acid oxidation in propofol infusion syndrome. Lancet 2001;357:606–7.

27. Lewis W. Cardiomyopathy in AIDS: a pathophysiological perspective. Prog Cardiovasc Dis 2000;43(2):151–70.

28. Lewis W, Haase CP, Raidel SM, et al. Combined antiretroviral therapy causes cardiomyopathy and elevates plasma lactate in transgenic AIDS mice. Lab Invest 2001;81(11):1527–36.

29. Powderly WG. Long-term exposure to lifelong therapies. J Acquir Immune Defic Syndr 2002;29(Suppl 1):S28–40.

30. Sacktor N. The epidemiology of human immunodeficiency virus-associated neurological disease in the era of highly active antiretroviral therapy. J Neurovirol 2002;8(Suppl 2):115–21.

31. Stankov MV, Behrens GM. HIV-therapy associated lipodystrophy: experimental and clinical evidence for the pathogenesis and treatment. Endocr Metab Immune Disord Drug Targets 2007;7(4):237–49.

32. Milinkovic A, Martinez E. Current perspectives on HIV-associated lipodystrophy syndrome. J Antimicrob Chemother 2005;56(1):6–9.

33. Balasubramanyam A, Sekhar RV, Jahoor F, et al. Pathophysiology of dyslipidemia and increased cardiovascular risk in HIV lipodystrophy: a model of 'systemic steatosis'. Curr Opin Lipidol 2004;15(1):59–67.
34. Moyle G. Anaemia in persons with HIV infection: prognostic marker and contributor to morbidity. AIDS Rev 2002;4(1):13–20.
35. Luther J, Glesby MJ. Dermatologic adverse effects of antiretroviral therapy: recognition and management. Am J Clin Dermatol 2007;8(4):221–33.
36. World Health Organization. WHO case definitions of HIV for surveillance and revised clinical staging and immunological classification of HIV related disease in adult and children. World Health Organization. Geneva (Switzerland): WHO Press; 2007. Available at: http://www.who.int/hiv/pub/guidelines/HIVstaging150307.pdf.
37. Evron S, Glezerman M, Harow E, et al. Human immunodeficiency virus: anesthetic and obstetric considerations. Anesth Analg 2004;98:503–11.
38. Panlilio AL, Cardo DM, Grohskoph LA, et al. Updated U.S. Public Health Service guidelines for the management of occupational exposures to HIV and recommendations for postexposure prophylaxis. MMWR Recomm Rep 2005;54:1–17.
39. American Cancer Society. Cancer facts & figures 2013. Atlanta (GA): American Cancer Society; 2013.
40. Huettemann E, Sakka SG. Anaesthesia and anti cancer chemotherapeutic drugs. Curr Opin Anaesthesiol 2005;18:307–14.
41. Arain MR, Buggy DJ. Anaesthesia for cancer patients. Curr Opin Anaesthesiol 2007;20:247–53.
42. Cormier JN, Pollock RE. Principles of surgical cancer care. In: Shaw A, Reidel B, Burton A, editors. Acute care of the cancer patient. London: Taylor and Francis Group; 2005. p. 17–30.
43. Thorosian MH. Nutrition and cancer. In: Bland KI, Daly JM, Karakousis CP, editors. Surgical oncology: contemporary principles and practice. New York: McGraw-Hill; 2001. p. 472–9.
44. Weesner KM, Bledsoe M, Chauvenet A, et al. Exercise echocardiography in the detection of anthracycline cardiotoxicity. Cancer 1991;68(2):435–8.
45. Thorne AC, Orazem JP, Shah NK, et al. Isoflurane versus fentanyl: hemodynamic effects in cancer patients treated with anthracycline. J Cardiothorac Vasc Anesth 1993;7(3):307–11.
46. Burrows FA, Hickey PR, Colan S. Peroperative complications in patients with anthracycline chemotherapeutic agents. Can Anaesth Soc J 1985;32(2):149–57.
47. Gorton H, Wilson R, Robinson A, et al. Survivors of childhood cancers: implications for obstetric anaesthesia. Br J Anaesth 2000;85(6):911–3.
48. Zaniboni A, Prabhu S, Audisio RA. Chemotherapy and anaesthetic drugs: too little is known. Lancet Oncol 2005;6(3):176–81.
49. Pai VB, Nahata MC. Cardiotoxicity of chemotherapeutic agents: incidence, treatment, and prevention. Drug Saf 2000;22:263–302.
50. Berliner S, Rahima M, Sidi Y, et al. Acute coronary events following cisplatin-based chemotherapy. Cancer Invest 1990;8(6):583–6.
51. Meinardi MT, Gietema JA, van der Graaf WT, et al. Cardiovascular morbidity in long-term survivors of metastatic testicular cancer. J Clin Oncol 2000;18(8): 1725–32.
52. Alter P, Herzum M, Soufi M, et al. Cardiotoxicity of 5-fluorouracil. Cardiovasc Hematol Agents Med Chem 2006;4(1):1–5.
53. Perik PJ, de Korte MA, van Veldhuisen DJ, et al. Cardiotoxicity associated with the use of trastuzumab in breast cancer patients. Expert Rev Anticancer Ther 2007;7(12):1763–71.

54. Telli ML, Hunt SA, Carlson RW, et al. Trastuzumab-related cardiotoxicity: calling into question the concept of reversibility. J Clin Oncol 2007;25(23):3525–33.

55. Mitchell MS. Combinations of anticancer drugs and immunotherapy. Cancer Immunol Immunother 2003;52(11):686–92.

56. Owczuk R, Wujtewicz MA, Sawika W, et al. Is prolongation of the QTc interval during isoflurane anesthesia more prominent in women pretreated with anthracyclines for breast cancer? Br J Anaesth 2004;92(5):658–61.

57. Carver JR, Shapiro CL, Ng A, et al. American Society of Clinical Oncology clinical evidence review on the ongoing care of adult cancer survivors: cardiac and pulmonary late effects [see comment]. J Clin Oncol 2007;25(25):3991–4008.

58. Jules-Elysee K, White DA. Bleomycin-induced pulmonary toxicity. Clin Chest Med 1990;11:1–20.

59. Donat SM, Levy DA. Bleomycin associated pulmonary toxicity: is perioperative oxygen restriction necessary? J Urol 1998;160:1347–52.

60. Hopf HW, Rollins MD. Wounds: an overview of the role of oxygen. Antioxid Redox Signal 2007;9(8):1183–92.

61. Ghafoori P, Marks LB, Vujaskovic Z, et al. Radiation-induced lung injury. Assessment, management, and prevention. Oncology (Williston Park) 2008;22(1): 37–47 [discussion: 52–3].

62. Madani I, De Ruyck K, Goeminne H, et al. Predicting risk of radiation-induced lung injury. J Thorac Oncol 2007;2(9):864–74.

63. Floyd J, Mirza I, Sachs B, et al. Hepatotoxicity of chemotherapy. Semin Oncol 2006;33(1):50–67.

64. King PD, Perry MC. Hepatotoxicity of chemotherapy. Oncologist 2001;6(2): 162–76.

65. Harris CM, Blanchart RH. Bilateral recurrent laryngeal nerve palsy resulting from treatment with vincristine. J Oral Maxillofac Surg 2006;64(4):738–9.

66. Praveen CV, DeLord CF. Bilateral vocal fold paralysis following treatment with vincristine. J Laryngol Otol 2006;120(5):423.

67. Hebl JR, Horlocker TT, Pritchard DJ. Diffuse brachial plexopathy after interscalene blockade in a patient receiving cisplatin chemotherapy: the pharmacologic double crush syndrome. Anesth Analg 2001;92(1):249–51.

68. Organ Procurement and Transplantation Network (OPTN), Scientific Registry of Transplant Recipients (SRTR). OPTN/SRTR 2011 annual data report. Rockville (MD): Department of Health and Human Services, Health Resources and Services Administration, Healthcare Systems Bureau, Division of Transplantation; 2012.

69. 2009 Annual Report of the US Organ Procurement and Transplantation Network and the Scientific Registry of Transplant Recipients: Transplant Data 1999-2008. Rockville (MD): US Department of Health and Human Services, Health Resources and Services Administration, Healthcare Systems Bureau, Division of Transplantation.

70. Crapo JD, Harmsen AG, Sherman MP, et al. Pulmonary immunobiology and inflammation in pulmonary diseases. Am J Respir Crit Care Med 2000;162: 1983–6.

71. de Marie S. Diseases and drug-related interventions affecting host defense. Eur J Clin Microbiol Infect Dis 1993;12(Suppl 1):36–41.

72. Hauser AB, Stinghen AE, Kato S, et al. Characteristics and causes of immune dysfunction related to uremia and dialysis. Perit Dial Int 2008;28:S183–7.

73. Kato S, Chmielewski M, Honda H, et al. Aspects of immune dysfunction in end-stage renal disease. Clin J Am Soc Nephrol 2008;3:1526–33.

74. Mukherjee S, Mukherjee U. A comprehensive review of immunosuppression used for liver transplantation. J Transplant 2009.
75. Hammel L, Sebranek J, Hevesi Z. The anesthetic management of adult patients with organ transplants undergoing nontransplant surgery. Adv Anesth 2010;28: 211–44.
76. Kallwitz ER. Metabolic syndrome after liver transplantation: preventable illness or common consequence? World J Gastroenterol 2012;18(28):3627–34.
77. Neskovic V. Preoperative assessment of the immunocompromised patient. Acta Chir Iugosl 2011;58(2):185–92.
78. Whiting J. Perioperative concerns for transplant recipients undergoing non-transplant surgery. Surg Clin North Am 2006;86:1185–94.
79. Brown CJ, Buie WD. Perioperative stress dose steroids: do they make a difference? J Am Coll Surg 2001;193(6):678–86.
80. Kostopanagiotou G, Sidiropoulou T, Pyrsopoulos N, et al. Anesthetic and perioperative management of intestinal and multivisceral allograft recipient in nontransplant surgery. Transpl Int 2008;21:415–27.
81. Kostopanagiotou G, Smyrniotis V, Arkadopoulos N, et al. Anesthetic and perioperative management of adult transplant recipients in nontransplant surgery. Anesth Analg 1999;89:613–22.

Patients with Disorders of Thrombosis and Hemostasis

Andrea Orfanakis, MD[a],*, Thomas DeLoughery, MD[b]

KEYWORDS

- Coagulation • Thrombosis • Hemostasis • Perioperative management

KEY POINTS

- A thorough bleeding history of all patients is recommended during the preoperative interview, which may elucidate a previously unknown disorder of the hematologic system. The interview should investigate occurrences of skin and mucosal bleeding, bleeding following minor trauma or injury, bleeding with prior surgical procedures, excessive bleeding in menses and labor, bleeding at birth, and any history of prior transfusion.
- The most common disorders of hemostasis include the hemophilias (A and B) and von Willebrand disease. The risks of perioperative bleeding in this group can be minimized by careful planning and coordination. The mainstay of treatment is factor replacement for each disorder's respective deficiency. It is important to coordinate these efforts with Hematology or pharmacy services to ensure adequate factor is available at the time of surgery.
- The disorders of thrombosis are many and preoperative planning is important to minimize the risk of venous or arterial thrombotic event. Patients may often present on oral antithrombotic therapy and the preoperative physician will need to manage these agents with either cessation or continuation and possible bridging therapy. This article offers a guide to the management of anticoagulants in the perioperative setting.

INTRODUCTION

Surgery, by definition, is a challenge to the hemostatic system. In addition, a surgical procedure may provoke inappropriate venous or arterial thrombosis, such as is suggested historically by Virchow's triad (**Table 1**). For these reasons, proper functioning of the hematologic system is integral in a successful and safe perioperative period. Patients with a disorder of either coagulation or hemostasis, therefore, present an exciting challenge to the preoperative physician. Diagnosis of a hematologic disorder may be more or less occult. A proper bleeding and clotting history can serve to elucidate such a disorder and is therefore paramount to the preoperative workup. For those

[a] Department of Anesthesiology and Perioperative Medicine, Oregon Health and Science University, Portland, OR, USA; [b] Division of Hematology/Oncology, Department of Medicine, Oregon Health and Science University, Portland, OR, USA
* Corresponding author.
E-mail address: orfanaka@ohsu.edu

Med Clin N Am 97 (2013) 1161–1180
http://dx.doi.org/10.1016/j.mcna.2013.07.004
0025-7125/13/$ – see front matter © 2013 Elsevier Inc. All rights reserved.

Table 1 Obtaining a bleeding history	
Mucosal bleeding	Epistaxis, gingival bleeding with oral care Purpura, hematoma, or petechiae and the location and incidence of events
Bleeding in infancy or birth	Inappropriate bleeding at birth from the scalp or following heel stick, circumcision, or immunization
Bleeding associated with trauma or surgery	Bleeding following minor surgery particularly if a blood transfusion was required Response to minor injury, such as with shaving, minor joint or muscle sprain including duration of active bleeding
Menses and childbirth in the woman	Menorrhagia including number of tampons or pads used per day and duration of menses Bleeding after childbirth and whether a blood transfusion was necessary
Medications of interest	Prior transfusion history Nonsteroidal anti-inflammatory medications Oral anticoagulants Over-the-counter medications, supplements, and herbal remedies

patients with a previously diagnosed disorder of the hematologic system, appropriate laboratory investigation and a concise therapeutic plan for the day of surgery can help to minimize risks in the perioperative period.

SCREENING FOR BLEEDING DISORDERS

The bleeding history is the first step in identifying the patient at increased risk for abnormal clotting.[1] Many patients will present preoperatively to their physician consultant with no prior surgical or hematologic history and this is particularly true in the pediatric population. In many cases, the patient's hemostatic system has previously been challenged through a surgical procedure but this is not investigation enough to indicate a normal hemostatic system, if no complications occurred.[2] In all cases the bleeding history is the critical first step in evaluation.

A high yield set of questions in this regard should include coverage of several important topics, namely, skin and mucosal bleeding, bleeding following trauma or surgery, menorrhagia and labor in the woman, bleeding with dental work, medications of interest, bleeding during birth or childhood, and finally, any diagnosed hematologic disorder.[3]

A thorough history can be helpful in eliciting information suggestive of a bleeding diathesis. The physician should inquire about a history of epistaxis and the frequency of events including any need for cauterization of a nasal vessel or the need for transfusion. Oral bleeding can also be clinically important such as that which occurs with tooth brushing or flossing. Inquire about skin findings such as hematoma and petechiae and their size and location. The patient should be asked if hematomas are located in expected areas such as lower extremities or unexpected locations such as the torso and upper arms. The amount of between bleeding after trauma or minor injury should be ascertained and whether the patient ever experiences spontaneous bleeding, the duration of bleeding episodes, and whether bleeding responds to simple measures, such as holding pressure, with cessation or clot formation. Minor dermatologic or dental procedures, such as biopsy or tooth extractions, are a lesser challenge to the hemostatic system so it is important to determine if the patient has bled abnormally after these interventions. If the patient has previously undergone surgery, increased bleeding complications and whether the patient received a transfusion should be inquired about. It is important to also understand the type of surgery during which this occurred. If the patient is female, information should be gathered regarding extent of bleeding during menses and labor, if applicable. The patient or family members may be aware of the birth history. If so, scalp bleeding, bleeding following circumcision, bleeding following heel stick, and subcutaneous bleeding or hematoma in an extremity following immunization should be inquired about.[4] A family history of bleeding should be obtained in a similar fashion. Finally, a thorough medication list, including prescribed pharmaceuticals, "over-the-counter" agents, herbal remedies, and supplements, should be gathered. Non-steroidal anti-inflammatory medications, antiplatelet agents, rheumatologic medications, and any anticoagulant use should be specifically asked about.

A physical examination may deliver further information. Special attention should be paid to the mucous membranes (of the eyes, nose, and mouth), the skin (paying attention to pressure points of the back, hips, and elbows), any current petechiae or hematomas, and swelling of joints and muscles that might indicate prior bleeding. If the patient is hospitalized, intravenous sites, chest tube and drain insertion sites, and bandages should also be examined for excessive bleeding.[3] The medical care team should be asked about increased bleeding during interventions. In the case of a patient with a known hematologic disorder, it is appropriate to receive consultation from the patient's hematologist before surgery. Common hematologic disorders and their perioperative management are also discussed later in this article.

If the history is positive for excess bleeding or clinical suspicion is high, laboratory testing is warranted. If the history is entirely negative and the surgical procedure is low or moderate risk for bleeding, it is prudent not to pursue further testing. Routine preoperative testing without a clinical suspicion (positive bleeding history or known anticoagulant use) has not demonstrated an ability to predict blood loss at the time of surgery nor identify occult disease.[1,5] In the case of a high-risk procedure, additional laboratory testing is appropriate regardless of the results of the bleeding history.

PREOPERATIVE COAGULATION LABORATORY TESTING
Indication

If the history is positive for excess bleeding or clinical suspicion is high, laboratory testing is warranted. If the history is entirely negative and the surgical procedure has low or moderate risk for bleeding, it is reasonable not to pursue further testing. Routine preoperative testing without a clinical suspicion (positive bleeding history or known anticoagulant use) has not been shown to predict blood loss at the time of surgery nor identify occult disease.[1] In the case of a high-risk procedure, additional laboratory testing is appropriate regardless of the results of the bleeding history.

Recommended Laboratory Testing

Before ordering coagulation laboratory tests, it is important to understand each test's diagnostic scope and limitations. Discussed are the most common initial coagulation laboratory tests in use today (**Table 2**).

Laboratory Analysis of Secondary Hemostasis

The prothrombin time (PT) is an in vitro analysis of the extrinsic and final common pathways. This test is best for identifying factor VII deficiency and also used to guide

Table 2
Laboratory tests of coagulation

Laboratory Test	Indication	Abnormal in Disease States
Prothrombin time (PT)	Test of the extrinsic and final common pathways	Factor VII deficiency with high sensitivity Factor II, V, or X deficiency with lesser sensitivity Accidental heparin overdose Synthetic liver disease Vitamin K deficiency Poor nutritional state Consumptive coagulopathy Disseminated intravascular coagulation Fibrinogen deficiency
Activated partial thromboplastin (aPTT)	Test of the intrinsic and final common pathways	Factor XII, XI, IX, VIII, or fibrinogen deficiency Factor II, V, or X deficiency with lesser sensitivity Presence of coagulation factor inhibitor Fibrinogen deficiency Lupus anticoagulant
Platelet count	Circulating platelet number	Thrombocytopenia Idiopathic thrombocytopenic purpura Myeloproliferative disorders Splenic sequestration Liver disease Bernard-Soulier syndrome Pseudothrombocytopenia
Platelet function analysis	Assessment of primary hemostasis and platelet function	von Willebrand disease Presence of IIb/IIIa inhibitor Glanzmann thrombasthenia

the dosing of vitamin K antagonists toward the goal of anticoagulation. The PT test involves adding calcium and thromboplastin (an activator of the extrinsic pathway) to patient plasma and measuring the time in seconds to clot formation. In the past, interlaboratory variation had been a problem, prompting the development of the international normalized ratio (INR). The thromboplastin reagents produced by various manufacturers each have their own intrinsic sensitivity to clotting factors. Each manufacturer supplies the laboratory with a sensitivity index, which is calculated based on the exposure of healthy subjects to the specific manufacturer's reagent and the calculated mean of the resultant PTs. The INR is designed for interlaboratory reagent system comparison of warfarin-treated patients as opposed to assessment of other pathophysiologic states or to predict surgical bleeding.[4,6]

The PT reagents are most sensitive to deficiencies in factor VII and less so to deficiencies of factors in the final common pathway (II, V, X, and fibrinogen). In fact, significant fibrinogen deficiency (<80 mg/dL) needs to be present before the PT is prolonged. If hypofibrinogenemia is a concern for the clinician, the fibrinogen level should be ordered separately.

Limitations of the PT include false positive results secondary to a variety of factors. Each laboratory tube is designed for a specific volume of patient blood. Too much or too little volume will result in an erroneous PT because the tube citrate-to-plasma calcium ratio must be exact. For example, patient polycythemia, with a hematocrit greater than 55%, will lead to decreased plasma volumes added to the tube and disruption of the intended citrate-to-plasma calcium ratio, producing an artificially prolonged PT. Excess administered unfractionated heparin or low-molecular-weight heparin (LMWH) can prolong the PT by antithrombin-mediated inhibition of factor II in the common pathway. Because heparin use is ubiquitous in the hospital setting, a prolonged PT, which does not match a clinical scenario, should alert the physician to possible heparin contamination.

Activated partial thromboplastin time (aPTT) is an in vitro test of the intrinsic and final common pathways. Intrinsic pathway factors include XII, XI, IX, VIII, and also prekallikrein and high-molecular-weight kininogen, while common pathway factors include II, V, X, and fibrinogen. The aPTT is indicated for analysis of factor function and monitoring of anticoagulation therapy. The aPTT is a measure of time to clot following exposure of patient plasma to a phospholipid. The term partial thromboplastin specifically refers to the absence of tissue factor in this assay, therefore isolating the analysis of the intrinsic pathway.

Limitations of the aPTT overlap somewhat with the PT. Again, the citrate-to-patient plasma ratio is important to maintain with correct blood volume addition to laboratory tubes. The aPTT is highly affected by the presence of heparin (hence its use to monitor anticoagulation with heparin); therefore, accidental contamination with this medication could provide false positive results. Antiphospholipid antibodies, such as lupus anticoagulant, will prolong the aPTT in the laboratory while leading to inappropriate thrombosis in vivo. The clinician should consider this diagnosis when the aPTT is prolonged without a clinically relevant explanation.[4,6]

Interpretation of test results

Isolated prolonged PT (with normal aPTT) Prolongation of the PT suggests a defect of the extrinsic pathway. A congenital deficiency of factor VII is the most common, whereas isolated congenital deficiencies of factor V or X are very rare and, if severe, will also elevate the aPTT. Factor VII, with its short circulating half-life, can be an early marker of a general coagulopathy such as in the surgical setting associated with factor consumption or the medical setting of disseminated intravascular coagulation. Chronic stable systemic disease state may also lead to prolonged PT. Because all coagulation factors except factor VIII are synthesized in the liver, liver disease will prolong PT. Poor nutritional state leading to vitamin K deficiency will similarly prolong PT because of poor production of vitamin K–dependent factors II, VII, IX, and X. Vitamin K antagonists or deficiency in a patient with poor oral intake will prolong the PT.[7]

Isolated prolonged aPTT (with normal PT) Prolongation of the aPTT suggests a defect of the intrinsic or final common pathway. When the PT is normal, this suggests the defect is isolated to the intrinsic pathway alone. Prolongation may be due to decreased production or activity of one or more factors either congenitally or acquired. A factor deficiency may be of varying clinical significance. For instance, deficiencies of factors VIII, IX, or XI can produce significant hemorrhage spontaneously and following trauma, whereas factor XII, high-molecular-weight kininogen, and prekallikrein deficiencies are not clinically significant risks for bleeding. Acquired deficiencies of factors typically involve a systemic disease state or the presence of a factor inhibitor. Mixing studies will help to differentiate between them. Lupus anticoagulant can also prolong the aPTT in vitro while producing thrombosis in vivo.

If an isolated aPTT is prolonged, the next step is to perform a mixing study to distinguish between factor deficiency and the presence of factor inhibitor. If the mixing study is suggestive of a factor deficiency, then the clinically significant factors VIII, IX, and XI should be next measured.[7]

Prolonged PT and aPTT

Prolongation of both tests suggests a defect of both the extrinsic and the intrinsic pathways or the final common pathway or all 3 pathways. This defect is seen in generalized coagulopathy and the systemic disease state. Examples of these states may include consumptive coagulopathy, certain lymphoproliferative disorders that produce inhibitor-like reactions, or the ingestion of large doses of vitamin K antagonists or direct thrombin inhibitors. As both assays are dependent on adequate function of the final common pathway, a defect in a common pathway factor (II, V, X, fibrinogen) could also create this scenario. Causes attributable to fibrinogen are either a defect in quantity (hypofibrinogenemia) or function (dysfibrinogenemia) and can be analyzed further by fibrinogen-specific assays (see **Table 2**).[7]

Analysis of Primary Hemostasis

The platelet count as part of the complete blood count is a common preoperative test. Artifactual error is rare and occurs secondary to a size discrepancy or platelet activation during collection. Small nonplatelet particles may be counted as platelets, erroneously elevating the final count, whereas large platelets may be missed by the analyzer, producing an erroneously low count, which may occur in myeloproliferative disorders, Bernard-Soulier syndrome, a variety of congenital thrombocytopenias, or idiopathic thrombocytopenic purpura. Platelets may become activated during collection leading to clumping and therefore may be missed on final count; this may be termed pseudo-thrombocytopenia and is most often detected by the clinical laboratory.[8]

Bleeding time (BT) has fallen out of favor in recent years. The interlaboratory and reader variability are very high, whereas reproducibility is very low. It is now considered a poor predictor of increased surgical bleeding and may lead clinicians away from accurate diagnosis. BT is also a poor predictor of platelet function in the setting of aspirin or nonsteroidal anti-inflammatory medication use. The detailed bleeding history is a better predictor of impaired hemostasis when compared to the BT.

Platelet function analysis (PFA) is a test of whole blood platelet function. One such commercially available option is the Innovance PFA-200 (Siemens AG, Munich, Germany).[9] The testing method involves exposure of patient whole blood to 2 mediums or membranes, a collagen/adenosine diphosphate sample and a collagen/epinephrine sample, resulting in patient-specific platelet attachment, aggregation, and activation; the analysis will continue until a stable platelet plug is formed on the cartridge. The test can therefore assay for disorders of platelet adherence and aggregation. PFA can assess for von Willebrand disease (VWD), congenital platelet dysfunction, aspirin, or IIb/IIIa inhibitor exposure. The role of PFA in the evaluation of congenital platelet function defects is less well studied but will be abnormal with very impaired platelet function (see **Table 2**).

Specimen handling specific to this assay is important. Following collection, the specimen should be delivered promptly to the laboratory but not in a pneumatic tube system. Also, the specimen should not be centrifuged as is common with many coagulation tubes.

Platelet aggregation studies may be more sensitive but less specific for mild or rare disease states. These tests are best used and analyzed by a hematology consultant and therefore will not be discussed further.

DISORDERS OF HEMOSTASIS

The patient with a diagnosis of hypocoagulability will often present with a positive bleeding history but a subset of patients may appear asymptomatic if they are only heterozygous carriers of disease or have not had their hemostatic system sufficiently challenged previously. Ideally the bleeding history will tease out this subset of patients and appropriate laboratory testing will confirm the diagnosis. Preparing a patient with a known disorder of hemostasis to the hemostatic challenge of surgery is best done with a careful investigation of the extent of their disease, involvement of the patient's hematologist if possible, and coordination with the anesthesia provider, clinical pharmacist, and surgeon before the date of surgery. Discussed here are the most common disorders of hemostasis and their preoperative management.

Hemophilia A

Hemophilia A is an X-linked recessive disorder with an incidence of 1 in 5000 male births. Female carriers may show clinically significant effects in the cases of chromosome lionization or Turner syndrome. Simple female carriers may also exhibit subclinical symptoms of the disease. Hemophilia A results in a variable decrease, in some cases absence, of circulating factor VIII activity leading to a poor coagulation state. Factor VIII is a plasma glycoprotein synthesized largely in endothelial cells of the liver and also in a lesser degree by systemic endothelial cells. Factor VIII demonstrates a short circulating half-life in the absence of von Willebrand factor (VWF). VWF forms a covalent linkage with factor VIII, which prolongs its half-life by preventing enzymatic degradation. When coagulation is activated, thrombin cleaves the light chain of factor VIII, releasing activated factor VIII into circulation. Activated factor VIII then serves as a cofactor on phospholipid surfaces to activate factors V, X, and thrombin. A patient with hemophilia A would therefore lack the ability to generate adequate amounts of thrombin.[10]

Clinically, patients with hemophilia A exhibit delayed bleeding, either spontaneously or in response to trauma, and also hemorrhage into unexpected tissues such as muscle and joints. The severity of bleeding depends on the circulating factor activity. Patients are classified as having mild, moderate, or severe disease based on factor VIII activity levels of 5% to 40%, 1% to 5%, or less than 1%, respectively. A patient with mild or moderate disease will bleed inappropriately following trauma or intervention, whereas a patient with severe disease will bleed spontaneously.[10]

Diagnosis of Hemophilia A is made by assaying factor VIII activity. One clue is that most patients will demonstrate prolonged partial thromboplastin time. In most cases, a family history will be positive but in nearly 30% of new diagnoses, no family history was noted, possibly due to frequent spontaneous mutations of the gene for factor VIII. If a patient presents preoperatively with a diagnosis of Hemophilia A, the recommendation is for laboratory testing of factor VIII activity in addition to testing for the presence or absence of factor inhibitor. Management of Hemophilia A is based on the clinical situation. In general, patients and family members should be educated and counseled on safe management of the disease state, avoiding injury when possible, and presenting to medical professionals promptly when a hemorrhage does occur. Perioperatively, carriers of clinically mild disease should avoid being treated with blood products when applicable, using desmopressin (DDAVP), which leads to release of factor VIII and VWF from storage sites, and antifibrinolytics, such as tranexamic or aminocaproic acid, when appropriate such as in oral surgery. Management of Hemophilia A in the setting of hemorrhage or prophylaxis is centered on factor replacement therapy. Factor VIII concentrates are either plasma-derived highly purified proteins or recombinant product. Dosing factor replacement is based on the half-life of the product, size of the patient, and goal clotting factor activity. Not all perioperative states require equal clotting factor activity. Minor surgery may be managed with factor activity corrected to 70%, whereas major surgery or surgery in a high-risk location probably warrants correction of activity to 100% and maintenance of 70% activity for several days to a week following the operation. Of course, surgical methods to minimize and manage bleeding are recommended, such as electrocautery and compression dressings. If a patient presents with a diagnosis of Hemophilia, the preoperative physician is encouraged to contact their hospital pharmacy to ensure that factor replacement concentrates are made available at the time of surgery. In addition, it is recommended to consult a hematologist to engage in the planning of administration of these agents perioperatively (**Table 3**).[10]

A complication of Hemophilia A in 30% of patients is the development of inhibitor antibody to factor replacement proteins. Inhibitor antibodies can be strong deactivators of both endogenous and exogenous factor VIII. Inhibitor antibody titers are measured according to the Bethesda assay and expressed in Bethesda units (BU). Greater than 5 BU is considered clinically severe inhibitor titer and can impact patient therapy substantially. Hemorrhage in the setting of high antibody titer presence requires alternative therapies. Factor eight inhibitor bypass activity (Baxter Healthcare Corporation, Deerfield, IL, USA) is a plasma-derived prothrombin complex concentrate designed for use specifically in this clinical application as well as recombinant activated factor VII. Both products carry a risk of inappropriate thrombosis including myocardial infarction and should be reserved for patients with clinically significant factor inhibitor antibody titers. In some cases desensitization therapy with exposure to chronic high doses of factor VIII, in the nonhemorrhagic state, has been successful in eradicating the antibody. If the presence of factor inhibitor is noted on the preoperative laboratory assessment of a patient with Hemophilia A, the recommendation is again that the preoperative physician obtain a hematology consult and coordinate with the hospital pharmacy to ensure that appropriate factor replacement agents are made available at the time of surgery.[10]

Hemophilia B

Hemophilia B is an X-linked recessive congenital deficiency of factor IX. Factor IX is a vitamin K–dependent protein produced by the hepatocytes of the liver. It is a serine protease, which is released into circulation in its inactive form. Tissue factor and factor VII activate factor IX, which in turn activates factor VIII. Together activated factors IX and VIII serve as cofactors on the phospholipid surface, ultimately activating

Table 3 Perioperative management of hemophilia		
Disease Type	**Preoperative Screening**	**Therapy**
Hemophilia A	Clinical history Factor VIII level and activity Factor VIII inhibitor level in Bethesda units	Recombinant factor VIII or plasma-derived factor VIII concentrate
Hemophilia A with inhibitor	Bleeding and transfusion history Factor VIII inhibitor level in Bethesda units	Recombinant factor VIIa Factor eight inhibitor bypass activity (Baxter)
Hemophilia B	Clinical history Factor IX level and activity Factor IX inhibitor level in Bethesda units	Recombinant factor IX or plasma-derived factor IX concentrate
Hemophilia B with inhibitor	Bleeding and transfusion history Factor IX inhibitor level in Bethesda units	Recombinant factor VIIa

thrombin. Patients with Hemophilia B are unable to generate adequate amounts of thrombin.[10]

The incidence of Hemophilia B is 1 in 25,000 male births. Again, in the same manner as described with Hemophilia A, female births may be clinically affected. Severity of disease is classified based on factor activity level to be mild, moderate, or severe correlating with 5% to 40% activity, 1% to 5% activity, or less than 1% activity, respectively. Patients may present with spontaneous bleeding in the case of severe disease or bleeding following trauma in the lesser disease states. Bleeding at the time of birth such as intracranially or from heel sticks or immunization sites is a common presentation. Older individuals will experience excessive bruising, joint, and mouth bleeds and may bleed excessively if hemostatically challenged with a surgery or intervention. Female carriers may present with menorrhagia and also surgical or trauma-related bleeding excesses.[10]

If a patient presents with a diagnosis of Hemophilia, the preoperative physician is encouraged to contact their hospital pharmacy to ensure that factor replacement concentrates are made available at the time of surgery. In addition, it is recommended to consult a hematologist to engage in the planning of administration of these agents perioperatively.

Management of Hemophilia B is similar to Hemophilia A. The mainstay of therapy is factor replacement. Factor IX is given either in a prophylactic setting to prevent future bleeding or as a demand therapy in response to hemorrhage. Hemorrhage should be treated promptly and should not be delayed by imaging or laboratory studies, to prevent long-term sequelae such as degenerative joint disease in the setting of hemarthrosis. Factor replacement therapy is from either plasma-derived concentrates or recombinant factor. Minor surgery may be managed with factor activity corrected to 70%, whereas major surgery or surgery in a high-risk location probably warrants correction of activity to 100% and maintenance of 70% activity for several days to a week following the operation. Surgical methods to minimize and manage bleeding are recommended, such as electrocautery and compression dressings (see **Table 3**).[10]

Development of inhibitory antibodies in Hemophilia B is rare compared with Hemophilia A and is approximately 3% in hemophilia B versus nearly 30% in Hemophilia A. Anaphylactoid reactions to exogenous factor IX are more common and certainly concerning. There is an association between anaphylactoid reaction and development of high antibody inhibitor titers. Inhibitor antibody titers are measured according to the Bethesda assay and expressed in Bethesda units. Greater than 5 BU is considered a clinically alarming inhibitor titer and can impact patient therapy substantially. Hemorrhage in the setting of high antibody titer presence requires alternative therapies. Activated recombinant factor VII is the therapy of choice in this clinical setting. If the presence of factor inhibitor is noted on the preoperative laboratory assessment of a patient with Hemophilia B, the recommendation is again that the preoperative physician obtain a hematology consult and coordinate with the hospital pharmacy to ensure that appropriate factor replacement agents are made available at the time of surgery.[10]

VWD

VWD is the most common inherited bleeding disorder. The incidence is approximately 0.1% to 1%. Type 1 and 2 VWD are autosomal-dominant in inheritance, whereas type 3 is recessive. Patients may also develop an acquired deficiency in the setting of systemic disease such as myeloproliferative disorders. Inherited VWD disproportionately presents clinically in women of child-bearing age due to the hemostatic challenges of menstruation and child birth but is genetically present in men and women equally. The VWF is a large protein stored and secreted from both megakaryocytes and endothelial cells. VWF functions as a carrier protein for factor VIII and aids in the formation of a link between the platelet surface glycoprotein Ib and collagen of the endothelial matrix effectively bridging platelet to blood vessel wall. VWD classification divides patients into 3 major groups: partial quantitative deficiency (type 1), qualitative deficiency (type 2), and total deficiency (type 3). VWD type 2 is further classified into 4 variants (2A, 2B, 2M, 2N).[11,12]

Type 1 VWD accounts for the largest percentage of persons affected, approximately 75% of cases. Type 1 is a quantitative defect with VWF binding normally but in low quantity, manifesting clinically as low antigen levels and activity. In addition, factor VIII levels may be low due to the role of VWF and carrier protein for factor VIII.[12]

Type 2A VWD is a qualitative variant in which VWF-platelet adhesion is decreased. The genetic mutation responsible also effects assembly and secretion of the large subunits of the VWF protein sometimes placing the subunits at increased susceptibility to proteolysis. Type 2B VWD is a qualitative defect, which leads to a pathologic increase in platelet-VWF binding. Patients may also present with a mild thrombocytopenia and the platelet count may decrease significantly in the setting of a hemostatic challenge or stress. Interestingly, this type of VWD will respond to the antibiotic ristocetin with increased platelet aggregation in vitro, which can be used as a diagnostic method. Type 2N VWD is defective in its factor VIII binding domain preventing stabilization of the complex and ultimately leading to low factor VIII activity. This variant is often misdiagnosed as Hemophilia A, but the clinical picture will fit more closely with VWD as well as its autosomal-dominant inheritance.[12]

Type 3 VWD is characterized by complete absence of VWF. Type 3 is inherited in an autosomal-recessive manner (either homozygous or compound heterozygous). In type 3 VWD factor VIII activity will also be very low.[12]

Acquired von Willebrand syndrome (AVWS) may present similarly to VWD in the current state, whereas the past personal and family histories are often negative for bleeding. AVWS may occur spontaneously or secondary to systemic disease. Associated diseases include monoclonal gammopathies, myeloproliferative disorders, valvular and congenital heart disease, autoimmune disorders, and hypothyroidism.[12]

Clinically the patient with VWD may present with a positive bleeding history often centered around mucocutaneous bleeding. Younger patients and those with no history of hemostatic challenge may not always present with remarkable symptom history. Despite this reality, the bleeding history remains a valuable tool in identifying patients with VWD.[12]

Often common coagulation laboratory tests may be normal. For instance, the aPTT will be prolonged only if factor VIII activity is less than 40%, easily preventing a large number of VWD patients from being diagnosed by this test. More specific screening for VWD includes VWF antigen, VWF ristocetin cofactor activity, factor VIII activity, and VWF multimers analysis. If a diagnosis of VWD is known or suspected, the preoperative physician should initiate an investigation to classify the type of VWD further using the laboratory tests outlined above. A hematology consult is also recommended to plan for therapy on the day of surgery.[12]

The diagnosis of VWD is considered certain when VWF is less than 30%. Those patients in the range of 30% to 50% are under suspicion of VWD but their diagnosis is not clear without a supporting clinical picture of bleeding. Patients with a positive bleeding history and a VWF level greater than 50% may still carry the disease and their laboratory levels may have been affected by one or more modulating factors. Factors that impact VWD testing include ABO blood type with lower levels seen in type O blood, and elevated levels seen with aging, presence of stress or acute disease, menses, pregnancy, and exercise.[12]

In the case of ABO blood type, type O blood is associated with lower levels of VWF compared with other groups. VWF is also an acute phase reactant and may elevate in response to stress. A patient with normally low VWF levels may present as "normal" if the laboratory sample is drawn during a period of stress such as in acute illness or psychologic stress of hospitalization or laboratory testing. Pregnancy, mid menstrual cycle, and exercise may also elevate VWF, producing a similar scenario. With all of these modulating factors present, correlation with symptoms of bleeding is important to make the diagnosis. The differential diagnosis of VWD should also entertain other disorders that affect primary hemostasis, mainly inherited platelet function disorders such as platelet-type VWD or Glanzmann thrombasthenia, and vascular bleeding disorders such as Ehlers Danlos or Marfan syndrome.[12]

Management of VWD is focused on 3 main principles: increase the release of endogenous stores of VWF, supplementation with plasma-derived concentrates of exogenous VWF, and employment of hemostatic agents that do not consume VWF. Unlike in hemophilia, VWD is rarely managed with prophylactic replacement therapy; rather demand therapy and preoperative optimization are the strategies of choice. Minor bleeding, such as oral bleeding or epistaxis, may be managed by using the first and third principles (**Table 4**).[11]

DDAVP is a synthetic derivative of vasopressin but lacks vasoconstrictive properties. DDAVP stimulates release of VWF from the Weibel-Palade bodies of endothelial cells. Due to the additional role played by VWF, a noticeable increase in factor VIII will also occur following DDAVP administration. DDAVP also enhances GP IIbIIIa interaction and platelet microparticle release. DDAVP is available in intravenous, oral, and intranasal forms. The intravenous route is preferred in surgical bleeding and hemorrhage. The recommended dose of DDAVP is 0.3 µg/kg diluted in 30 mL of saline and administered over 30 minutes. Peak effect will occur 30 to 90 minutes following infusion completion. DDAVP is appropriate for minor bleeding in type 1 and some type 2 VWD, although its use is contraindicated in type 2B with concern for both thrombocytopenia and thrombosis. Complications of DDAVP use, particularly repeated use, include blood pressure changes, tachyphylaxis, and rarely,

Table 4		
von Willebrand disease classification and therapy		
Disease Type	**Definition**	**Suggested Therapy**
Type 1	Low protein level	Desmopressin
Type 2	Abnormal protein structure	Desmopressin
Type 2A	Abnormal protein structure leading to lower levels of high weight multimers	Desmopressin (only effective in 10%), Factor VIII concentrate or recombinant Factor VIII
Type 2B	Abnormal protein structure with increased binding of Gp Ib leading to lower levels of high weight multimers	Factor VIII concentrate or recombinant Factor VIII
Type 2N	Lack of Factor VIII binding site leading to low Factor VIII levels	Desmopressin
Type 2M	Abnormal protein structure but normal multimer size	Factor VIII concentrate or recombinant Factor VIII
Type 3	No von Willebrand factor or factor VIII in circulation	Factor VIII concentrate or recombinant Factor VIII

hyponatremia or seizures. Because DDAVP does have antidiuretic properties, free water should be limited after giving this drug.[11,12]

Minor bleeding may also be managed with antifibrinolytic therapy, namely, aminocaproic acid or tranexamic acid. Antifibrinolytics inhibit the conversion of plasminogen to plasmin, inhibit fibrinolysis, and stabilize formed clot. This therapy is available orally or intravenously and in the case of tranexamic acid is available in topical form, which is particularly useful for management of oral bleeding in the form of a "swish and spit" solution, although not currently available in the United States.[12]

If a patient presents for preoperative evaluation with a diagnosis of VWD, it is recommended that the health care provider obtain a hematology consult and coordinate with the hospital pharmacy to ensure that the von Willebrand factor replacement therapies will be available on the day of surgery. Major bleeding or high-risk surgery with suspected high hemostatic challenge is best managed with replacement of VWF in addition to antifibrinolytic therapy. Replacement therapies include Humate-P (CSL Behring, King of Prussia, PA, USA) and Alphanate SD/HT (Grifols, Orange, CA, USA). These therapies are both plasma-derived concentrates from donor-pooled plasma. The goal of VWF replacement in hemorrhage or major surgery is to achieve VWF-ristocetin cofactor activity greater than 50% during the immediate perioperative period and continued for several days followed by maintenance of activity at a slightly lower level for days to weeks postoperatively, to support proper healing.[11]

Antifibrinolytic therapy may also be useful in the perioperative period. Aminocaproic acid may be initiated with a loading dose immediately preoperatively followed by continuous infusion or serial bolus dosing intraoperatively and postoperatively for several days. Tranexamic acid is also of utility and is given on a similar repeat basis, but without a loading dose.[12]

In the case of AVWS, the mainstay of treatment is to eliminate or modulate the underlying disorder. Treatment with VWF and factor VIII products may be used for acute bleeding. Immunomodulation with intravenous immune globulin or plasma exchange has been used to eliminate antibody mediated AVWS.[12]

DISORDERS OF THROMBOSIS

The preoperative clinician will encounter a variety of patients at increased risk of thrombosis. Perioperative assessment and management are patient-centered and driven by the pathophysiology of each specific thrombophilia. The most notable will include factor V Leiden (FVL) mutation, prothrombin gene mutation, protein C and S deficiency, antiphospholipid antibody syndrome (APS), antithrombin (AT) deficiency, and malignancy.

Classically, an increased risk of thrombosis has been viewed according to Virchow's triad. The supposition is that one or more of the following, blood stasis, vascular endothelial injury, or increased number or alternative function of coagulation factors, will drive the pathogenesis of thrombosis. In addition, the coagulation system can be viewed in a constant homeostatic balance of coagulation and anticoagulation, which is a reminder that coagulation is a natural and necessary process for organ maintenance, repair, and growth. When functioning properly, permanent coagulation will occur at the site of tissue injury and only when out of balance does venous or arterial thrombosis occur.

FVL

FVL is a genetic mutation (Arg506Gln) that leads to resistance on part of activated factor V to be inactivated by activated protein C. Proteins C and S function as negative feedback to limit the extent of coagulation. When factor V activity continues in an unlimited fashion, increased thrombin is generated and inappropriate thrombosis occurs. FVL leads to venous thrombosis with symptomatic venous thrombosis, including deep venous thrombosis and pulmonary embolus, the possible presenting diagnosis. FVL is the most common of the thrombophilias, occurring in approximately 5% of the North American population. FVL is an autosomal-inherited mutation affecting heterozygous individuals and homozygous individuals more significantly. When clinically suspected, FVL may be diagnosed through activated protein C sensitivity testing. Because additional mutations, other than FVL, may provide resistance to activated protein C, further molecular testing (polymerase chain reaction) is recommended to verify the diagnosis.[13]

Management is aimed at primary and secondary prevention. A patient with asymptomatic FVL does not require routine prophylaxis. Patients who develop venous thromboembolism (VTE) with FVL commonly are exposed to a secondary insult at the time of the event. Secondary insults may include obesity, oral contraceptives, hormone replacement, travel or prolonged immobilization, smoking, pregnancy, or surgery. Primary prevention should therefore be focused on education and counseling to modulate or eliminate these secondary insults, or to prepare appropriately as in the case of pregnancy and surgery.[13]

Treatment of a first time VTE is similar to any patient with VTE who does not have FVL. The recommendation is for anticoagulation with a vitamin K antagonist to a goal INR 2–3 for 3 months. Surprisingly, although FVL is a risk factor for thrombosis, it is not (even in the homozygous state) a major risk factor for recurrence.[13]

If a patient presents preoperatively with a diagnosis of FVL and without a thrombosis history, no changes need to be made preoperatively. Postoperatively it is important for the surgical team to be vigilant for signs and symptoms of thrombosis and to consider initiating prophylactic therapy in the form of unfractionated heparin, LMWH, or one of the new direct oral anticoagulants, as soon as possible. If a patient presents preoperatively with a diagnosis of VTE in the setting of FVL and on anticoagulation, the decision to withhold therapeutic anticoagulation must be based on the risk for operative bleeding. A low bleeding risk procedure may not require cessation of anticoagulation at all. A moderate-risk or high-risk surgery for bleeding warrants withholding anticoagulation. Management of common anticoagulants is discussed later in this article.[13]

Protein C or S Deficiency

Proteins C and S are vitamin K–dependent factors involved in the process of anticoagulation. They are activated by the presence of coagulation and serve as a negative feedback mechanism. The protein C/S complex inhibits factors Va and VIIIa. A deficiency of either or both protein C and S eliminates the negative feedback mechanism and leads to inappropriate thrombosis without clot degradation. Patients are at risk for VTE with protein C or S deficiency and profound thrombophilia with both C and S deficiency. Testing for deficiencies in protein C or S can be completed through assays of function or quantitative measure. For activity level, patient blood is exposed to either thrombin activating agents or snake venom and the aPTT is measured. Because the aPTT depends on many factor participants in the intrinsic pathway, false results may occur as a result of another factor deficiency, from exposure to exogenous anticoagulation such as heparin or warfarin, or any systemic state known to prolong the laboratory aPTT. Protein C or S deficiency can be of the qualitative or quantitative variety. Both activity and levels may be needed for accurate diagnosis.[14]

Management is aimed at primary or secondary prophylaxis. Primary prophylaxis when no surgery is planned should involve counseling about lifestyle modification to avoid secondary prothrombotic states such as seen in obesity, oral contraceptives use, hormone replacement therapy, travel or prolonged immobilization, smoking, pregnancy, or surgery. Patients with asymptomatic protein C or S deficiency do not automatically require chemoprophylaxis. However, patients presenting with a known diagnosis who are to be exposed to a secondary insult such as surgery should be considered high risk for VTE and chemoprophylaxis with unfractionated heparin, LMWH, or new direct oral anticoagulants, instituted as soon as possible postoperatively.

Recommendation for treatment of VTE in the setting of known protein C or S deficiency is oral anticoagulation, such as with warfarin, to a goal INR 2–3 for 3 months if the event was provoked such as in the case of surgery or prolonged immobilization. Patients with idiopathic thrombosis are candidates for longer duration of therapy, particularly after surgical interventions because they are at high risk of recurrence.[14]

If a patient presents preoperatively with a diagnosis of protein C or S deficiency and without a thrombosis event, no changes need to be made preoperatively. Postoperatively it is important for the surgical team to be vigilant for signs and symptoms of thrombosis and to consider initiating prophylactic therapy in the form of unfractionated heparin or LMWH as soon as possible. If a patient presents preoperatively with a diagnosis of VTE in the setting of protein C or S deficiency and on anticoagulation, the decision to withhold therapeutic anticoagulation must be based on the risk for operative bleeding. A low bleeding risk procedure may not require cessation of anticoagulation at all. A moderate-risk or high-risk surgery for bleeding warrants withholding anticoagulation. Suggestions for the management of patients on common anticoagulants are provided later in this article.[14,15]

APS

APS is an antibody-mediated thrombophilia. Patients with APS are at risk for a variety of morbid events including venous and arterial thrombosis presenting as stroke, myocardial infarct, miscarriage, placental insufficiency and preterm labor, valvular disease, renal infarct, thrombocytopenia, hemolytic anemia, and cognitive dysfunction. Antiphospholipid antibodies modulate activity of endothelial cells, monocytes, platelets, and the complement cascade, culminating in a prothrombotic state. These antibodies may also interfere with inactivation of procoagulation factors and therefore present a resistance to fibrinolysis. Thrombotic events typically occur in younger patients without additional risk factors. Clinically, patients will present with a major thrombotic event, such as stroke, before the age of 50. Of patients presenting with a cerebral infarct before the age of 50, approximately 1 in 5 will demonstrate antiphospholipid antibodies. Patients presenting with stroke but over the age of 70 have a much lower likelihood of antibody positivity. Women may present at a younger age with a history of multiple miscarriages. Of those with this history, about 10% are diagnosed with APS. Another group disproportionately affected is of those patients with systemic lupus erythematosus (SLE). About 40% of patients with SLE will have antiphospholipid antibodies but less than half of those will experience thrombotic events. If APS is diagnosed in a patient with SLE, the prognosis is poor.[16,17]

The thrombosis associated with APS differs from the congenital thrombophilias in that the event may occur in any tissue bed: vessel, skin, brain, muscle, kidney, heart valve, retina, placenta, and bone. The clinical examination may be particularly revealing in this population.[17]

Management is based on primary versus secondary prevention. For known carriers of APS who are asymptomatic, the recommendation is low-dose aspirin or no therapy if the patient has any contraindication to aspirin. Primary prophylaxis in those patients with a risk factor such as SLE with known antibody positivity is hydroxychloroquine plus low-dose aspirin. For obstetric APS patients, aspirin-only therapy is appropriate but in women with APS and miscarriages, the addition of heparin is indicated.[18]

Management of patients who have already experienced a thrombotic event is typically oral anticoagulation, such as with vitamin K antagonists, to a goal INR 2–3 indefinitely. In patients with breakthrough thrombosis, LMWH is used. The addition of an antiplatelet agent is recommended by some practitioners for those patients with a recent stroke. High-risk patients would also include those with known APS who are slated for surgery or are hospitalized or immobilized.[18]

A patient presenting preoperatively with a diagnosis of APS while on anticoagulation is a complicated medical case. As this patient is at high risk for both venous and arterial thrombosis, the additional stimulus of surgery and possible immobilization will typically place them in the extremely high-risk category for thrombosis. Most patients with APL will present preoperatively already on anticoagulation. The recommendation for surgery is to continue anticoagulation if the risk for operative bleeding is low. In the case of moderate-risk to high-risk surgery, a therapeutic bridge, with an agent such as LMWH, up until the point of surgery, is suggested if the patient is already on oral anticoagulation. Management of patients on oral anticoagulation including suggestions for bridging therapy is discussed at the end of this article.[18]

AT Deficiency

AT is a serine protease inhibitor, synthesized in the liver, that functions to inactivate factors IIa and Xa and less so factors IXa, XIa, and XIIa. The activity of AT is accelerated by the presence of heparin or heparin-like substances. Conversely, when AT is lowered in quantity or activity, a patient will confer a relative resistance to heparin. In addition, AT interacts with the endothelium to enhance release of interleukins producing an anti-inflammatory effect. AT deficiency is an inherited disorder with a population prevalence of 1 in 500 to 1 in 5000. Either the quantity is lowered (type 1) or the activity is reduced (type 2). Liver disease and nephrotic syndrome can also lead to an acquired AT deficiency. Patients with AT deficiency are at significant risk for VTE often in the deep veins. Additional venous systems are not immune to this disease state. Patients may present with VTE of the brain, mesentery, hepatic, renal, and retinal systems. A patient's typical first presentation will be between the third to fifth decades of life. Female carriers may also present with miscarriage in any term of pregnancy.[19]

Diagnosis of AT deficiency is through an assay of AT activity. It is ideal to wait 12 weeks from the time of a thrombotic event to pursue testing including an additional several days after completion of heparin therapy. Testing in the immediate period surrounding VTE can produce spurious results. If the repeated functional assays are positive, an antigen assay to determine AT level is pursued to classify the type of AT deficiency further.[19]

Management of AT deficiency is divided into primary prophylactic and secondary prophylactic therapy. An asymptomatic individual does not require oral anticoagulation prophylaxis, because the risk of bleeding will far outweigh the benefit of prevention of a potential perioperative thrombosis. In addition, most primary VTE events, in this population, were associated with a thrombophilic challenge or temporary risk factor. Surgery is the classic example. A patient with AT deficiency presenting preoperatively should receive VTE prophylaxis postoperatively and should receive AT concentrates before surgery and several days afterward. Secondary prophylactic therapy is similar to patients without an AT deficiency diagnosis and relies on the use of heparin, both unfractionated and low molecular weight, as a bridge to oral anticoagulation with warfarin to a goal INR 2–3. Patients with a single VTE event are at increased risk of a secondary event and anticoagulation has been shown to lower that risk. For this reason, long-term anticoagulation is recommended.[19]

If a patient presents preoperatively, while on therapeutic anticoagulation, the recommendation is to continue anticoagulation if the risk for operative bleeding is low. In the case of moderate-risk to high-risk surgery, a therapeutic bridge, with an agent such as LMWH, up until the point of surgery, is suggested if the patient is already on oral anticoagulation.[19] The management of patients on oral anticoagulation including appropriate bridging therapy is discussed at the end of this article.

Hypercoagulability in Malignancy

Cancer-associated VTE is a well-known risk of the systemic disease state. VTE may even be the initial presentation of an occult malignancy. Malignancy is of particular concern if the VTE occurs bilaterally or in an unexpected vascular bed. Thrombosis is the second leading cause of death in this patient population after the malignancy itself. The morbidity caused by VTE is greater in the population with cancer compared with the noncancer cohort.[20]

The pathophysiology of cancer-associated VTE is a multisystem insult. The tumor cells themselves exert a prothrombotic effect, while also interacting through monocytes and endothelial cells to support the prothrombotic state. Tumor cells are able to activate coagulation proteases to enhance the tumor's mobility and invasive qualities. In addition, tumor cells express tissue factor leading to increased generation of thrombin. A more complicated mechanism via angiogenesis promotes the growth of defective endothelial layers within tumor vessels to promote the up-regulation of vascular endothelial growth factor further, thereby supporting unrestricted future growth. Finally, vascular endothelial growth factor up-regulates the expression of tissue factor. The immune system's interaction, via monocytes or macrophages, with tumor cells results in the release of tumor necrosis factor, interleukins, and activation of platelets, all of which support a thrombogenic state. Compounding this predisposition to thrombosis, the common therapies available for cancer, namely surgery and chemotherapy, are also prothrombotic. Hormone therapy and blood product transfusion also can enhance the development of thrombosis.[20]

Primary prevention of thrombosis in the patient with cancer is particularly important in those patients presenting for cancer surgery. Surgery for cancer as compared with noncancer has a 3 times increased risk for VTE and this risk persists for many weeks postoperatively. Prophylactic therapy should be instituted as soon as possible postoperatively and in some cases intraoperatively. Unfractionated heparins and LMWH are the mainstay of prophylactic therapy in this patient group.[20]

The recommendation for treatment of VTE in a patient with cancer is 6 months of LMWH therapy and should be extended until cancer therapy is completed. Vitamin K antagonists, such as warfarin, are more difficult to dose in this population because of the need for repeated cessation of anticoagulation as well as changes in nutritional status, infection, and drug-drug interactions. For patients who experience recurrent VTE while on LMWH, it is recommended to increase the dose or a move to twice daily dosing of LMWH.[20]

PERIOPERATIVE MANAGEMENT OF THE ANTICOAGULATED PATIENT

The perioperative physician will encounter many patients on antithrombotic therapy. Antithrombotic therapy is a complicated area of medicine with few randomized controlled trials to support strong recommendations. The goal of management is to limit the period of withholding anticoagulation based on 2 important aspects of the clinical scenario: the patient's specific thrombotic risk and the surgical risk for bleeding. These recommendations are based on the most recent CHEST guidelines in combination with the senior authors' personal practice.[21–25]

Recommendations for patients anticoagulated with warfarin[22,23]

1. Do not withhold warfarin in low-bleeding-risk surgical procedures where local hemostatic strategies may be sufficient to limit bleeding.
2. Stop warfarin 5 days before moderate-risk or high-risk scheduled/elective surgery.
3. Replace warfarin with a bridging therapy alternative such as LMWH in cases of patients with mechanical heart valve, atrial fibrillation with history of stroke, or CHADS2 score of 4 or greater. Patients with recent (>3 months) venous thrombosis or severe thrombophilia such as APS or cancer should also be bridged. LMWH should be stopped 24 hours before surgery and full-dose LMWH should be restarted no sooner than 48 hours after surgery.
4. Resume warfarin 12 to 24 hours postoperatively or when optimal hemostasis is achieved.

Recommendations for patients anticoagulated with Dabigatran[24]

1. Withhold Dabigatran 24 hours before surgery in a patient with normal creatinine clearance. Withhold Dabigatran 48 hours before surgery if the patient's creatinine clearance is 30 to 50 mL/min. Withhold Dabigatran more than 3 days for a creatinine clearance less than 30 mL/min.
2. Withhold Dabigatran 2 to 4 days before high-risk bleeding procedures such as cardiothoracic surgery or intracranial or spinal surgery.
3. Resume Dabigatran 24 to 48 hours postoperatively and when optimal hemostasis is achieved.

Recommendations for patients anticoagulated with Rivaroxaban[24]

1. Withhold Rivaroxaban 24 hours before surgery in a patient with normal creatinine clearance. Withhold Rivaroxaban more than 48 hours in a patient with creatinine clearance less than 50 mL/min.
2. Resume Rivaroxaban 24 hours postoperatively and when optimal hemostasis is achieved.

Recommendations for patients anticoagulated with Apixaban[24]

1. Withhold Apixaban 24 hours before surgery in a patient with normal creatinine clearance. Withhold Apixaban more than 48 hours in a patient with creatinine clearance less than 50 mL/min.
2. Resume Apixaban 24 hours postoperatively and when optimal hemostasis is achieved.

Recommendations for patients on antiplatelet therapy (prevention of secondary cardiovascular event)[25]

No Stent
1. Continue aspirin therapy but withhold clopidogrel for 7 to 10 days in the case of minor surgical procedure such minor dental, dermatologic, or cataract surgery.
2. Withhold aspirin and clopidogrel therapy 7 to 10 days before moderate-risk or high-risk surgery in patients with a low risk for cardiovascular event.
3. Continue aspirin therapy but withhold clopidogrel 10 days before surgery, for the patient at moderate to high risk of cardiovascular event presenting for noncardiac surgery.

4. In the patient presenting for coronary artery bypass graft surgery, continue aspirin therapy but withhold clopidogrel 5 days before surgery.

Stent

1. In the patient with coronary stents, delay surgery for a minimum of 6 weeks after placement of a bare-metal stent and 6 months after placement of a drug-eluting stent.
2. If this cannot be avoided, continue both aspirin and clopidogrel therapy around the time of surgery.
3. Resume antiplatelet therapy postoperatively when adequate hemostasis is achieved, preferably within 24 to 48 hours. Clopidogrel may take days to reach peak effectiveness. Consider a loading dose in the patient at high risk of arterial thrombotic event when not taking clopidogrel.

Stent—Bare-Metal

1. Delay, if possible, surgery for 6 weeks. Continue aspirin unless the procedure is high risk for bleeding.
2. If surgery is necessary within the 6-week period, continue both antiplatelet agents.

Stent—Drug-Eluting

1. Delay, if possible, surgery for 6 to 12 months.
2. If surgery is necessary within the 12-month period, continue both antiplatelet agents.
3. Close coordination with cardiology consultants is recommended as degree of risk from discontinuing antiplatelet agents depends on both the type of stent, the drug-eluting versus bare-metal, and the patient's specific risk factors and coronary anatomy.

SUMMARY

The perioperative physician is likely to encounter patients with various degrees of thrombosis or hemostasis. For those patients without a prior hematologic diagnosis, the bleeding history will be paramount in elucidating occult disease and furthering an appropriate workup and should therefore be included in any perioperative visit. For those patients with a known disorder of thrombosis or hemostasis, including patients on chronic anticoagulation, the preoperative visit is the critical step in planning for a surgical intervention. For this reason, it is recommended that any patient with a known hematologic disorder be seen by their perioperative physician well in advance of surgery to ensure a safe perioperative period. The most important aspect to management of these patients is careful preparation and communication. Patients will require clear verbal and written instruction on preoperative testing, management of anticoagulation, and appropriate follow-up or hematology referral for consultation. Surgical pharmacies may require time to obtain and stock appropriate pharmacologic agents. Anesthesiology and surgical services will benefit from clear communication on the perioperative plan for management of these disorders. Patients with these disorders can safely proceed through surgery following careful preparation by all parties involved.

REFERENCES

1. Chee YL, Crawford JC, Watson HG, et al. Guidelines on the assessment of bleeding risk prior to surgery or invasive procedure. British Committee for Standards in Haematology. Br J Haematol 2008;140:496–504.

2. Favaloro EJ. Clinical utility of the PFA-100. Semin Thromb Hemost 2008;34: 709–33.
3. Rodeghiero F, Tosetto A, Castaman G. How to estimate bleeding risk in mild bleeding disorders. J Thromb Haemost 2007;5:157–66.
4. Gill JC, Shapiro A, Valentino LA, et al. von Willebrand factor/factor VIII concentrate (Humate-P) for management of elective surgery in adults and children with von Willebrand disease. Haemophilia 2011;17:895–905.
5. Koscielny J, Ziemer S, Radtke H, et al. A practical concept for preoperative identification of patients with impaired primary hemostasis. Clin Appl Thromb Hemost 2004;10:195–204.
6. Kamal A, Tefferi A, Pruthi RK. How to interpret and pursue an abnormal prothrombin time, activated partial thromboplastin time, and bleeding time in adults. Mayo Clin Proc 2007;82:864–73.
7. Lippi G, Favaloro E, Salvagno GL, et al. Laboratory assessment and perioperative management of patients on antiplatelet therapy: from the bench to the bedside. Clin Chim Acta 2009;405:8–16.
8. Gabriel P, Mazoit X, Ecoffey C. Relationship between clinical history, coagulation tests, and perioperative bleeding during tonsillectomies in pediatrics. J Clin Anesth 2000;12:288–91.
9. Chee YL, Greaves M. Role of coagulation testing in predicting bleeding risk. Hematol J 2003;4:373–8.
10. Eckman M, Erban JK, Singh SK, et al. Screening for the risk for bleeding or thrombosis. Ann Intern Med 2003;138:W15–24.
11. United Kingdom Haemophelia Centre Doctors' Organisation. Guidelines on the selection and use of therapeutic products to treat haemophilia and other hereditary bleeding disorders. Haemophilia 2003;9:1–23.
12. Nichols WL, Hultin MB, James AH, et al. von Willebrand disease (VWD): evidence-based diagnosis and management guidelines, the National Heart, Lung, and Blood Institute (NHLBI) expert panel report (USA). Haemophilia 2008;14:171–232.
13. Shaheen K, Alraies MC, Alrayes AH, et al. Factor V Leiden: how great is the risk of venous thromboembolism? Cleve Clin J Med 2012;4:265–72.
14. De Stefano V, Rossi E, Za T, et al. Prophylaxis and treatment of venous thromboembolism in individuals with inherited thrombophilia. Semin Thromb Hemost 2006;8:767–80.
15. Castoldi E, Hackeng T. Regulation of coagulation by protein S. Curr Opin Hematol 2008;15:529–36.
16. Ruiz-Irastorza G, Crowther M, Branch W, et al. Antiphospholipid syndrome. Lancet 2010;376:1498–509.
17. Giannakopoulos B, Krilis S. The pathogenesis of antiphospholipid syndrome. N Engl J Med 2013;368:1033–44.
18. Pengo V, Denas G, Benzato A, et al. Secondary prevention in thrombotic antiphospholipid syndrome. Lupus 2012;21:734–5.
19. Patnaik MM, Moll S. Inherited antithrombin deficiency: a review. Haemophilia 2008;14:1229–39.
20. Barsam SJ, Patel R, Arya R. Anticoagulation for prevention and treatment of cancer-related venous thromboembolism. Br J Haematol 2013;5:1–14.
21. Guyatt GH, Akl EA, Crowther M. Executive summary: antithrombotic therapy and prevention of thrombosis, 9th ed: American College of Chest Physicians evidence-based clinical practice guidelines. Chest 2012;141:7S–47S.
22. Douketis JD, Spyropoulos AC, Spencer FA, et al. Perioperative management of antithrombotic therapy. Chest 2012;141:e326s–50s.

23. Ortel T. Perioperative management of patients on chronic antithrombotic therapy. Blood 2012;120:4699–705.

24. Weitz JI, Eikelboom JW, Samama MM. New antithrombotic drugs. Chest 2012; 141:e120s–51s.

25. Chassot PG, Delabays A, Spahn DR. Perioperative antiplatelet therapy: the case for continuing therapy for patients at risk for myocardial infarction. Br J Anaesth 2007;99:316–28.

Patients Requiring Perioperative Nutritional Support

T. Miko Enomoto, MD[a], Dawn Larson, MD[a],
Robert G. Martindale, MD, PhD[b],*

KEYWORDS

- Perioperative nutrition • Malnutrition classifications • Immune-modulating nutrition
- Omega-3 fatty acids • Arginine • Preoperative carbohydrate loading

KEY POINTS

- Malnutrition is associated with significantly increased surgical morbidity and mortality.
- Malnutrition can result from inadequate nutrients, excessive consumption of nutrients during pathologic processes, or a combination of these factors.
- Therapeutic nutritional interventions beginning before surgery and continuing through the perioperative period can improve outcomes.
- Feeding the gastrointestinal tract is vastly preferable to parenteral feeding.

PREOPERATIVE SCREENING

The common goal of a preoperative evaluation is to optimize patient outcome.[1] Outpatient evaluations are becoming more prevalent, and this is an opportune time to intervene. Of the criteria for a thorough evaluation, nutrition is perhaps overlooked secondary to more tangible objectives, such as cardiac clearance and preoperative risk stratification. Patients undergoing elective surgery may be malnourished for a variety of reasons, including metabolic consequences of neoplastic disease, swallowing dysfunction, poor access to adequate nutrition, or alimentary track dysfunction. Ideally, these patients at risk are identified during a preoperative evaluation and a nutrition plan is implemented before surgery. A myriad of studies have shown the association of malnutrition and poor surgical outcome.[2–8] This outcome includes not only increased overall mortality but also morbidity such as increased hospital stay, admissions to the intensive care unit (ICU), delayed wound healing, and infectious

Funding Sources: T.M. Enomoto, unrestricted research grant, Actelion Pharmaceuticals.
Conflict of Interest: None.
[a] Department of Anesthesiology and Perioperative Medicine, Oregon Health & Science University, 3181 Southwest Sam Jackson Park Road, UHS-2, Portland, OR 97239, USA; [b] Department of Surgery, Oregon Health & Science University, 3181 Southwest Sam Jackson Park Road, L223A, Portland, OR 97239, USA
* Corresponding author.
E-mail address: martindr@ohsu.edu

Med Clin N Am 97 (2013) 1181–1200
http://dx.doi.org/10.1016/j.mcna.2013.07.003
medical.theclinics.com

complications via multiple mechanisms. Poor nutritional status has been ascribed to decreased survival in patients who have cancer.[9] In surgical patients, poor nutritional status is associated with a potential for increased rate of major morbidity, cancer recurrence, reoperations, and hospital readmissions.[10,11] For inpatients, the Joint Commission requires nutrition screening to be initiated within 24 hours of admission and a full assessment performed of at-risk patients.[12] No guidelines are available for when and how to evaluate and manage nutritional therapy in the preoperative setting.

The potential to screen and intervene in the preoperative setting is ideal, and several well-designed trials have shown benefit from preoperative enteral nutritional supplementation.[1] Recently, a randomized prospective trial of more than 1000 patients were assessed using a simple screening tool. Those patients deemed to be at high nutritional risk were then randomized to nutritional intervention versus standard of care.[13] Enteral nutritional intervention decreases major morbidity by 50% in those identified to be at risk.

The benefits of preoperative nutritional optimization do not seem to extend to parenteral supplementation. Most studies in which preoperative parenteral nutrition (PN) was given yielded no benefit and in some cases worsened the outcome.[14]

MALNUTRITION

The traditional concept of malnutrition brings to mind one associated with low body mass index (BMI) and decreased muscle mass; however, several categories have been proposed that take into account both chronic and acute states of inflammation-associated disease and injury. Because of heterogeneity in the medical literature as to what constitutes malnutrition and the best way to categorize it, an international guideline committee was formed under the auspices of the American Society for Parenteral and Enteral Nutrition (ASPEN) and European Society for Parenteral and Enteral Nutrition (ESPEN) congresses (**Table 1**). Recognition that malnutrition requires an imbalance of nutrient intake with metabolic demands has led to a reconceptualization of malnutrition to include situations of reduced nutrition intake, as well as states involving accelerated or increased catabolism from inflammation associated with chronic or acute disease. From the ASPEN and ESPEN congresses, 3 categories of malnutrition based on cause have been proposed (**Table 2**).[15–17]

To standardize the criteria for adult malnutrition based on these etiologic categories, the Academy of Nutrition and Dietetics and ASPEN developed a consensus statement designed to incorporate both the nutrition status and the inflammatory

Table 1 ASPEN clinical characteristics to support malnutrition: 2 or more of the following 6 characteristics	
Clinical Characteristic	**Malnutrition Context**
Insufficient energy intake Weight loss	Acute illness/injury
Loss of muscle mass Loss of subcutaneous fat	Chronic illness
Fluid retention Diminished handgrip strength	Social/environmental

Data from White JV, Guenter P, Jensen G, et al. Consensus statement: Academy of Nutrition and Dietetics and American Society for Parenteral and Enteral Nutrition: characteristics recommended for the identification and documentation of adult malnutrition (undernutrition). JPEN J Parenter Enteral Nutr 2012;36(3):275–83.

Table 2 Cause of malnutrition	
Starvation-related malnutrition	Chronic starvation without inflammation is often classically seen in anorexia nervosa, poor access to food, and famines and can be reversed with standard nutritional supplementation
Chronic disease-related malnutrition	This exists in the setting of chronic illnesses that impose sustained inflammation of mild to moderate degree such as organ failure, cancer, autoimmune disorders, or sarcopenic obesity, in which muscle loss occurs in the setting of obesity
Acute disease-related or injury-related malnutrition	This is categorized by marked inflammation, as in the case of major infection, burns, trauma, or neurologic injury

Data from Jensen GL, Mirtallo J, Compher C, et al. Adult starvation and disease-related malnutrition: a proposal for etiology-based diagnosis in the clinical practice setting from the international consensus guideline committee. JPEN J Parenter Enteral Nutr 2010;34(2):156–9.

disease–associated component. Because it is difficult to assign a single parameter, the committee proposed the following characteristics for an appropriate nutrition assessment:

Nutrition assessment has been defined by ASPEN as consisting of the following: medical, nutrition, and medication histories; physical examination; anthropometric measurements; and laboratory data.[18] There are a variety of nutrition screening and assessment tools; essentially, these may consist of physical examination and historical data such as weight loss history, fat store loss, muscle wasting and BMI, as well as laboratory data such as albumin, prealbumin, and cholesterol levels and lymphocyte count.[19]

Other nutritional assessments such as the Nutritional Risk Screening 2002 guides the practitioner to initiate a nutritional care plan in the perioperative period on patients meeting sufficient scores based on weight loss, reduced intake, and illness.[20] The NUTRIC (Nutrition Risk in the Critically Ill) score attempts to quantify the risk of morbidity in critically ill patients that could be modified by nutritional intervention. Here, the following variables are assessed: age, APACHE (Acute Physiology And Chronic Health Evaluation) II, SOFA (Sequential Organ Failure Assessment), comorbidities, length of hospital and ICU stay, and interleukin 6.[21]

PREOPERATIVE NUTRITION
Starvation-Related Malnutrition

Starvation-related malnutrition from a global health perspective has roots in areas of famine. In more developed countries, starvation-related malnutrition is more often seen in medical conditions such as anorexia nervosa or unintentional starvation, as occurs in the geriatric population, caused by inadequate access to macronutrients, severe gastrointestinal (GI) dysfunction, or neglect. Preoperative addition of a balanced macronutrient high-protein supplement is useful to initiate as far in advance of surgery as possible, although in this severely malnourished population, the time needed to see benefit from supplementation is unknown (estimated minimum of 2–4 weeks). Abnormalities such as hypokalemia, hypophosphatemia, hypocalcemia, and hypomagnesemia should be addressed. Total body stores are commonly depleted, and preoperative repletion has been shown to decrease postoperative complications, including cardiac arrhythmias and metabolic issues.

For severely malnourished patients, refeeding syndrome can occur when carbohydrate-rich fluids are provided too rapidly. Categorized by the hallmark of hypophosphatemia, as well as hypokalemia, hypomagnesemia, and volume overload, this syndrome can be life threatening.[22,23] For chronically ill and severely malnourished patients, preoperative admission for nutrition and electrolyte management and monitoring may be indicated.

For those deemed malnourished, specialized preoperative nutritional support should be initiated orally, enterally, or rarely, parenterally with therapeutic intent. ASPEN and the Society of Critical Care Nutritional Guidelines (SCCM) guidelines state that for those who cannot take adequate calories on oral supplementation alone, enteral nutrition should be considered and is preferred over PN if the GI tract is functional.[24]

Although initial guidelines have advocated the use of artificial nutritional support (enteral preferred to parenteral) if preoperative weight loss has occurred (>10%) or oral intake is not expected for more than 7 to 10 days postoperatively (ASPEN), there has been interest in supporting preoperative and postoperative nutrition orally for all comers to elective surgery regardless of nutritional status.[25] Furthermore, certain studies have investigated the progressive notion of supplementing diets preoperatively, as well as throughout the postoperative period, suggesting that there may be less weight loss, fewer minor complications, and cost efficiency.[26]

Geriatric Nutrition

Attention to appropriate preoperative nutrition in the geriatric population becomes even more critical because of increased risk resulting from multiple physiologic changes associated with aging, multiple medications, relative decrease in activity, and high incidence of sarcopenia.[27]

In developed countries, up to 15% of community elderly, 23% to 62% of hospitalized elderly, and up to 85% of nursing home elderly are malnourished.[28] Inadequate energy intake may have a variety of causes, including mechanical (ie, dysphagia), dementia, or other neurologic conditions, as well as poor dentition or ill-fitting dental appliances. Social factors such as isolation or poor access to nutritious foods or depression can limit intake. Medication side effects (polypharmacy) are one of the major causes for poor nutrition intake.[29] Age-associated changes in smell and taste, as well as medically recommended restricted diets (low salt, fat, or sugar) dramatically influence appetite.[30] In relation to preoperative preparation, this demographic is more likely to have other mitigating disease processes, such as infections, cancers, congestive heart failure, renal disease, or chronic pulmonary disease. Furthermore, the elderly are at risk for sarcopenia and decreased functional performance because of changes in hormonal status, insulin resistance, protein intake, and physical activity. Although the typical 0.8 g protein/kg body weight per day is the recommended dietary allowance, this may not be adequate for those at risk for lean muscle loss in aging and increasing this to 1.5 g protein/kg/d may be beneficial to function.[31] Oral caloric-rich and protein-rich supplements are available as adjuncts to boost energy intake if needed, and it is important to address other factors that contribute to poor intake, as mentioned earlier. Compared with standard care groups, cohorts who receive oral supplements combined with resistance exercise yield better muscle retention of protein, with resulting improvements in postoperative recovery.[32–34]

Nutritional Support in Obesity

Worldwide obesity has nearly doubled[35] since 1980 and 35.7% of US adults are obese.[36] Obesity leads to a myriad of health comorbidities, including hypertension, coronary artery disease, cerebrovascular disease, cancer, obstructive sleep apnea, and osteoarthritis. Moreover, obesity is more than a structural issue with body mass; it is also a multisystem proinflammatory disorder. Adipose tissue releases humoral substances such as adipokines, tumor necrosis factor α (TNF-α), leptin, and adiponectin, leading to inflammation.[37] Metabolic syndrome has been recognized as an important entity associated with abdominal obesity, accelerated cardiovascular disease, and type II diabetes, as well as an increased risk of malignancies.[37–39]

Although obesity is most commonly associated with macronutrient excess, it is reported that at least 15% to 20% of obese patients may be nutritionally deficient in at least 1 micronutrient. If vitamin D is considered, up to 60% of obese patients are deficient in at least 1 micronutrient or macronutrient.[40–42] Obese patients are categorized in the malnutrition category of chronic disease with inflammation. Other common deficiencies, especially in those who have had bariatric surgery, include ferritin, iron, folic acid, zinc, and selenium, vitamin B_6 and vitamin B_{12}.[40–42] This deficiency may be particularly pertinent in surgical patients, because zinc, selenium, and vitamin C are critical for normal wound healing. Preoperative assessment and correction of micronutrients should be considered at least 4 to 6 weeks before undergoing elective surgery.[43] Furthermore, previously obese patients who have undergone bariatric surgery are even more likely to have macronutrient and micronutrient deficiencies, which should be screened for before elective surgery. Sarcopenic obesity is a common occurrence in the postbariatric surgical population; this results in dramatic increase in perioperative morbidity, including increased need for postoperative ventilator support, increased duration of ICU stay, and worsening infectious complications.[44]

Immunonutrition Supplementation

Disease-related malnutrition states, either chronic or acute, are known to benefit from traditional caloric and protein supplementation. There is a growing body of evidence to support the use of specific immune-modulating and metabolism-modulating nutrients delivered at a level higher than that needed for normal cell metabolism. Multiple recent large prospective randomized clinical trials, which have assessed the role of treating patients with immune-modulating and metabolically modulating nutrients, have reported a decrease in infectious complications as well as decreased length of hospital and ICU stay, although no mortality benefit has been shown.[45] The inflammatory response of surgery predisposes to immune dysfunction and, in turn, the risk of infections may be increased and worsened if patients are already ill or malnourished. Of the myriad of nutrients studied, arginine, glutamine, fish oils, and nucleic acids seem to have the most published literature supporting the value of preoperative supplementation. Arginine has been a popular area of research, given its promising results as a nutritional supplement. Arginine is considered a semiessential amino acid, which becomes essential in times of significant stress, when intake normally decreases dramatically. Arginine is vital in protein synthesis, intermediary metabolism, and as a substrate for nitric oxide (NO) synthase (NOS) (inducible NOS [iNOS], endothelial NOS [eNOS], neuronal NOS [nNOS]). NOS derivatives regulate vascular dilatation and regional blood flow, T-cell function and maturation, as well as being an intermediate metabolite in the urea cycle.[46,47] Perioperative arginine supplementation has been reported to decrease perioperative infections and has been implicated in increased survival in certain malignancies. In the population with head and neck cancer, arginine supplementation is associated with improved long-term survival and long-term disease-specific survival.[48,49] Multiple mechanisms have been proposed for the noted benefit of supplemental arginine in decreasing infections, including regulating T-cell function, enhancing NO production to improve neutrophil and macrophage phagocytic activity, as well as intracellular bacterial killing. Recently, arginine has been shown to enhance maturation of myeloid-derived suppressor cells and to enhance tissue perfusion via improved cardiac output.[50–52] A potential explanation has been proposed to explain the influence of arginine in cancer, in that arginine levels are reduced in cancer and perioperative arginine supplementation may affect survival.[49]

Many formulations of nutritional supplements have been developed, but those containing omega-3 fatty acids (eicosanoic acid [EPA] and docohexanoic acid [DHA]), arginine, and RNA seem to have the most published literature to support use in the surgical patient. In a meta-analysis, Drover and colleagues[45] concluded that a nutritional therapy containing omega-3 fatty acids and arginine in both the preoperative and postoperative period in high-risk surgical patients was associated with a substantial reduction in infections and length of stay.[53] Many of these studies emphasize the importance of initiation of these immune and metabolically active supplements 5 to 7 days before surgery to optimize the reduction in postoperative infections, morbidity, length of stay,[45,51,54,55] and inflammatory markers.[56,57]

Preoperative preparation of the patient with specific metabolically and immune-active agents gained support after several landmark studies by Gianotti and colleagues.[58,59] These studies showed that metabolic preparation for surgery was possible by supplementing the regular diet with arginine, fish oils, DHA, EPA, and an RNA diet for 5 to 7 days preoperatively. By following this protocol, major perioperative morbidity could be reduced by approximately 50% in patients undergoing resection for malignancy of the esophagus, stomach, or pancreas. This benefit was noted in both the well-nourished and malnourished patient populations, indicating a paradigm shift from the concept that correction of malnutrition alone was the important factor.[59] These studies introduced the concept of metabolic preparation before surgical insult. The patients consumed 750 mL to 1 L per day of the metabolic-modulating formula in addition to their regular diet. In a recent systematic review of the evidence including 35 studies, Drover and colleagues[45] reported that these arginine-containing nutritional supplements yielded a significant benefit in decreasing infectious complications across the several surgical specialties included. These investigators also reported a decrease in length of hospital stay. The fish oils have multiple mechanisms, which could explain the beneficial effects seen in the surgical patient, including attenuating the metabolic response to stress, altering gene expression to minimize proinflammatory cytokine production, beneficially modifying the T helper type 1 (Th1) to Th2 lymphocyte population to decrease the inflammatory response, increasing production of the antiinflammatory lipid compounds resolvins and protectins, and regulating bowel motility via vagal efferents.[60–63]

Preoperative Carbohydrate Loading

The well-engrained dogma of preoperative fasting is being called into question in light of increasing evidence that postoperative insulin resistance is harmful and can be ameliorated by avoidance of preoperative fasting and carbohydrate loading. Preoperative fasting induces metabolic stress, impairs optimal mitochondrial functioning, obligates the host to use lean tissue, and contributes to insulin resistance.[64–66] In cardiac surgery patients, insulin resistance correlates with increased incidence of major complications, including death.[67] Multiple recent studies using an isotonic carbohydrate and electrolyte drink administered the night before surgery and then 3 hours preoperatively seem to attenuate some of these responses.[68–70] The theory, which is supported by animal and clinical studies, supports the hypothesis that maximum glycogen storage during surgery in patients allows carbohydrate to be used for energy and protects the lean body tissue from degradation.[71] This carbohydrate loading concept has been incorporated into enhanced recovery after surgery protocols.[72] Although the results have been exciting, more studies are needed to change current nil-by-mouth standard of care guidelines.

INTRAOPERATIVE NUTRITION
Total PN

Although enteral feeding is the preferred route of nutrition, in certain situations, patients may be unable to tolerate enteral feedings secondary to anatomic issues, such as bowel discontinuity and high-output proximal fistula or motility disorders, and total PN (TPN) may be necessary preoperatively and postoperatively. TPN provides hypertonic glucose, amino acids, lipids, electrolytes, trace elements, and minerals. Patients in the perioperative periods receiving TPN should be managed by a multidisciplinary team, with frequent adjustment of the prescription. Major complications of TPN are infections, intravascular catheter complications, and metabolic abnormalities. Abrupt discontinuation of these solutions during the intraoperative period can lead to significant hypoglycemia. One option is to continue TPN at its full rate during the intraoperative period, but care must be taken to avoid inadvertent bolus of the TPN solution. If TPN is continued during surgery, serial serum glucose levels should be followed closely to prevent hyperglycemia, with the added insulin resistance from the stress of surgical procedures. Alternatively, the infusion rate can be reduced to half the night before surgery and discontinued. When TPN is stopped in the immediate preoperative period, a 5% or 10% dextrose solution should be started preoperatively. Because serum glucose, potassium, and phosphate levels may be affected, these should be measured preoperatively and replaced before surgery. Hypophosphatemia can be a problem for patients receiving TPN, particularly with solutions that are phosphate-free, and may manifest as serious side effects. Severe hypophosphatemia can cause cardiac failure, tachypnea, seizures, and shifting of the oxygen dissociation curve to the left.[73]

Continuous Enteral Nutrition

Patients receiving enteral nutrition before surgery often have their feedings held before surgery and procedures for several unpredicted hours, often resulting in a significant calorie deficit. This concept of continuous enteral feedings throughout the perioperative period was first studied in patients suffering from burns, in whom caloric intake was vital, given their markedly increased metabolic rate. These patients were successfully fed intraoperatively without an increase in infections or aspiration, resulting in better caloric intake.[74] Although there are not many studies regarding the validity and safety of this treatment in nonvisceral surgical procedures, the feasibility of implementing a reduced fasting protocol in mechanically ventilated patients with trauma was performed, and no increase in adverse outcomes was found, paving the way for further randomized studies; particularly in patients who come to the operating room with a protected airway (intubated or tracheostomy).[75]

Postoperative Nutrition

Among the most important factors affecting outcome and recovery from surgical trauma are preoperative nutritional status and the patient's metabolic response to the surgical insult. This situation was clearly shown in the large preoperative risk assessment study performed by the US Department of Veterans Affairs. This prospective trial included more than 87,000 patients from 44 separate medical centers, with more than 60 variables collected on each patient. This study reported that the single most valuable predictor of poor outcome was a serum albumin less than 3.0 g/dL.[1] The benefits of preoperative preparation for the nutritionally at-risk population were shown in a recent study by Jie and colleagues.[13] In this trial, high-risk patients were identified and nutritionally supplemented preoperatively, resulting in a 50% reduction in postoperative morbidity.

After surgery, nutritional goals at the most basic level should be to provide caloric support for wound healing and to avoid excessive loss of lean body mass. As our understanding of nutritional therapy progresses, these goals have broadened to include modulating the immune response, optimizing glucose control, attenuating the hypermetabolic response to surgery, and providing micronutrients and macronutrients to optimize healing and recovery. Previously well-nourished patients undergoing minor surgery with expected short hospital stay derive little if any clinical or metabolic benefit from early postoperative nutrition therapy. On the other hand, most patients undergoing major surgery with anticipated extended stay in the hospital and ICU yield significant benefits. In addition, those at moderate to severe nutrition risk in the preoperative setting realize significant benefits from attention to early enteral nutrition. Whether a benefit from nutrition therapy is realized depends on factors such as route and timing of delivery, content of nutrient substrate, and efforts to promote patient mobility. Recent data support a preoperative assessment and nutritional intervention if the patient meets high-risk criteria.[13,58]

Enteral nutrition is clearly superior to PN for supporting most postoperative patients and should always be the first choice for nutrient delivery, when feasible.[24,76]

Prolonged periods of fasting are associated with breakdown of the barrier function of the GI tract, atrophy of the endothelial microvilli, and decrease in the mass of gut-associated lymphoid tissue (GALT).[77] These changes are associated with increased risk of bowel dysfunction, infection, and sepsis,[78,79] and reverse with reinstitution of luminal delivery of nutrition.[80]

Early enteral nutrition has been associated with reduced infections, shorter hospital stays, and reduced mortality, not only in the elective surgical population,[81] but also in the critically ill.[82,83] Proposed mechanisms for these effects center around maintenance of the barrier functions of the GI tract: both the structural integrity and immunologic function.

The GI tract is the largest immune organ in the body, because of the resident GALT. Regulation of the mucosal-associated lymphoid tissue throughout the body is via the GALT. Dendritic cells and macrophage-presenting cells communicate in the gut and then distribute to every epithelial-based immune tissue. Greater than 80% of the immunoglobulin-producing ability of the body resides in the GI tract. The physical barrier function of the gut requires maintenance of epithelial tight junctions and secretory capabilities of the mucosal cells, which in turn requires luminal exposure to nutrients.[77] Enteral nutrition also augments visceral blood flow and enhances local and systemic immune response.[82–84]

Postoperative Ileus

Postoperative ileus is such a common complication of abdominal surgery that it is considered a physiologic response of the bowel to surgical trauma. Kalff and colleagues[85] characterized the pathophysiology of ileus in an elaborate series of experiments. Initially, the endothelium expresses intracellular adhesion molecule 1 (ICAM-1), which binds receptors on macrophages, allowing them to migrate into the bowel muscularis. Once there, the macrophages set up inflammatory changes mediated by cytokines and other kinetically active substances, subsequently leading to a loss of coordinated peristalsis.

Historically, surgical dogma prescribed waiting for signs of return of bowel function (ie, bowel sounds, flatus, defecation) before initiation of enteral intake. Evidence does not support this practice.[86] Although early enteral nutrition has not been conclusively shown to decrease or shorten postoperative ileus,[87] its safety has been shown in many postoperative populations, even after major abdominal surgeries.[88] Early initiation of enteral feeding has been shown to have many benefits, including preservation of the villous architecture of the GI lumen, GALT, tight junctions, and IgA production.[89]

Elective Surgery

Patients able to eat of their own volition should be allowed to do so in the early postoperative period, essentially as soon as postoperative nausea, caused either by anesthesia or surgical manipulation, has subsided. Intake of normal food has been shown to be safe as early as 4 hours after colorectal surgery,[87,90] and within 24 hours after gastrectomy.[91,92] In the well-nourished patient recovering from minor elective surgery, resumption of a standard healthy diet is encouraged.

GI intolerance presenting as nausea, abdominal distension, increased gastric residual volume, abdominal pain, or diarrhea represents one of the largest barriers to delivery of goal calories. Promotility agents such as erythromycin and metoclopramide are useful in some series, but are typically not required in the routine postoperative setting. Alvimopan, a peripheral opioid antagonist, may be helpful in preventing opioid-induced bowel dysmotility.[93] No current large series supports the routine use of promotility agents, and use of promotility agents should be considered only once mechanical bowel obstruction has been ruled out, when adequate perfusion of bowel is likely, and all other metabolic causes for the dysmotility have been addressed. The most common reason for postoperative dysmotility is electrolyte abnormality.[94]

Several studies support the use of protocol-driven perioperative regimens that prioritize preoperative recognition and treatment of malnutrition, early postoperative enteral nutrition, glycemic control, and use of immunonutrition in improving patient outcomes after elective colorectal surgery.[95–97] More complex decisions are needed when the patient is not able to take in nutrition of their own volition, when there is intolerance to enteral feeding because of mechanical or functional disease, when the patient had preexisting malnutrition, and when the patient is critically ill.

The Critically Ill Surgical Patient

Nutritional therapy in the critically ill is confounded by patient heterogeneity. Nonetheless, guiding principles are emerging from a growing body of literature, which are applicable across the spectrum of critical illness (burn, trauma, surgical, and medical) and have been summarized in guidelines published by SCCM and ASPEN.[24,76]

Although the optimal time to initiate nutrition seems to be as early as possible in the well-resuscitated elective surgical patient, there are concerns about feeding in the critically ill population. Multiple factors need to be considered, including patient age, preexisting nutritional status, premorbid conditions, metabolic state, organ perfusion, and function. Although the situation is rare, concern for inducing mesenteric ischemia with enteral feeding in the underresuscitated patient on high-dose vasoconstrictors remains. Although there is evidence that enteral feeding in patients requiring vasopressors may be beneficial, this requires attention to details and close observation.[98,99] In the critically ill patient with evidence of decreased organ perfusion, enteral and PN should be withheld during the initial resuscitation phase.

HOW TO FEED
Tube Feeding

In the patient unable to take in adequate nutrition of their own volition, routine practice is to place a feeding tube, either nasogastric or nasojejunal. Feeding postpyloric was initially believed to be associated with less risk for GI intolerance and aspiration because of delivery of nutrient postpylorically, thereby not influenced by the decreased gastric motility. Two randomized controlled trials have since shown that there is no significant advantage to feeding distal to the stomach.[100,101] Davies and colleagues[101] reported similar caloric delivery, rates of pneumonia, diarrhea, and mortality between ventilated patients in the nasogastric group compared with the nasojejunal group. A slightly higher rate of minor GI hemorrhage was noted in the nasojejunal group.

Parenteral Versus Enteral Nutrition

Hundreds of experimental and clinical studies over the past 3 decades have consistently shown that enteral nutrition is superior to PN in the critically ill patient. Enteral nutrition has been reported to maintain and stimulate the protective effects of the GALT and preserve GI mucosal structure and function,[102–111] as well as support commensal organisms and limit the overgrowth of pathogenic bacteria.[112] Clinical outcome studies are consistent with basic science findings, which show better outcomes with respect to infection, organ failure, and hospital length of stay with enteral nutrition.[15,25,103–105,107] These results should be interpreted with some caution, because many of the early comparison studies were performed in the 1980s and early 1990s. There have been several areas of advancement in clinical care since that time, including improved glycemic control, reduction or elimination of proinflammatory omega-6 fatty acids, and enactment of protocols to limit central line–associated bloodstream infections. Even so, in the era of tight glycemic control and better central line care techniques, no evidence exists that PN results in improved outcomes over enteral nutrition in critically ill medical or surgical patients. As a consequence, all major nutrition organizations and critical care societies support enteral nutrition over parenteral whenever possible.[24,113–115]

WHAT TO FEED
Hypercaloric Feeding

The initial catabolic phase that immediately follows every surgery or traumatic insult leads to loss of lean body mass. In the early use of PN, it was believed that hypercaloric nutrient delivery might protect the lean body mass from catabolism. Most believe that hypercaloric feeding results in hepatic steatosis and hyperglycemia and increases the risk of infectious complications. The hyperdynamic response to surgical stress continues even in the face of adequate supply of enterally or parenterally delivered protein and calories. The concept of using specific nutrients delivered at levels higher than that needed for normal cell metabolism, which could alter this hyperdynamic response, was proposed in the late 1980s.[116] This strategy has now been verified to benefit and has become the standard of care for critically ill, traumatized, and surgical patients.[76]

SPECIFIC NUTRIENTS IN SURGERY
Fish Oil and Omega-3 Fatty Acids

Fish oil supplementation in various medical and surgical diseases has shown positive benefit. It is now well reported using various human models that appropriate use of omega-3 fatty acids can partially attenuate the hypermetabolic response to surgery, minimize the loss of lean body tissue, prevent oxidative injury, and favorably modulate the inflammatory response.[62,117] The mechanisms for these reported benefits are numerous and beyond the scope of this article but include alterations of the metabolic response to stress by changes in cell membrane phospholipids, alterations in gene expression, and modulation of endothelial expression of ICAM-1, E-selectin, and other endothelial receptors that regulate vascular integrity and function. In addition, EPA and DHA, the 20 and 22 carbon omega-3 fatty acids, undergo metabolic conversion in vivo to form resolvins, docosatrienes, and neuroprotectins. These are potent active effectors for the resolution of inflammation.[118] Resolvins regulate polymorphonuclear neutrophil transmigration. Docosanoids and neuroprotectins are both derived from DHA and have potent neuroprotective properties. Neuroprotectin D1 has been found to reduce brain infarct volume by half in an animal ischemia-reperfusion model.[119] The protective and antiinflammatory effects of these compounds are clearly important from an evolutionary basis, because they are highly conserved among species, from fish to mammals.[120] As the cellular and subcellular mechanisms of these lipid based compounds has become better elucidated, it is now accepted that resolution of inflammation is an active process rather than a passive time-dependent process, as was previously believed.[121] It is also becoming increasingly apparent that omega-3 fatty acids modulate this process. Recently, enterally delivered fish oils have also been shown to have a regulatory influence on the vagus nerve. The vagus facilitates multiple complex regulatory processes and interactions between the central nervous system and the innate and adaptive immune system. Fish oils dampen the inflammatory response mediated by the vagal fibers.[122] Incorporating the fatty acids DHA and EPA should be a part of routine ICU nutritional therapy, with multiple benefits reported and essentially no downside.[123]

Arginine

As discussed earlier, arginine is a semiessential amino acid and there is increasing support for its administration in the perioperative period. It is a prominent intermediate in several key processes: polyamine synthesis, which regulates cell growth and proliferation; proline synthesis, which is essential for normal wound healing and collagen synthesis; nitric oxide production (via eNOS, iNOS, nNOS) for regulation of microvascular perfusion; and modulation of lymphocyte proliferation and differentiation.[52] De novo synthesis and dietary intake are commonly reduced in times of stress and critical illness. In surgical, trauma, and ICU settings, the supply of arginine is decreased, whereas the cellular demand is dramatically increased, driven primarily by the upregulation of arginase and iNOS.[124]

In the past, controversy surrounded the use of arginine in the ICU setting.[110,125] The theory and speculation that arginine pose a potential threat to the critically ill patient are based on the observation that septic patients have upregulated iNOS and that supplementing additional arginine could result in excess nitric oxide production, with consequent vasodilation in a population already at risk of hemodynamic compromise. An alternative, equally valid argument is that cellular oxygenation is inadequate during septic shock and additional NO is a compensatory mechanism to increase oxygen delivery to relatively ischemic cells.[126] In the past 4 years, at least 5 studies have addressed this issue and support the benefit of arginine administration in the septic patient, or at least show no harm.[127–130] The mechanistic data have become even more complex with the discovery that asymmetric dimethyl arginine (ADMA) is involved in inhibiting NO synthase enzyme activity. ADMA is a posttranslational protein modification that is noted to increase in plasma during catabolic events when endogenous protein is being broken down. ADMA is a potent inhibitor of iNOS, and the ADMA/arginine ratio is critical to cardiac and vascular function. Added arginine supports increased cardiac output and tissue perfusion by altering the ADMA/arginine ratio.[128]

Glutamine

Over the past 3 decades, glutamine has been reported to offer a myriad of benefits in the medical, surgical, and trauma patient. These benefits include maintenance of acid-base balance, serving as the primary fuel for rapidly proliferating cells (ie, enterocytes, granulation tissue, and lymphocytes), and the rate limiting amino acid for the synthesis of endogenous antioxidant glutathione, attenuation of insulin resistance during stress, and a key substrate for hepatic gluconeogenesis.[131] Glutamine is a major regulator of heat shock protein production in numerous tissue beds.[132] Heat shock proteins are vital in the surgical stressed model, because this intracellular chaperone protein protects the cell from subsequent stress or insult, especially in the surgically stressed individual.[132]

Probiotics

Probiotics are living microbial organisms, which are believed to benefit human health through the prevention or attenuation of specific disease states. Probiotics have been used to prepare fermented food products to prevent spoilage in many cultures for hundreds of years. More recently, probiotics have been shown to benefit digestive functions and augment the immune system.[133]

Increasing evidence supports the influence of the intestinal microbial environment on physiology, nutritional status, immune function, and overall health status of the host. Admission to the hospital, surgical suite, and ICU is all associated with invasive techniques that eliminate or dramatically alter host natural barriers. Surgical and medical treatments or interventions may include the use of multiple medications that alter GI motility, luminal pH, systemic blood flow, and oxygenation. The widespread use of broad-spectrum antibiotics in hospital patients, along with delivery of nutrients via parenteral route or via highly refined enteral formulae, make the changes in the GI tract flora even more complex.[134] Within minutes of a surgical procedure or ICU admissions, the microbiome becomes dramatically altered. The acute or chronic stress on the host induced by illness, surgery, or trauma also causes significant changes to the mucosal microenvironment, including pH, redox potential, and mucosal energy supply.[112] These stress-induced gut mucosal changes result in increased virulence in the endogenous bacteria, which facilitate attachment and invasion of the host epithelial barrier.[135]

Data from randomized prospective studies suggest treatment benefits from delivering probiotics to manipulate the host microbiota in various surgical settings for prevention of nosocomial infections. Strong supportive data are now available for use of probiotics in prevention of antibiotic-associated diarrhea, *Clostridium difficile* diarrhea, and ventilator-associated pneumonia.[136,137] Optimal timing, formulation, and dose are still in question. Many now believe that the use of probiotics will be a part of routine surgical and ICU care in the near future. Not all species of probiotics have the same influence in disease states. Current probiotics in the surgical setting should be used under protocols with understanding for the potential downside of these live species.

SUMMARY

The disease states benefiting from metabolic modulation by nutritional means are wide ranging and spread over several organ systems. These nutrients discussed in this article, either alone or in combination, have been shown to attenuate the incidence and severity of acute lung injury, decrease adverse cardiac events in the postoperative setting, and enhance early recovery from GI surgery and trauma. Not only have clinical studies shown benefit in shortening total hospital and ICU length of stay, they have also reported reduced hospital infection rates and decreased mortality.[116,138] Although the data overwhelmingly support the use of metabolically active nutrients as a concept, the dose, timing of delivery, and duration of this therapy is not yet clear. As trials continue, these data should become available.

The concept of pharmaconutrition is now clearly accepted by many physicians globally as yet another tool in the toolbox for the perioperative physician. Subsequent studies will further elaborate which patient populations will maximally benefit. The use of fish oils, arginine, glutamine, and other metabolically active nutrients is now a major part of trauma and critical care nutrition protocols, as noted by SCCM, ASPEN, and ESPEN guidelines. All 3 of these major societies have given an A grade to the use of immune-active and metabolically active agents in specific populations.[24,76,108] Whether nutrients are used in combination or individually, these agents should be part of the perioperative physician's armamentarium for improving outcome and cost-effective care. For optimal outcome for the surgical patient, nutrition should be a part of the initial evaluation and assessment. Overt malnutrition should be treated in the preoperative period if time and disease state permit. The concept of metabolic manipulation for patients undergoing major surgical procedures given before surgical insult has gained acceptance globally.

REFERENCES

1. Daley J, Khuri SF, Henderson W, et al. Risk adjustment of the postoperative morbidity rate for the comparative assessment of the quality of surgical care: results of the National Veterans Affairs Surgical Risk Study. J Am Coll Surg 1997; 185(4):328–40.
2. Bruun LI, Bosaeus I, Bergstad I, et al. Prevalence of malnutrition in surgical patients: evaluation of nutritional support and documentation. Clin Nutr 1999;18(3): 141–7.
3. Gallagher C, Voss A, Finn S. Malnutrition and clinical outcomes: the case for medical nutrition therapy. J Am Diet Assoc 1996;96:361–6, 369.
4. Awad S, Lobo DN. What's new in perioperative nutritional support? Curr Opin Anaesthesiol 2011;24(3):339–48.
5. Schiesser M, Kirchhoff P, Muller MK, et al. The correlation of nutrition risk index, nutrition risk score, and bioimpedance analysis with postoperative complications in patients undergoing gastrointestinal surgery. Surgery 2009;145(5): 519–26.
6. Mullen JL. Consequences of malnutrition in the surgical patient. Surg Clin North Am 1981;61(3):465–87.
7. Correia MI, Waitzberg DL. The impact of malnutrition on morbidity, mortality, length of hospital stay and costs evaluated through a multivariate model analysis. Clin Nutr 2003;22(3):235–9.
8. Dempsey DT, Mullen JL, Buzby GP. The link between nutritional status and clinical outcome: can nutritional intervention modify it? Am J Clin Nutr 1988; 47(Suppl 2):352–6.
9. Dewys WD, Begg C, Lavin PT, et al. Prognostic effect of weight loss prior to chemotherapy in cancer patients. Eastern Cooperative Oncology Group. Am J Med 1980;69(4):491–7.

10. Kathiresan AS, Brookfield KF, Schuman SI, et al. Malnutrition as a predictor of poor postoperative outcomes in gynecologic cancer patients. Arch Gynecol Obstet 2011;284(2):445–51.

11. Kudsk KA. Enteral feeding and bowel necrosis: an uncommon but perplexing problem. Nutr Clin Pract 2003;18(4):277–8.

12. Fischer S, Bader A, Sweitzer BJ. Perioperative evaluation. In: Miller RD , editor. Miller's anesthesia. 7th edition. Philadelphia (PA): Churchill Livingstone; 2009. p. 1042–3.

13. Jie B, Jiang ZM, Nolan MT, et al. Impact of preoperative nutritional support on clinical outcome in abdominal surgical patients at nutritional risk. Nutrition 2012;28(10):1022–7.

14. Perioperative total parenteral nutrition in surgical patients. The Veterans Affairs Total Parenteral Nutrition Cooperative Study Group. N Engl J Med 1991; 325(8):525–32.

15. Taylor SJ, Fettes SB, Jewkes C, et al. Prospective, randomized, controlled trial to determine the effect of early enhanced enteral nutrition on clinical outcome in mechanically ventilated patients suffering head injury. Crit Care Med 1999; 27(11):2525–31.

16. Jensen GL, Mirtallo J, Compher C, et al. Adult starvation and disease-related malnutrition: a proposal for etiology-based diagnosis in the clinical practice setting from the international consensus guideline committee. JPEN J Parenter Enteral Nutr 2010;34(2):156–9.

17. White JV, Guenter P, Jensen G, et al. Consensus statement: Academy of Nutrition and Dietetics and American Society for Parenteral and Enteral Nutrition: characteristics recommended for the identification and documentation of adult malnutrition (undernutrition). JPEN J Parenter Enteral Nutr 2012;36(3): 275–83.

18. American Society for Parenteral and Enteral Nutrition (ASPEN). Board of directors and clinical practice committee. Definition of terms, style, and conventions used in ASPEN. Board of directors–approved documents. Available at: www. nutritioncare.org/Library.aspx. Updated 2010. Accessed July 2, 2013.

19. Mueller C, Compher C, Ellen DM, American Society for Parenteral and Enteral Nutrition (ASPEN) Board of Directors. ASPEN clinical guidelines: nutrition screening, assessment, and intervention in adults. JPEN J Parenter Enteral Nutr 2011;35(1):16–24.

20. Kondrup J, Allison SP, Elia M, et al, Educational and Clinical Practice Committee, European Society of Parenteral and Enteral Nutrition (ESPEN). ESPEN guidelines for nutrition screening 2002. Clin Nutr 2003;22(4):415–21.

21. Heyland DK, Dhaliwal R, Jiang X, et al. Identifying critically ill patients who benefit the most from nutrition therapy: the development and initial validation of a novel risk assessment tool. Crit Care 2011;15(6):R268.

22. Mehanna HM, Moledina J, Travis J. Refeeding syndrome: what it is, and how to prevent and treat it. BMJ 2008;336(7659):1495–8.

23. Fuentebella J, Kerner JA. Refeeding syndrome. Pediatr Clin North Am 2009; 56(5):1201–10.

24. McClave SA, Martindale RG, Vanek VW, et al. Guidelines for the provision and assessment of nutrition support therapy in the adult critically ill patient: Society of Critical Care Medicine (SCCM) and American Society for Parenteral and Enteral Nutrition (ASPEN). JPEN J Parenter Enteral Nutr 2009;33(3): 277–316.

25. Windsor AC, Kanwar S, Li AG, et al. Compared with parenteral nutrition, enteral feeding attenuates the acute phase response and improves disease severity in acute pancreatitis. Gut 1998;42(3):431–5.

26. Smedley F, Bowling T, James M, et al. Randomized clinical trial of the effects of preoperative and postoperative oral nutritional supplements on clinical course and cost of care. Br J Surg 2004;91(8):983–90.

27. Paddon-Jones D, Short KR, Campbell WW, et al. Role of dietary protein in the sarcopenia of aging. Am J Clin Nutr 2008;87(5):1562S–6S.

28. Morley JE. Anorexia of aging: physiologic and pathologic. Am J Clin Nutr 1997; 66(4):760–73.

29. Jyrkka J, Mursu J, Enlund H, et al. Polypharmacy and nutritional status in elderly people. Curr Opin Clin Nutr Metab Care 2012;15(1):1–6.

30. Zadak Z, Hyspler R, Ticha A, et al. Polypharmacy and malnutrition. Curr Opin Clin Nutr Metab Care 2013;16(1):50–5.

31. Wolfe RR, Miller SL, Miller KB. Optimal protein intake in the elderly. Clin Nutr 2008;27(5):675–84.

32. Valkenet K, van de Port IG, Dronkers JJ, et al. The effects of preoperative exercise therapy on postoperative outcome: a systematic review. Clin Rehabil 2011; 25(2):99–111.

33. Mayo NE, Feldman L, Scott S, et al. Impact of preoperative change in physical function on postoperative recovery: argument supporting prehabilitation for colorectal surgery. Surgery 2011;150(3):505–14.

34. Li C, Carli F, Lee L, et al. Impact of a trimodal prehabilitation program on functional recovery after colorectal cancer surgery: a pilot study. Surg Endosc 2013; 27(4):1072–82.

35. World Health Organization. Fact sheet no. 311, obesity and overweight. Available at: www.who.int/mediacentre/factsheets/fs311/en/. Accessed March 14, 2013.

36. Centers for Disease Control. Overweight and obesity. Available at: www.cdc. gov/obesity/data/adult.html. Accessed March 14, 2013.

37. Oda E. Metabolic syndrome: its history, mechanisms, and limitations. Acta Diabetol 2012;49(2):89–95.

38. Nicolucci A. Epidemiological aspects of neoplasms in diabetes. Acta Diabetol 2010;47(2):87–95.

39. World Health Organization. The international classification of adult underweight, overweight and obesity according to BMI. Available at: http://apps.who.int/bmi/index.jsp?introPage=intro_3.html. Accessed May 15, 2013.

40. Damms-Machado A, Friedrich A, Kramer KM, et al. Pre- and postoperative nutritional deficiencies in obese patients undergoing laparoscopic sleeve gastrectomy. Obes Surg 2012;22(6):881–9.

41. Toh SY, Zarshenas N, Jorgensen J. Prevalence of nutrient deficiencies in bariatric patients. Nutrition 2009;25(11–12):1150–6.

42. Valentino D, Sriram K, Shankar P. Update on micronutrients in bariatric surgery. Curr Opin Clin Nutr Metab Care 2011;14(6):635–41.

43. Cullen A, Ferguson A. Perioperative management of the severely obese patient: a selective pathophysiological review. Can J Anaesth 2012;59(10):974–96.

44. Tsai S. Importance of lean body mass in the oncologic patient. Nutr Clin Pract 2012;27(5):593–8.

45. Drover JW, Dhaliwal R, Weitzel L, et al. Perioperative use of arginine-supplemented diets: a systematic review of the evidence. J Am Coll Surg 2011;212(3):385–99, 399.e1.

46. Barbul A. Arginine: biochemistry, physiology, and therapeutic implications. JPEN J Parenter Enteral Nutr 1986;10(2):227–38.

47. Popovic PJ, Zeh HJ 3rd, Ochoa JB. Arginine and immunity. J Nutr 2007; 137(6 Suppl 2):1681S–6S.

48. Buijs N, van Bokhorst-de van der Schueren MA, Langius JA, et al. Perioperative arginine-supplemented nutrition in malnourished patients with head and neck cancer improves long-term survival. Am J Clin Nutr 2010;92(5):1151–6.

49. Vissers YL, Dejong CH, Luiking YC, et al. Plasma arginine concentrations are reduced in cancer patients: evidence for arginine deficiency? Am J Clin Nutr 2005;81(5):1142–6.

50. Raber P, Ochoa AC, Rodriguez PC. Metabolism of L-arginine by myeloid-derived suppressor cells in cancer: mechanisms of T cell suppression and therapeutic perspectives. Immunol Invest 2012;41(6–7):614–34.

51. Braga M. Perioperative immunonutrition and gut function. Curr Opin Clin Nutr Metab Care 2012;15(5):485–8.

52. Marik PE, Flemmer M. Immunonutrition in the surgical patient. Minerva Anestesiol 2012;78(3):336–42.

53. Marimuthu K, Varadhan KK, Ljungqvist O, et al. A meta-analysis of the effect of combinations of immune modulating nutrients on outcome in patients undergoing major open gastrointestinal surgery. Ann Surg 2012;255(6):1060–8.

54. Marik PE, Zaloga GP. Immunonutrition in high-risk surgical patients: a systematic review and analysis of the literature. JPEN J Parenter Enteral Nutr 2010; 34(4):378–86.

55. Braga M, Gianotti L, Radaelli G, et al. Perioperative immunonutrition in patients undergoing cancer surgery: results of a randomized double-blind phase 3 trial. Arch Surg 1999;134(4):428–33.

56. Giger U, Buchler M, Farhadi J, et al. Preoperative immunonutrition suppresses perioperative inflammatory response in patients with major abdominal surgery–a randomized controlled pilot study. Ann Surg Oncol 2007;14(10):2798–806.

57. Braga M, Gianotti L, Cestari A, et al. Gut function and immune and inflammatory responses in patients perioperatively fed with supplemented enteral formulas. Arch Surg 1996;131(12):1257–64 [discussion: 1264–5].

58. Gianotti L, Braga M, Nespoli L, et al. A randomized controlled trial of preoperative oral supplementation with a specialized diet in patients with gastrointestinal cancer. Gastroenterology 2002;122(7):1763–70.

59. Braga M, Gianotti L, Nespoli L, et al. Nutritional approach in malnourished surgical patients: a prospective randomized study. Arch Surg 2002;137(2):174–80.

60. Calder PC. Omega-3 polyunsaturated fatty acids and inflammatory processes: nutrition or pharmacology? Br J Clin Pharmacol 2013;75(3):645–62.

61. Lee HN, Surh YJ. Therapeutic potential of resolvins in the prevention and treatment of inflammatory disorders. Biochem Pharmacol 2012;84(10):1340–50.

62. Calder PC. Mechanisms of action of (n-3) fatty acids. J Nutr 2012;142(3):592S–9S.

63. Spite M, Norling LV, Summers L, et al. Resolvin D2 is a potent regulator of leukocytes and controls microbial sepsis. Nature 2009;461(7268):1287–91.

64. Awad S, Constantin-Teodosiu D, Macdonald IA, et al. Short-term starvation and mitochondrial dysfunction–a possible mechanism leading to postoperative insulin resistance. Clin Nutr 2009;28(5):497–509.

65. Awad S, Stephenson MC, Placidi E, et al. The effects of fasting and refeeding with a 'metabolic preconditioning' drink on substrate reserves and mononuclear cell mitochondrial function. Clin Nutr 2010;29(4):538–44.

66. Ljungqvist O. Modulating postoperative insulin resistance by preoperative car-bohydrate loading. Best Pract Res Clin Anaesthesiol 2009;23(4):401–9.
67. Sato H, Carvalho G, Sato T, et al. The association of preoperative glycemic con-trol, intraoperative insulin sensitivity, and outcomes after cardiac surgery. J Clin Endocrinol Metab 2010;95(9):4338–44.
68. Nygren J, Soop M, Thorell A, et al. Preoperative oral carbohydrate administra-tion reduces postoperative insulin resistance. Clin Nutr 1998;17(2):65–71.
69. Soop M, Nygren J, Myrenfors P, et al. Preoperative oral carbohydrate treatment attenuates immediate postoperative insulin resistance. Am J Physiol Endocrinol Metab 2001;280(4):E576–83.
70. Li L, Wang Z, Ying X, et al. Preoperative carbohydrate loading for elective sur-gery: a systematic review and meta-analysis. Surg Today 2012;42(7):613–24.
71. Awad S, Stephens F, Shannnon C, et al. Perioperative perturbations in carnitine metabolism are attenuated by preoperative carbohydrate treatment: another mechanism by which preoperative feeding may attenuate development of post-operative insulin resistance. Clin Nutr 2012;31(5):717–20.
72. Gustafsson UO, Ljungqvist O. Perioperative nutritional management in digestive tract surgery. Curr Opin Clin Nutr Metab Care 2011;14(5):504–9.
73. Roizen MF. Anesthetic implications of concurrent diseases. In: Miller RD, editor. Miller's anesthesia. 7th edition. Philadelphia: Churchill Livingstone; 2009. p. 1077–8.
74. Jenkins ME, Gottschlich MM, Warden GD. Enteral feeding during operative pro-cedures in thermal injuries. J Burn Care Rehabil 1994;15(2):199–205.
75. Pousman RM, Pepper C, Pandharipande P, et al. Feasibility of implementing a reduced fasting protocol for critically ill trauma patients undergoing opera-tive and nonoperative procedures. JPEN J Parenter Enteral Nutr 2009;33(2):176–80.
76. Martindale RG, McClave SA, Vanek VW, et al. Guidelines for the provision and assessment of nutrition support therapy in the adult critically ill patient: Society of Critical Care Medicine and American Society for Parenteral and Enteral Nutri-tion: executive summary. Crit Care Med 2009;37(5):1757–61.
77. Buchman AL, Moukarzel AA, Bhuta S, et al. Parenteral nutrition is associated with intestinal morphologic and functional changes in humans. JPEN J Parenter Enteral Nutr 1995;19(6):453–60.
78. Hotchkiss RS, Karl IE. The pathophysiology and treatment of sepsis. N Engl J Med 2003;348(2):138–50.
79. Doig GS, Heighes PT, Simpson F, et al. Early enteral nutrition reduces mortality in trauma patients requiring intensive care: a meta-analysis of randomised controlled trials. Injury 2011;42(1):50–6.
80. Sands KE, Bates DW, Lanken PN, et al. Epidemiology of sepsis syndrome in 8 academic medical centers. JAMA 1997;278(3):234–40.
81. Osland E, Yunus RM, Khan S, et al. Early versus traditional postoperative feeding in patients undergoing resectional gastrointestinal surgery: a meta-analysis. JPEN J Parenter Enteral Nutr 2011;35(4):473–87.
82. Marik PE, Zaloga GP. Early enteral nutrition in acutely ill patients: a systematic review. Crit Care Med 2001;29(12):2264–70.
83. Zaloga GP, Roberts PR, Marik P. Feeding the hemodynamically unstable patient: a critical evaluation of the evidence. Nutr Clin Pract 2003;18(4):285–93.
84. Sacks GS, Kudsk KA. Maintaining mucosal immunity during parenteral feeding with surrogates to enteral nutrition. Nutr Clin Pract 2003;18(6):483–8.

85. Kalff JC, Turler A, Schwarz NT, et al. Intra-abdominal activation of a local inflammatory response within the human muscularis externa during laparotomy. Ann Surg 2003;237(3):301–15.

86. Caddell KA, Martindale R, McClave SA, et al. Can the intestinal dysmotility of critical illness be differentiated from postoperative ileus? Curr Gastroenterol Rep 2011;13(4):358–67.

87. Han-Geurts IJ, Hop WC, Kok NF, et al. Randomized clinical trial of the impact of early enteral feeding on postoperative ileus and recovery. Br J Surg 2007;94(5): 555–61.

88. Suehiro T, Matsumata T, Shikada Y, et al. Accelerated rehabilitation with early postoperative oral feeding following gastrectomy. Hepatogastroenterology 2004;51(60):1852–5.

89. Fukatsu K, Kudsk KA. Nutrition and gut immunity. Surg Clin North Am 2011; 91(4):755–70, vii.

90. Lassen K, Soop M, Nygren J, et al. Consensus review of optimal perioperative care in colorectal surgery: enhanced recovery after surgery (ERAS) group recommendations. Arch Surg 2009;144(10):961–9.

91. Andersen HK, Lewis SJ, Thomas S. Early enteral nutrition within 24 h of colorectal surgery versus later commencement of feeding for postoperative complications. Cochrane Database Syst Rev 2006;(4):CD004080.

92. Lewis SJ, Egger M, Sylvester PA, et al. Early enteral feeding versus "nil by mouth" after gastrointestinal surgery: systematic review and meta-analysis of controlled trials. BMJ 2001;323(7316):773–6.

93. Vaughan-Shaw PG, Fecher IC, Harris S, et al. A meta-analysis of the effectiveness of the opioid receptor antagonist alvimopan in reducing hospital length of stay and time to GI recovery in patients enrolled in a standardized accelerated recovery program after abdominal surgery. Dis Colon Rectum 2012; 55(5):611–20.

94. Doorly MG, Senagore AJ. Pathogenesis and clinical and economic consequences of postoperative ileus. Surg Clin North Am 2012;92(2):259–72, viii.

95. Varadhan KK, Neal KR, D'ejong CH, et al. The enhanced recovery after surgery (ERAS) pathway for patients undergoing major elective open colorectal surgery: a meta-analysis of randomized controlled trials. Clin Nutr 2010;29(4): 434–40.

96. Fearon KC, Ljungqvist O, Von Meyenfeldt M, et al. Enhanced recovery after surgery: a consensus review of clinical care for patients undergoing colonic resection. Clin Nutr 2005;24(3):466–77.

97. Barr J, Hecht M, Flavin KE, et al. Outcomes in critically ill patients before and after the implementation of an evidence-based nutritional management protocol. Chest 2004;125(4):1446–57.

98. Wells DL. Provision of enteral nutrition during vasopressor therapy for hemodynamic instability: an evidence-based review. Nutr Clin Pract 2012;27(4):521–6.

99. Khalid I, Doshi P, DiGiovine B. Early enteral nutrition and outcomes of critically ill patients treated with vasopressors and mechanical ventilation. Am J Crit Care 2010;19(3):261–8.

100. White H, Sosnowski K, Tran K, et al. A randomised controlled comparison of early post-pyloric versus early gastric feeding to meet nutritional targets in ventilated intensive care patients. Crit Care 2009;13(6):R187.

101. Davies AR, Morrison SS, Bailey MJ, et al. A multicenter, randomized controlled trial comparing early nasojejunal with nasogastric nutrition in critical illness. Crit Care Med 2012;40(8):2342–8.

102. Runyon BA, Squier S, Borzio M. Translocation of gut bacteria in rats with cirrhosis to mesenteric lymph nodes partially explains the pathogenesis of spontaneous bacterial peritonitis. J Hepatol 1994;21(5):792–6.

103. Moore FA, Feliciano DV, Andrassy RJ, et al. Early enteral feeding, compared with parenteral, reduces postoperative septic complications. The results of a meta-analysis. Ann Surg 1992;216(2):172–83.

104. Moore FA, Moore EE, Jones TN, et al. TEN versus TPN following major abdominal trauma–reduced septic morbidity. J Trauma 1989;29(7):916–22 [discussion: 922–3].

105. Kudsk KA, Croce MA, Fabian TC, et al. Enteral versus parenteral feeding. Effects on septic morbidity after blunt and penetrating abdominal trauma. Ann Surg 1992;215(5):503–11 [discussion: 511–3].

106. Grahm TW, Zadrozny DB, Harrington T. The benefits of early jejunal hyperalimentation in the head-injured patient. Neurosurgery 1989;25(5):729–35.

107. Kalfarentzos F, Kehagias J, Mead N, et al. Enteral nutrition is superior to parenteral nutrition in severe acute pancreatitis: results of a randomized prospective trial. Br J Surg 1997;84(12):1665–9.

108. McClave SA. Nutrition in the ICU, part 1: enteral feeding–when and why? J Critical Illness 2001;16(4):197–204.

109. Groos S, Hunefeld G, Luciano L. Parenteral versus enteral nutrition: morphological changes in human adult intestinal mucosa. J Submicrosc Cytol Pathol 1996; 28(1):61–74.

110. Hadfield RJ, Sinclair DG, Houldsworth PE, et al. Effects of enteral and parenteral nutrition on gut mucosal permeability in the critically ill. Am J Respir Crit Care Med 1995;152(5 Pt 1):1545–8.

111. Hernandez G, Velasco N, Wainstein C, et al. Gut mucosal atrophy after a short enteral fasting period in critically ill patients. J Crit Care 1999;14(2): 73–7.

112. Morowitz MJ, Babrowski T, Carlisle EM, et al. The human microbiome and surgical disease. Ann Surg 2011;253(6):1094–101.

113. Cerra FB, Benitez MR, Blackburn GL, et al. Applied nutrition in ICU patients. A consensus statement of the American College of Chest Physicians. Chest 1997; 111(3):769–78.

114. Heyland DK, Dhaliwal R, Drover JW, et al, Canadian Critical Care Clinical Practice Guidelines Committee. Canadian clinical practice guidelines for nutrition support in mechanically ventilated, critically ill adult patients. JPEN J Parenter Enteral Nutr 2003;27(5):355–73.

115. Singer P, Berger MM, Van den Berghe G, et al. ESPEN guidelines on parenteral nutrition: intensive care. Clin Nutr 2009;28(4):387–400.

116. Hegazi RA, Wischmeyer PE. Clinical review: optimizing enteral nutrition for critically ill patients–a simple data-driven formula. Crit Care 2011;15(6):234.

117. Lubbers T, Kox M, de Haan JJ, et al. Continuous administration of enteral lipid- and protein-rich nutrition limits inflammation in a human endotoxemia model. Crit Care Med 2013;41(5):1258–65.

118. Ji RR, Xu ZZ, Strichartz G, et al. Emerging roles of resolvins in the resolution of inflammation and pain. Trends Neurosci 2011;34(11):599–609.

119. Serhan CN, Arita M, Hong S, et al. Resolvins, docosatrienes, and neuroprotectins, novel omega-3-derived mediators, and their endogenous aspirin-triggered epimers. Lipids 2004;39(11):1125–32.

120. Calder PC. Omega-3 fatty acids and inflammatory processes. Nutrients 2010; 2(3):355–74.

121. Buckley CD, Gilroy DW, Serhan CN, et al. The resolution of inflammation. Nat Rev Immunol 2013;13(1):59–66.
122. Kiecolt-Glaser JK. Stress, food, and inflammation: psychoneuroimmunology and nutrition at the cutting edge. Psychosom Med 2010;72(4):365–9.
123. Munroe C, Frantz D, Martindale RG, et al. The optimal lipid formulation in enteral feeding in critical illness: clinical update and review of the literature. Curr Gastroenterol Rep 2011;13(4):368–75.
124. Zhu X, Pribis JP, Rodriguez PC, et al. The central role of arginine catabolism in T-cell dysfunction and increased susceptibility to infection after physical injury. Ann Surg 2013. [Epub ahead of print].
125. Suchner U, Heyland DK, Peter K. Immune-modulatory actions of arginine in the critically ill. Br J Nutr 2002;87(Suppl 1):S121–32.
126. Zhou M, Martindale RG. Arginine in the critical care setting. J Nutr 2007; 137(6 Suppl 2):1687S–92S.
127. Luiking YC, Poeze M, Ramsay G, et al. Reduced citrulline production in sepsis is related to diminished de novo arginine and nitric oxide production. Am J Clin Nutr 2009;89(1):142–52.
128. Visser M, Vermeulen MA, Richir MC, et al. Imbalance of arginine and asymmetric dimethylarginine is associated with markers of circulatory failure, organ failure and mortality in shock patients. Br J Nutr 2012;107(10):1458–65.
129. Kao CC, Bandi V, Guntupalli KK, et al. Arginine, citrulline and nitric oxide metabolism in sepsis. Clin Sci (Lond) 2009;117(1):23–30.
130. Gough MS, Morgan MA, Mack CM, et al. The ratio of arginine to dimethylarginines is reduced and predicts outcomes in patients with severe sepsis. Crit Care Med 2011;39(6):1351–8.
131. Al Balushi RM, Cohen J, Banks M, et al. The clinical role of glutamine supplementation in patients with multiple trauma: a narrative review. Anaesth Intensive Care 2013;41(1):24–34.
132. Wischmeyer PE. Glutamine: the first clinically relevant pharmacological regulator of heat shock protein expression? Curr Opin Clin Nutr Metab Care 2006; 9(3):201–6.
133. Gee AC, Kiraly L, McCarthy MS, et al. Nutrition support and therapy in patients with head and neck squamous cell carcinomas. Curr Gastroenterol Rep 2012; 14(4):349–55.
134. Bengmark S. Integrative medicine and human health–the role of pre-, pro- and synbiotics. Clin Transl Med 2012;1(1):6.
135. Zaborina O, Zaborin A, Romanowski K, et al. Host stress and virulence expression in intestinal pathogens: development of therapeutic strategies using mice and *C. elegans*. Curr Pharm Des 2011;17(13):1254–60.
136. Johnston BC. Probiotics for the prevention of *Clostridium difficile*-associated diarrhea. Ann Intern Med 2013;158(9):706–7.
137. Gu WJ, Deng T, Gong YZ, et al. The effects of probiotics in early enteral nutrition on the outcomes of trauma: a meta-analysis of randomized controlled trials. JPEN J Parenter Enteral Nutr 2013;37(3):310–7.
138. Santora R, Kozar RA. Molecular mechanisms of pharmaconutrients. J Surg Res 2010;161(2):2C88–294.

Patients with Chronic Pain

Joseph Salama-Hanna, MBBS[1], Grace Chen, MD*

KEYWORDS

- Preoperative evaluation • Opioid tolerance • Postoperative pain
- Multimodal analgesia • Multidisciplinary pain treatment • Preoperative opioid abuse
- Buprenorphine

KEY POINTS

- Preoperative assessment and treatment of chronic pain and its comorbidities are essential to assure a positive operative outcome and smooth recovery.
- Multimodal analgesia can decrease postoperative pain, increase patient satisfaction, and reduce opioid requirements and may help avoid the development of chronic pain.
- If there is adequate preoperative time, multidisciplinary treatment of chronic pain to minimize catastrophizing, anxiety, deconditioning, and medication tolerance can improve perioperative outcomes in chronic pain patients.
- Special situations, such as patients with intrathecal drug delivery systems and patients who are on buprenorphine, may warrant coordination of care with subspecialists.

OVERVIEW

Chronic pain afflicts more than 100 million Americans,[1] making it approximately 4 times more common than diabetes and 10 times more common than cancer. The Institute of Medicine recognizes ongoing pain as a disease, with far-reaching physiologic, psychological, and emotional implications that are frequently inadequately assessed and treated. These issues are often in the forefront when a chronic pain patient presents for surgery, requiring individualized assessment and preparation to assure effective postoperative pain control and a seamless recovery. Surgical patient satisfaction and pain control have been shown to correlate closely. One study, by Hanna and colleagues,[2] of 4349 patients found that surgical patient satisfaction was significantly improved when their pain was well treated.

Chronic pain patients undergoing surgery often experience more postoperative pain and consume more opioids than patients without chronic pain.[3,4] Possible

Disclosures: None.

Department of Anesthesiology and Perioperative Medicine, Oregon Health & Science University, 3303 Southwest Bond Avenue, Portland, OR 97239, USA

[1] Present address: Henry Ford Hospital, 2799 West Grand Boulevard, Detroit, MI 48202, USA.

* Corresponding author.

E-mail address: cheng@ohsu.edu

factors contributing to increased postoperative pain include increased preoperative pain, anxiety, age, and type of surgery. The type of surgery, age, and psychological distress are significant predictors for analgesic consumption.[5] Psychological variables, including anxiety, depression, and patients overwhelmed by out-of-proportion fear—all predictors of increased postoperative pain, are more common in chronic pain patients.[6,7] Effectively managing these issues requires a multidisciplinary approach incorporating multimodal analgesic approaches initiated prior to incision, thus emphasizing the importance of effective preoperative evaluation and planning.

IMPORTANT CONCEPTS

Acute pain accompanies trauma and injury (such as surgery) and typically resolves as tissues heal. In contrast, chronic pain can be defined as ongoing pain that extends beyond the typical period of healing and adversely affects the function and well being of the individual.[8] Chronic pain is a complex biopsychosocial disease process with accompanying changes in physiology that promote ongoing pain. Chronic pain is associated with depression, anxiety, deconditioning, poor sleep, increased medication use, and increased use of health services. Chronic pain and its comorbidities are associated with poor postoperative pain control, and patients who come into surgery without chronic pain are more likely to develop chronic postsurgical pain when perioperative pain is not well controlled. Chronic pain is a national problem, having an impact on more than 100 million Americans and costing the US economy more than $600 million per year.[1]

Out of the approximately 40 million surgical procedures performed each year in North America, 10% to 15% of patients continue to have ongoing pain 1 year later because they develop chronic postsurgical pain. This process of transition from acute pain to chronic pain is complex and poorly understood. In a given individual, there is likely interplay between genetic, biologic, psychological, and social-environmental factors that leads to ongoing pain.[9,10]

Demographically, younger female patients seem an increased risk group for developing chronic postsurgical pain.[11] Patients with anxiety, depression, or other chronic pain; those with longer preoperative opioid requirements[12]; or those who have out-of-proportion fear[13] or are less optimistic about their postoperative pain and outcomes have more postoperative pain and may be at increased risk for developing chronic pain.[14–16] Although not routinely performed clinically, preoperative assessment of pain perception by assessing sensitivity to pressure or other stimuli that reflect physiologic and processing changes is associated with more postoperative pain.[17–19] Patients with poor pain control in the hours and days after surgery are more likely to have ongoing chronic pain.[20]

Another quantifiable factor associated with a more challenging postoperative pain experience is the use of long-term opioids to treat chronic pain. Patients with opioid prescription for preoperative pain are likely to have more pain and increased opioid requirements. Given these identifiable factors associated with both increased acute pain and chronic postsurgical pain, it is clear that preoperative evaluation is helpful in identifying patients at increased risk for this complication of surgery. This is particularly true for chronic pain patients who often manifest many of these risk factors as part of their pain syndrome. For example, patients with neuropathic pain associated with diabetes have increased anxiety, depression, and sleep disturbance.[21] Additionally, many chronic pain syndromes are treated with opioids, which pose special challenges in the perioperative period.

In the forefront of perioperative pain control is the concept of multimodal analgesia—the practice of implementing together several pharmaceutical and nonmedication treatments to reduce postoperative pain and enhance recovery. Multimodal analgesia shifts the focus away from opioids to a host of treatments that can reduce pain by complementary mechanisms of action. The common theme of these treatments is that by reducing the physiologic response to the intense nociceptive (pain) stimulus of surgery, pain is reduced. Related concepts include pre-emptive analgesia (initiating treatment before the surgery to reduce pain after surgery) and preventive analgesia (a broader time frame for intervention including the entire perioperative period). Overwhelming evidence shows that multimodal strategies improve clinical outcomes. For chronic pain patients, this is of increased importance, and the therapy likely has enhanced benefit if doses and strategies are individualized.[22,23] This multimodal analgesia review suggests a 5-step approach to optimize the preoperative care of patients who suffer from chronic pain.

Step One: Preoperative Evaluation of Chronic Pain Patients

According to the International Association for the Study of Pain, pain is defined as an unpleasant subjective physical and emotional experience.[24] Acute pain tends to be adaptive and signals impending or ongoing tissue damage.

Chronic pain (excluding cancer pain) persists beyond the expected period of recovery. The exact pathway of transformation is the focus of intensive study. The process seems to begin in the periphery with up-regulation of cyclooxygenase-2 and interleukin 1β–sensitizing first-order neurons, which eventually sensitize second-order spinal neurons, a process that requires activating N-methyl-D-aspartic acid (NMDA) receptor-channel activity. Prostaglandins, endocannabinoids, a variety of ion channels, microglia, and scavenger cells have all been implicated in the transformation of acute to chronic pain.[25] Clinically, intense uncontrolled pain seems to be a risk factor for the development of postoperative chronic pain, making pre-emptive analgesia important for chronic pain prevention.[26,27]

In the United States, pain is termed, *the fifth vital sign*, emphasizing its importance in patient care, and is often recorded on a numeric rating scale.[28] More sophisticated and function-focused instruments, such as the Brief Pain Inventory, are also used. To optimize postoperative recovery and patient satisfaction, physicians and midlevel providers who evaluate patients for surgery should inquire about pain and document pain intensity, location, functional impairment, and concomitant medication use for treatment. Like cardiopulmonary disease, patients' chronic pain can significantly affect surgical outcome and patient satisfaction. One European study found that of factors of nociception, depression and anxiety, and activities of daily living, only pain caused dissatisfaction with surgical care.[29] Patients who have their chronic pain, anxiety, and depression under reasonable control are in the best position to cope effectively with the additional stress of acute postoperative pain and have a lower risk of developing new chronic pain.

If depression or anxiety is not well controlled, it is reasonable to consider either additional pharmacotherapy or appropriate psychotherapy. Beyond the medical preparations for surgery, patient education is an important aspect of optimizing surgical recovery, with patients who participate in preoperative education experiencing less pain and anxiety along with better recovery.[30,31] Patients who have realistic expectations, understand how to report their pain, and understand their options for treatment have less anxiety and are able to play a more active role in their recovery. The earlier this education process starts, the more likely they are to effectively implement it during the stresses of the perioperative period. Providers seeing patient pre-operatively should discuss a patient's fears and concerns, explain perioperative routines, and provide education for optimal use of patient-controlled analgesia (PCA) and other analgesic methods, such as regional analgesia. Patients may receive additional information during the preanesthetic evaluation, including educational materials they can take home with them for review. A clear evaluation of chronic pain risk factors and concise patient preparation are fundamentally important to optimize surgical outcome and patient satisfaction.

Step Two: Pain Specialist Preoperative Evaluation of the Patient on Opioids

Millions of people are prescribed long-term opioid therapy for the treatment of chronic pain and opioid abuse had been rising steadily over the decade, with unintentional opioid overdose deaths rising from 1/100,000 in 1970 to 10/100,000 in 2007.[32,33] The majority of these patients use their medications as prescribed by their health care providers. Some patients, however, have issues of abuse and addiction. For all patients on any type of opioid therapy, the main goals of opioid therapy are the same: avoid withdrawal, account for tolerance, avoid unnecessary dose escalation, provide reasonable postoperative pain control, and avoid opioid overdose. If patients understand these opioid goals, they are more likely to actively participate and fear may be allayed.[34]

Chronic opioid use alters physiology and the body's future response to the ongoing use of opioids. Long-term opioid use has been linked to endocrine derangements, such as sex hormone deficiency and cortisol deficiency.[35] Some studies suggest that patients exposed to opioids may have increased sensitivity for pain, thus exhibiting opioid-induced hyperalgesia.[7,36] Patients who suffer from substance abuse may benefit from psychiatric treatment and stabilization of their psychological state before elective surgery.

In addition to simply tallying preoperative opioid use, it is appropriate for a preoperative pain consultation to assess for opioid misuse and addiction to improve the care of patients in the vulnerable preoperative time period. If opioid addiction is suspected, a team approach involving the primary care provider, anesthesiologist, surgeon, pain specialist, and addiction specialist (psychiatry) facilitates achieving successful pain management without unintended long-term complications of addiction relapse (**Table 1**).

Many addiction-screening tools are available, including the Screening Tool for Addiction Risk, to identify opioid abuse potential in chronic pain patients. Patients who have an opioid abuse problem often display an overwhelming focus on opioid issues during preoperative pain clinic visits and clinicians should have a high index of suspicion for opioid abuse in those who exhibit such behavior. Patients with opioid abuse or misuse, those who often request early refills or escalate drug use in the absence of an acute change in medical condition, and young white male patients tend to be the most susceptible population for prescription opioid abuse.[37] In addition, an addictionologist should be consulted for patients who are identified as opioid abusers and have self-insight and a sincere desire to stop abusing.

If surgery needs to proceed without delay, multimodal analgesia, including acetaminophen, nonsteroidal anti-inflammatory drugs (NSAIDs), regional blocks, antidepressants, anticonvulsants, muscle relaxants, α-adrenergic agonists, or benzodiazepines, should be considered.[38] Patients should be monitored for opioid withdrawal if not offered opioids. If patients receive opioids in the acute postoperative setting, tapering the opioids should be implemented when a patient's acute pain is expected to subside. The most important factor in the perioperative care of a patient who suffers from opioid addiction is to establish a support structure for the patient to cope with the

Table 1
Substance use disorders and their definitions

Substance Use Disorder	Related Definitions
Addiction	Commonly used term meaning the aberrant use of a specific psychoactive substance in a manner characterized by loss of control, compulsive use, preoccupation, and continued use despite harm; pejorative term, replaced in the *DSM-IV11* in a nonpejorative way by the term, *substance use disorder*, with psychological and physical dependence
Dependence	1. Psychological dependence: need for a specific psychoactive substance either for its positive effects or to avoid negative psychological or physical effects associated with its withdrawal 2. Physical dependence: a physiologic state of adaptation to a specific psychoactive substance characterized by the emergence of a withdrawal syndrome during abstinence, which may be relieved in total or in part by readministration 3. One category of psychoactive substance use disorder
Chemical dependence	A generic term relating to psychological and/or physical dependence on one or more psychoactive substances
Substance use disorders	Term of *DSM-IV13* comprising 2 main groups: 1. Substance dependence disorder and substance abuse disorder 2. Substance-induced disorders (eg, intoxication, withdrawal, delirium, and psychotic disorders)
Tolerance	A state in which an increased dosage of a psychoactive substance is needed to produce a desired effect. Cross-tolerance: induced by repeated administration of one psychoactive substance that is manifested toward another substance to which an individual has not been recently exposed.
Withdrawal syndrome	The onset of a predictable constellation of signs and symptoms after the abrupt cessation of the drug
Polydrug dependence	Discontinuation of, or a rapid decrease in, dosage of a psychoactive substance
Recovery	A process of overcoming both physical and psychological dependence on a psychoactive substance with a commitment to sobriety
Abstinence	Nonuse of any psychoactive substance
Maintenance	Prevention of craving behavior and withdrawal symptoms of opioids by long-acting opioids (eg, methadone, buprenorphine)
Substance abuse	Use of a psychoactive substance in a manner outside of sociocultural conventions

Abbreviation: DSM-IV, Diagnostic and Statistical Manual of Mental Disorders (Fourth Edition).

stresses of the disease that necessitated the surgery, the preexisting addiction challenge, and the new stress of postoperative pain with exposure to the substance of abuse.

Step Three: Formulating a Perioperative Analgesic Plan

Formulating and communicating the plan for multidisciplinary preoperative treatment and multimodal perioperative pain control[39] to patients and care teams help alleviate patient anxiety and improve care.[32] Initiating treatment before surgical incision requires planning and is associated with the best outcomes (**Fig. 1**).

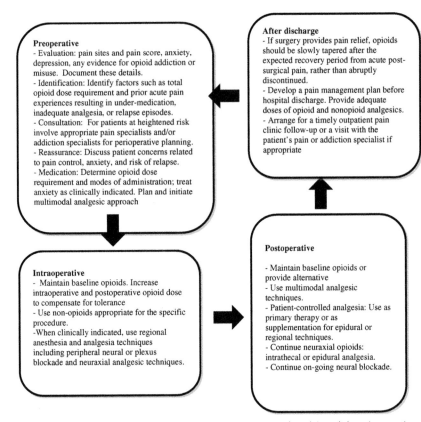

Preoperative
- Evaluation: pain sites and pain score, anxiety, depression, any evidence for opioid addiction or misuse. Document these details.
- Identification: Identify factors such as total opioid dose requirement and prior acute pain experiences resulting in under-medication, inadequate analgesia, or relapse episodes.
- Consultation: For patients at heightened risk involve appropriate pain specialists and/or addiction specialists for perioperative planning.
- Reassurance: Discuss patient concerns related to pain control, anxiety, and risk of relapse.
- Medication: Determine opioid dose requirement and modes of administration; treat anxiety as clinically indicated. Plan and initiate multimodal analgesic approach

After discharge
- If surgery provides pain relief, opioids should be slowly tapered after the expected recovery period from acute post-surgical pain, rather than abruptly discontinued.
- Develop a pain management plan before hospital discharge. Provide adequate doses of opioid and nonopioid analgesics.
- Arrange for a timely outpatient pain clinic follow-up or a visit with the patient's pain or addiction specialist if appropriate

Intraoperative
- Maintain baseline opioids. Increase intraoperative and postoperative opioid dose to compensate for tolerance
- Use non-opioids appropriate for the specific procedure.
- When clinically indicated, use regional anesthesia and analgesia techniques including peripheral neural or plexus blockade and neuraxial analgesic techniques.

Postoperative
- Maintain baseline opioids or provide alternative
- Use multimodal analgesic techniques.
- Patient-controlled analgesia: Use as primary therapy or as supplementation for epidural or regional techniques.
- Continue neuraxial opioids: intrathecal or epidural analgesia.
- Continue on-going neural blockade.

Fig. 1. Plan for multidisciplinary preoperative treatment and multimodal perioperative pain control.

Step Four: Specifics to Execute the Plan; the Key is Multimodal Analgesia

Multimodal analgesia optimizes analgesia and minimizes functionally limiting side effects. In the perioperative period, the use of steroids, such as dexamethasone; anticonvulsants, such as gabapentin; acetaminaphen; NSAIDs, such as celecoxib; and ketamine has been shown to be opioid sparing. A recent study of multilevel spine surgery patients demonstrated that, compared with a historic group of patients receiving usual care, multimodal analgesia significantly reduced opioid consumption, improved postoperative mobilization, and was associated with concomitant low levels of nausea, sedation, and dizziness.[40] Many other studies show multimodal analgesia has opioid-sparing properties concomitant with reduction of opioid side effects.[41]

The orally administered medications with the best evidence for reducing postoperative pain and opioid requirements are the NSAIDs, acetaminophen, and gabapentin/pregabalin.[42–44] Despite the desire to have patients nothing by mouth prior to transport to the operating room, it is common to administer a combination of oral medications (eg, acetaminophen, NSAID, and pregabalin) in the preoperative holding area. Initiating treatment with these medications the night before surgery is also an option that can provide adequate pre-emptive analgesia. In addition to the analgesic effects, gabapentin is an anxiolytic, with demonstrated efficacy in anxious patients undergoing surgery.[45] Standard preoperative doses for gabapentin are typically 600 mg to 1200 mg and, for acetaminophen, 650 mg to 1000 mg.

The nonopioid intravenous (IV) analgesic with the most impact seems to be ketamine, an anesthetic agent that is an NMDA receptor antagonist.[46,47] Ketamine reduces pain and opioid requirements and is particularly helpful in opioid-tolerant patients.[48] Ketamine is often given as a bolus dose prior to incision and may be continued through the operation and at times into the postoperative period.

Regional and neuraxial blocks with local anesthetics and opioids are key components of effective multimodal analgesia. Options include a field block or wound infiltration[49] (before or after incision), neuraxial analgesia (epidural or intrathecal often combined with an opioid), and peripheral nerve/plexus blockade (divisions of brachial plexus, lumbar plexus, and femoral nerve). Simple use of local anesthetic at the surgical site may reduce pain and opioid requirements, and contraindications or adverse effects are rare, making this option widely applicable.[50,51] For patients who are not candidates for neuraxial or peripheral nerve analgesic techniques, IV lidocaine infusion may reduce pain and opioid requirements while enhancing recovery.[52–55]

Neuraxial analgesia

Neuraxial analgesia (intrathecal or epidural) involves the delivery of local anesthetic and/or opioid to the spinal cord and surrounding nerve tissues to decrease pain at the spinal level.[56] Epidural analgesia with local anesthetic and opioid combination delivered via an indwelling catheter and continued into the postoperative period is the best-studied neuraxial technique. Particularly in high-risk patients, epidural analgesia can reduce pain and improve patient outcomes and is often used for many surgical procedures.[57–59] For opioid-tolerant patients, special attention is required for success, including a multimodal analgesia plan. One of the rare but potentially devastating complications of neuraxial analgesia is hematoma formation in the spinal canal. Anticoagulation and coagulation abnormalities are major risk factors for this complication. Readers are encouraged to refer to the American Society of Regional Anesthesia and Pain Medicine[60] guidelines if neuraxial therapy is expected in an anticoagulated patient. Consensus guidelines are recommendations and specific decisions on nerve blocks in patients on anticoagulants should be made on an individual basis. Optimal monitoring, adequate follow-up, and timely treatment should be practiced for patients taking anticoagulants and who had neuraxial or peripheral nerve blocks.

Patients should be educated regarding IV-PCA prior to surgery. The PCA is a programmable delivery system by which patients self-administer predetermined doses of analgesic medication, via the IV route, at the push of a button. The PCA can optimize drug delivery and improve satisfaction by enabling patients to titrate analgesia. Safe use of the PCA requires patients to control analgesic delivery. Increasing plasma concentrations of opioid usually causes sedation prior to causing clinically significant respiratory depression, but sedation usually impairs the ability of the patient to activate the PCA. Thus, it is important that patients are instructed to not allow family members or friends to activate the PCA while they are resting. In addition, each PCA pump is programmed to limit the amount of drug delivered. Thus, repeatedly pressing the activation button does not deliver an amount that exceeds the preset limit. This upper set limit may be enough, however, to cause apnea in an individual patient, if a family member or friend takes control of the control button while a patient is sleeping. Because the dose can be varied to accommodate patient needs, the IV-PCA is a reasonable choice for opioid-tolerant chronic pain patients. **Table 2** provides examples of guideline boluses and lockout intervals (time between the next dose of medication even if the PCA is activated) for different IV-PCA opioids.

Preoperative placement of a peripheral nerve block can be helpful in preventing postoperative pain. In adult patients, it is standard to place the nerve block under

Table 2
Sample bolus doses and lockout intervals for opioid IV

Drug	Bolus (mg)	Lockout Interval (min)
Fentanyl	0.015–0.05	3–10
Hydromorphone	0.1–0.5	5–15
Meperidine	5–15	5–15
Morphine	0.5–3	5–20
Oxymorphone	0.2–0.8	5–15
Remifentanil (labor)	0.5 µg/kg	2
Sufentanil	0.003–0.015	3–10

Data from Kong B, Ya Deau JT. Patient-controlled analgesia. In: Benzon HT, Fishman SM, Raja RT, et al, eds. Essentials of Pain Medicine, 3rd edition. Philadelphia: Saunders, 2011; with permission.

mild or moderate sedation. This practice allows patients to provide direct feedback to the provider placing the block, in the event that the block needle comes in contact with the target nerve. In addition, for patients who are thought to require several days of strong analgesia, local anesthetic can be continuously infused through a catheter positioned (usually with ultrasound) alongside the target nerve (referred to as continuous peripheral nerve block [CPNB]). Examples include femoral nerve catheters for knee surgery, paravertebral catheters for thoracotomy, and brachial plexus catheters for upper extremity orthopedic procedures. CPNB can reduce baseline pain, improve pain control with movement, facilitate recovery, and reduce opioid requirements.[61,62] For appropriate surgical procedures, CPNB is an important option for chronic pain patients undergoing surgery.[63,64]

Nonpharmacologic approaches

There are several approaches and techniques that have gained popularity in the chronic pain management field that may be helpful in perioperative pain management.[65] Physical modalities, including cooling, acupuncture, heat, and massage, are low-risk approaches that offer potential benefit. Among these, the best evidence is for transcutaneous electrical nerve stimulation (TENS). The TENS units are small portable devices that deliver electrical energy through the skin. There are more than 20 controlled trials of TENS for postoperative pain control with reasonable evidence to suggest an opioid-sparing effect.[66] Several cognitive techniques that offer the possibility of reducing anxiety and pain have been studied for postoperative pain control, including relaxation techniques, guided imagery, hypnosis, music, and positive suggestions. Given the low risk of these techniques, they are reasonable to suggest for chronic pain patients undergoing surgery.

Step Five: Special Situations that May Benefit from Acute Pain Specialist Referral for Preoperative Pain Optimization

Patients who suffer from special chronic pain conditions, especially those who are on multiple psychotropic medications, may benefit from a preoperative consult by a rheumatologist, psychiatrist, neurologist, or pain specialist. Special consideration should be given to the following patient situations.

Patients with intrathecal drug delivery systems

Intrathecal drug delivery systems (IDDSs)[67] should be interrogated preoperatively to assess proper functioning of the system and identify medication and dose. Cross tolerance of different opioids is unpredictable, even though there are approximate opioid conversion tables available. For example, patients may have improved response to fentanyl if the intrathecal pump is infusing hydromorphone. At the time of surgery, care should be taken to prevent surgical or regional anesthetic disruption of the intrathecal infusion. Electrocautery does not interfere with the device but there are case reports of the device being deactivated in patients undergoing an MRI. Intrathecal therapy should be continued (recognizing that abrupt cessation of baclofen as a baseline analgesic requirement is dangerous). Supplementation of appropriate doses of opioids, either orally or by using PCA for breakthrough pain as needed, is warranted. Because many patients with IDDS therapy are opioid tolerant, a multimodal analgesic approach is advisable.

Patients with arthritis

Osteoarthritis is usually treated with exercise, NSAIDs, and, in rare cases, opioids and surgery. Rheumatoid arthritis is treated with disease-modifying agents, biologic response modifiers, and steroids. If patients have recently been taking steroids, stress-dose steroids should be given perioperatively. Methotrexate is commonly prescribed to this group of patients. Because this drug can cause severe liver damage,[68] the status of liver function should be documented in the preoperative period. Multinational recommendations on pain management by pharmacotherapy should be followed in all patients with inflammatory arthritis in the preoperative period. For patients with arthritis, a multimodal analgesic technique is appropriate with continuation of their preoperative anti-inflammatory or disease-modifying agents as dictated by the specific surgical situation.

Patients with central pain syndrome

Central pain syndrome is a neurologic condition caused by damage to, or dysfunction of, the central nervous system, which includes the brain, brainstem, and spinal cord. Stroke, multiple sclerosis, tumors, epilepsy, brain/spinal cord trauma, or Parkinson disease may cause this syndrome.[69] If a patient presents with a diagnosis of central pain syndrome, investigating the underlying cause is recommended because this may have anesthetic implications. These patients may have a component of pain that is resistant to opioid therapy so management can be challenging. Multimodal analgesia is important, and often these patients are already taking gabapentin or pregabalin because these agents are considered first-line treatments.

Complex regional pain syndrome

The complex regional pain syndrome (CRPS) is a painful condition of a limb associated with physiologic changes and sensitivity to normally nonpainful stimuli. Because of this sensitivity to pain and because the inciting factor for CRPS is often trauma or surgery, it is important to provide aggressive multimodal analgesia to patients who already have the condition. Vitamin C (ascorbic acid) has potential to prevent CRPS, with specific evidence in wrist and foot/ankle surgery.[70,71] It is reasonable to suggest 500 mg of vitamin C for approximately 6 to 8 weeks for patients undergoing such procedures and for CRPS patients undergoing any surgical procedure.[72]

Fibromyalgia

Diagnostic criteria for fibromyalgia[73] include wide spread pain that lasts for at least 3 months; it is usually a diagnosis of exclusion. Treatment options include antidepressants, such as amitriptyline (a tricyclic antidepressant), venlafaxine in high doses (serotonin-norepinephrine reuptake inhibitors), duloxetine, and milnacipran (nonselective serotonin reuptake inhibitor). Anticonvulsants, mainly α-2-β ligands (gabapentin and pregabalin), are also used to effectively help with fibromyalgia pain. It should be emphasized that the current Food and Drug Administration–approved medications for fibromyalgia are pregabalin, duloxetinem, and milnacipran. Fibromyalgia patients have impaired diffuse noxious inhibitory control, a measurement of endogenous analgesia efficacy, which is predictive of more postoperative pain. Because these patients also have heightened responses to painful stimuli, postoperative pain control can be challenging. **Fig. 2** demonstrates different forms of soft tissue pain syndrome. It is important to differentiate among the different forms, because the clinical picture is sometimes confusing.

Preoperative evaluation of patients on buprenorphine

Buprenorphine is a partial μ-opioid receptor agonist and a κ-opioid receptor antagonist that has been used to treat pain and opioid addiction. To counteract potential abuse by injection, Subutex and Suboxone were formulated with the strategy of having buprenorphine in combination with the opioid receptor antagonist, naloxone, in a ratio of 4 to 1, for sublingual administration. Naloxone has poor bioavailability in the sublingual form and has high bioavailability if injected IV.[74] Suboxone and Subutex are the only Food and Drug Administration–approved office-based medications to treat opioid abuse. Patients are sometimes put on buprenorphine/naloxone formulations for chronic pain if they do not have previous addiction history. This is an off-label use. At the opioid receptor, buprenorphine has low intrinsic activity and high binding affinity and can induce withdrawal in opioid-dependent patients who are using full agonists.[75] Ceiling effect and poor bioavailability make buprenorphine safer for overdose potential than are opioid receptor full agonists. The maximal effects of buprenorphine seem to occur in the 16-mg to 32-mg dose range for sublingual tablets.[76] Preoperative pain, addiction history, and last dose of buprenorphine/naloxone should be reviewed before surgery. Previous experience with surgery and

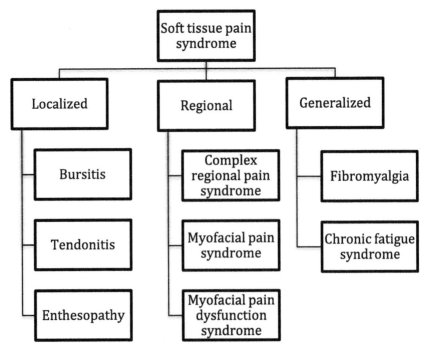

Fig. 2. Different forms of soft tissue pain syndrome.

buprenorphine/naloxone should also be checked because it can help with opioid dosing. If buprenorphine/naloxone had been stopped for greater than 5 days and switched to pure agonists, patients likely need increased doses of opioids preoperatively and perioperatively for adequate pain control. If buprenorphine/naloxone was not stopped preoperatively, increased doses can be used perioperatively for pain control. Patients may need to convert to methadone, a stronger, longer-acting opioid, if the surgery is painful and not likely treated by partial agonists. Intraoperatively, fentanyl may be an optimal choice due to its high opioid receptor affinity and ability to displace the partial agonist. If a pure opioid agonist was used intraoperatively and postoperatively, an addiction specialist may transition patients back onto a partial agonist when the acute postoperative period is over and pain subsided.

SUMMARY

Patients with chronic pain face many challenges in maintaining function and pain control in their day-to-day lives. The stresses of surgery, the accompanying postoperative pain, and altered physiology add to this challenge. Appropriate planning for surgery and implementation of an individualized multimodal analgesia strategy can reduce the pain and suffering after surgery for these patients and help speed their recovery.

REFERENCES

1. Institute of Medicine Report from the Committee on Advancing Pain Research, Care, and Education. Relieving pain in America, a blueprint for transforming prevention, care, education and research. Washington (DC): The National Academies Press; 2011.
2. Hanna MN, et al. Does patient perception of pain control affect patient satisfaction across surgical units in a tertiary teaching hospital. Am J Med Qual 2012; 27(5):411–6.
3. Bruce J, Thornton AJ, et al. Chronic preoperative pain and psychological robustness predict acute postoperative pain outcomes after surgery for breast cancer. Br J Cancer 2012;107(6):937–46.
4. Althaus A, Hinrichs-Rocker A, et al. Development of a risk index for the prediction of chronic post-surgical pain. Eur J Pain 2012;16(6):901–10.
5. Ip HY, et al. Predictors of postoperative pain and analgesic consumption: a qualitative systematic review. Anesthesiology 2009;111(3):657–77.
6. Angst MS, Clark JD. Opioid-induced hyperalgesia. A qualitative systematic review. Anesthesiology 2006;104(3):570–87.
7. Chu LF, Angst MS, Clark D. Opioid-induced hyperalgesia in humans. Molecular mechanisms and clinical considerations. Clin J Pain 2008;24(6):479–96.
8. American Society of Anesthesiologists Task Force on Chronic Pain Management, American Society of Regional Anesthesia and Pain Medicine. Practice guidelines for chronic pain management: an updated report by the American Society of Anesthesiologists Task Force on Chronic Pain Management and the American Society of Regional Anesthesia and Pain Medicine. Anesthesiology 2010;112:810–33.
9. Katz J, Seltzer Z. Transition from acute to chronic postsurgical pain: risk factors and protective factors. Expert Rev Neurother 2009;9(5):723–44.
10. Tammimaki A, Mannisto PT. Catechol-O-methyltransferase gene polymorphism and chronic human pain: a systematic review and meta-analysis. Pharmacogenet Genomics 2012;22(9):673–91.

11. Katz J, Poleshuck EL, Andrus CL, et al. Risk factors for acute pain and its persistence following breast cancer surgery. Pain 2005;119:16–25.

12. Zywiel MG, Stroh DA, Lee SY, et al. Chronic opioid use prior to total knee arthroplasty. J Bone Joint Surg Am 2011;93(21):1988–93.

13. Cohen L, Fouladi RT, Katz J. Preoperative coping strategies and distress predict postoperative pain and morphine consumption in women undergoing abdominal gynecologic surgery. J Psychosom Res 2005;58(2):201–9.

14. Caumo W, Schmidt AP, Schneider CN, et al. Preoperative predictors of moderate to intense acute postoperative pain in patients undergoing abdominal surgery. Acta Anaesthesiol Scand 2002;46(10):1265–71.

15. Theunissen M, Peters ML, et al. Preoperative anxiety and catastrophizing: a systematic review and meta-analysis of the association with chronic postsurgical pain. Clin J Pain 2012;28(9):819–41.

16. Powell R, Johnston M, Smith WC, et al. Psychological risk factors for chronic post-surgical pain after inguinal hernia repair surgery: a prospective cohort study. Eur J Pain 2012;16(4):600–10.

17. Werner MU, Mjobo HN, et al. Prediction of postoperative pain: a systematic review of predictive experimental pain studies. Anesthesiology 2010;112(6): 1494–502.

18. Brandsborg B, Dueholm M, Kehlet H, et al. Mechanosensitivity before and after hysterectomy: a prospective study on the prediction of acute and chronic postoperative pain. Br J Anaesth 2011;107(6):940–7.

19. Werner MU, Duun P, Kehlet H. Prediction of postoperative pain by preoperative nociceptive responses to heat stimulation. Anesthesiology 2004;100(1):115–9.

20. van Gulik L, Janssen LI, Ahlers SJ, et al. Risk factors for chronic thoracic pain after cardiac surgery via sternotomy. Eur J Cardiothorac Surg 2011;40(6): 1309–13.

21. Gore M, Brandenburg NA, Dukes E, et al. Pain severity in diabetic peripheral neuropathy (DPN) is associated with patient functioning, symptom levels of anxiety and depression, and sleep. J Pain Symptom Manage 2005;30(4): 374–85.

22. Woolf CJ, Salter MW. Neuronal plasticity: increasing the gain in pain. Science 2000;288:1765–9.

23. Watkins LR, Milligan ED, Maier SF. Spinal cord glia: new players in pain. Pain 2001;93:201–5.

24. Loeser JD, Treede RD. The Kyoto protocol of IASP basic pain terminology. Pain 2008;137(3):473–7.

25. Voscopoulos C, Lema M. When does acute pain become chronic? Br J Anaesth 2010;105(Suppl 1):i69–85.

26. Katz J, McCartney CJ. Current status of preemptive analgesia. Curr Opin Anaesthesiol 2002;15:435–41.

27. Pogatzki-Zahn EM, Zahn PK. From preemptive to preventive analgesia. Curr Opin Anaesthesiol 2006;19:551–5.

28. Lorenz KA, et al. How reliable is pain as the fifth vital sign? J Am Board Fam Med 2009;22(3):291–8.

29. Royse CF, et al. Predictors of patient satisfaction with anaesthesia and surgery care: a cohort study using the Postoperative Quality of Recovery Scale. Eur J Anaesthesiol 2013;30(3):106–10.

30. Crabtree TD, Puri V, Bell JM, et al. Outcomes and perception of lung surgery with implementation of a patient video education module: a prospective cohort study. J Am Coll Surg 2012;214(5):816–21.

31. Livbjerg AE, Froekjaer S, Simonsen O, et al. Pre-operative patient education is associated with decreased risk of arthrofibrosis after total knee arthroplasty: a case control study. J Arthroplasty 2013. [Epub ahead of print].
32. Mitra S, Sinatra RS. Perioperative management of acut pain in the opioid depnedant patient. Anesthesiology 2004;101:212–27.
33. Okie S. A flood of opioids, a rising tide of deaths. N Engl J Med 2010;363(21): 1981–5.
34. Kearney M, et al. Effects of preoperative education on patient outcomes after joint replacement surgery. Orthop Nurs 2011;30(6):391–6.
35. Rhodin A, Stridsberg M, Gordh T. Opioid endocrinopathy: a clinical problem in patients with chronic pain and long-term oral opioid treatment. Clin J Pain 2010; 26(5):374–80.
36. Célèrier E, Rivat C, Jun Y, et al. Long-lasting hyperalgesia induced by fentanyl in rats: preventive effect of ketamine. Anesthesiology 2000;92:465–72.
37. Sehgal N, Manchikanti L, Smith HS. Prescription opioid abuse in chronic pain: a review of opioid abuse predictors and strategies to curb opioid abuse. Pain Physician 2012;15(3):ES67–92.
38. Lewis M, Souki F. "The anesthetic implications of opioid addiction." Perioperative addiction. New York: Springer; 2012. p. 73–93.
39. Costantini R, et al. Controlling pain in the post-operative setting. Int J Clin Pharmacol Ther 2011;49(2):116.
40. Mathiesen O, et al. A comprehensive multimodal pain treatment reduces opioid consumption after multilevel spine surgery. Eur Spine J 2013;1–8.
41. Rasmussen ML, et al. Multimodal analgesia with gabapentin, ketamine and dexamethasone in combination with paracetamol and ketorolac after hip arthroplasty: a preliminary study. Eur J Anaesthesiol 2010;27(4):324–30.
42. Maund E, McDaid C, et al. Paracetamol and selective and non-selective non-steroidal anti-inflammatory drugs for the reduction in morphine-related side-effects after major surgery: a systematic review. Br J Anaesth 2011;106(3): 292–7.
43. Zhang J, Ho KY, et al. Efficacy of pregabalin in acute postoperative pain: a meta-analysis. Br J Anaesth 2011;106(4):454–62.
44. Clarke H, Bonin RP, et al. The prevention of chronic postsurgical pain using gabapentin and pregabalin: a combined systematic review and meta-analysis. Anesth Analg 2012;115(2):428–42.
45. Clarke H, Kirkham KR, Orser BA, et al. Gabapentin reduces preoperative anxiety and pain catastrophizing in highly anxious patients prior to major surgery: a blinded randomized placebo-controlled trial. Can J Anaesth 2013;60(5):432–43.
46. Laskowski K, Stirling A, et al. A systematic review of intravenous ketamine for postoperative analgesia. Can J Anaesth 2011;58(10):911–23.
47. Suzuki M. Role of N-methyl-D-aspartate receptor antagonists in postoperative pain management. Curr Opin Anaesthesiol 2009;22(5):618–22.
48. Gharaei B, Jafari A, et al. Opioid-sparing effect of preemptive bolus low-dose ketamine for moderate sedation in opioid abusers undergoing extracorporeal shock wave lithotripsy: a randomized clinical trial. Anesth Analg 2013;116(1): 75–80.
49. Ganapathy S, Brookes J, Bourne R. Local infiltration analgesia. Anesthesiol Clin 2011;29(2):329–42.
50. Scott NB. Wound infiltration for surgery. Anaesthesia 2010;65(Suppl 1):67–75.
51. Gupta A. Wound infiltration with local anaesthetics in ambulatory surgery. Curr Opin Anaesthesiol 2010;23(6):708–13.

52. Sun Y, Li T, et al. Perioperative systemic lidocaine for postoperative analgesia and recovery after abdominal surgery: a meta-analysis of randomized controlled trials. Dis Colon Rectum 2012;55(11):1183–94.

53. Kang JG, Kim MH, et al. Intraoperative intravenous lidocaine reduces hospital length of stay following open gastrectomy for stomach cancer in men. J Clin Anesth 2012;24(6):465–70.

54. Grigoras A, Lee P, et al. Perioperative intravenous lidocaine decreases the incidence of persistent pain after breast surgery. Clin J Pain 2012;28(7):567–72.

55. Vigneault L, Turgeon AF, et al. Perioperative intravenous lidocaine infusion for postoperative pain control: a meta-analysis of randomized controlled trials. Can J Anaesth 2011;58(1):22–37.

56. de Leon-Casasola OA, Lema MJ. Epidural bupivacaine/sufentanil therapy for postoperative pain control in patients tolerant to opioid and unresponsive to epidural bupivacaine/morphine. Anesthesiology 1994;80(2):303–9.

57. Manion SC, Brennan TJ. Thoracic epidural analgesia and acute pain management. Anesthesiology 2011;115(1):181–8.

58. Pottecher J, Falcoz PE, et al. Does thoracic epidural analgesia improve outcome after lung transplantation? Interact Cardiovasc Thorac Surg 2011;12(1):51–3.

59. Nishimori M, Low JH, et al. Epidural pain relief versus systemic opioid-based pain relief for abdominal aortic surgery. Cochrane Database Syst Rev 2012;(7):CD005059.

60. Horlocker TT, Wedel DJ, Rowlingson JC, et al. Regional anesthesia in the patient receiving antithrombotic or thrombolytic therapy. American Society of Regional Anesthesia and Pain Medicine evidence-basedguidelines. 3rd edition. Reg Anesth Pain Med 2010;35(2):226.

61. Bingham AE, Fu R, et al. Continuous peripheral nerve block compared with single-injection peripheral nerve block: a systematic review and meta-analysis of randomized controlled trials. Reg Anesth Pain Med 2012;37(6):583–94.

62. Ilfeld BM. Continuous peripheral nerve blocks: a review of the published evidence. Anesth Analg 2011;113(4):904–25.

63. Hurley RW, Cohen SP, Williams KA, et al. The analgesic effects of perioperative gabapentin on postoperative pain. A meta-analysis. Reg Anesth Pain Med 2006; 31:237–47.

64. Gilron I. Gabapentin and pregabalin for chronic neuropathic and early postsurgical pain. Current evidence and future directions. Curr Opin Anaesthesiol 2007; 20:456–72.

65. Srinivas P, Gan TJ. Perioperative pain management. Durham (NC): Department of Anesthesiology, Duke university Medical Center. CNS drugs 2007:185–211.

66. Bjordal JM, Johnson MI, et al. Transcutaneous electrical nerve stimulation (TENS) can reduce postoperative analgesic consumption. A meta-analysis with assessment of optimal treatment parameters for postoperative pain. Eur J Pain 2003;7(2):181–8.

67. Grider JS, Brown RE, Colclough GW. Perioperative management of patients with intrathecal durg delivery system for chronic pain. Anesth Analg 2008;107:1393–6.

68. Lindsay K, Gough A. Psoriatic arthritis, methotrexate and the liver. Rheumatology (Oxford) 2008;47:939–41.

69. Klit H, Nanna BF, Troels SJ. Central post-stroke pain: clinical characteristics, pathophysiology, and management. The Lancet Neurology 2009;857–68.

70. Besse JL, Gadeyne S, et al. Effect of vitamin C on prevention of complex regional pain syndrome type I in foot and ankle surgery. Foot Ankle Surg 2009;15(4):179–82.

71. Zollinger PE, Tuinebreijer WE, et al. Can vitamin C prevent complex regional pain syndrome in patients with wrist fractures? A randomized, controlled, multi-center dose-response study. J Bone Joint Surg Am 2007;89(7):1424–31.
72. Harden RN, Bruehl S. Proposed new diagnostic criteria for complex regional pain syndrome. Pain Med 2007;8(4):326–31.
73. Wolfe F, Häuser W. Fibromyalgia diagnosis and diagnostic criteria. Ann Med 2011;43(7):495–502. http://dx.doi.org/10.3109/07853890.2011.595734.
74. Bezchlibnyk-Butler KZ, Jeffries J, Virani A. Clinical handbook of psychotropic drugs. 17th edition. Cambridge (MA): Hogrefe & Huber Publishers; 2007.
75. Rosado J, Walsh SL, Bigelow GE, et al. Sublingual buprenorphine/naloxone precipitated withdrawal in subjects maintained on 100 mg of daily methadone. Drug Alcohol Depend 2007;90:261–9.
76. Ducharme S, Ronald F, Kathryn G. Update on the clinical use of buprenorphine In opioid-related disorders. Canadian Family Physician 2012;37–41.

Index

Note: Page numbers of article titles are in **boldface** type.

A

Med Clin N Am 97 (2013) 1217–1230
http://dx.doi.org/10.1016/S0025-7125(13)00139-9
0025-7125/13/$ – see front matter © 2013 Elsevier Inc. All rights reserved.

medical.theclinics.com

United States Postal Service

Statement of Ownership, Management, and Circulation
(All Periodicals Publications Except Requestor Publications)

1. Publication Title	2. Publication Number	3. Filing Date
Medical Clinics of North America	3 3 7 - 3 4 0	9/14/13

4. Issue Frequency	5. Number of Issues Published Annually	6. Annual Subscription Price
Jan, Mar, May, Jul, Sep, Nov	6	$241.00

7. Complete Mailing Address of Known Office of Publication (Not printer) (Street, city, county, state, and ZIP+4®)

Elsevier Inc.
360 Park Avenue South
New York, NY 10010-1710

Contact Person: Stephen Bushing
Telephone (Include area code): 215-239-3688

8. Complete Mailing Address of Headquarters or General Business Office of Publisher (Not printer)

Elsevier Inc., 360 Park Avenue South, New York, NY 10010-1710

9. Full Names and Complete Mailing Addresses of Publisher, Editor, and Managing Editor (Do not leave blank)

Publisher (Name and complete mailing address)

Linda Belfus, Elsevier, Inc., 1600 John F. Kennedy Blvd. Suite 1800, Philadelphia, PA 19103-2899

Editor (Name and complete mailing address)

Pamela Hetherington, Elsevier, Inc., 1600 John F. Kennedy Blvd. Suite 1800, Philadelphia, PA 19103-2899

Managing Editor (Name and complete mailing address)

Adrianne Brigido, Elsevier, Inc., 1600 John F. Kennedy Blvd. Suite 1800, Philadelphia, PA 19103-2899

10. Owner (Do not leave blank. If the publication is owned by a corporation, give the name and address of the corporation immediately followed by the names and addresses of all stockholders owning or holding 1 percent or more of the total amount of stock. If not owned by a corporation, give the names and addresses of the individual owners. If owned by a partnership or other unincorporated firm, give its name and address as well as those of each individual owner. If the publication is published by a nonprofit organization, give its name and address.)

Full Name	Complete Mailing Address
Wholly owned subsidiary of	1600 John F. Kennedy Blvd., Ste. 1800
Reed/Elsevier, US holdings	Philadelphia, PA 19103-2899

11. Known Bondholders, Mortgagees, and Other Security Holders Owning or Holding 1 Percent or More of Total Amount of Bonds, Mortgages, or Other Securities. If none, check box ☐ None

Full Name	Complete Mailing Address
N/A	

12. Tax Status (For completion by nonprofit organizations authorized to mail at nonprofit rates) (Check one)
The purpose, function, and nonprofit status of this organization and the exempt status for federal income tax purposes:
☐ Has Not Changed During Preceding 12 Months
☐ Has Changed During Preceding 12 Months (Publisher must submit explanation of change with this statement)

PS Form 3526, September 2007 (Page 1 of 3 (Instructions Page 3)) PSN 7530-01-000-9931 **PRIVACY NOTICE:** See our Privacy policy in www.usps.com

---

13. Publication Title		14. Issue Date for Circulation Data Below
Medical Clinics of North America		July 2013

15. Extent and Nature of Circulation		Average No. Copies Each Issue During Preceding 12 Months	No. Copies of Single Issue Published Nearest to Filing Date
a. Total Number of Copies (Net press run)		2,235	1,688
b. Paid Circulation (By Mail and Outside the Mail)	(1) Mailed Outside-County Paid Subscriptions Stated on PS Form 3541. (Include paid distribution above nominal rate, advertiser's proof copies, and exchange copies)	895	819
	(2) Mailed In-County Paid Subscriptions Stated on PS Form 3541 (Include paid distribution above nominal rate, advertiser's proof copies, and exchange copies)		
	(3) Paid Distribution Outside the Mails Including Sales Through Dealers and Carriers, Street Vendors, Counter Sales, and Other Paid Distribution Outside USPS®	453	455
	(4) Paid Distribution by Other Classes Mailed Through the USPS (e.g. First-Class Mail®)		
c. Total Paid Distribution (Sum of 15b (1), (2), (3), and (4))	►	1,348	1,274
d. Free or Nominal Rate Distribution (By Mail and Outside the Mail)	(1) Free or Nominal Rate Outside-County Copies Included on PS Form 3541	103	104
	(2) Free or Nominal Rate In-County Copies Included on PS Form 3541		
	(3) Free or Nominal Rate Copies Mailed at Other Classes Through the USPS (e.g. First-Class Mail)		
	(4) Free or Nominal Rate Distribution Outside the Mail (Carriers or other means)		
e. Total Free or Nominal Rate Distribution (Sum of 15d (1), (2), (3) and (4))	►	103	104
f. Total Distribution (Sum of 15c and 15e)	►	1,451	1,378
g. Copies not Distributed (See instructions to publishers #4 (page #3))		784	310
h. Total (Sum of 15f and g)	►	2,235	1,688
i. Percent Paid (15c divided by 15f times 100)		92.90%	92.45%

16. Publication of Statement of Ownership
☐ If the publication is a general publication, publication of this statement is required. Will be printed in the November 2013 issue of this publication. ☐ Publication not required

17. Signature and Title of Editor, Publisher, Business Manager, or Owner	Date
[signature] Stephen R. Bushing – Inventory Distribution Coordinator	September 14, 2013

I certify that all information furnished on this form is true and complete. I understand that anyone who furnishes false or misleading information on this form or who omits material or information requested on the form may be subject to criminal sanctions (including fines and imprisonment) and/or civil sanctions (including civil penalties).

PS Form 3526, September 2007 (Page 2 of 3)

Moving?

Make sure your subscription moves with you!

To notify us of your new address, find your **Clinics Account Number** (located on your mailing label above your name), and contact customer service at:

Email: journalscustomerservice-usa@elsevier.com

800-654-2452 (subscribers in the U.S. & Canada)
314-447-8871 (subscribers outside of the U.S. & Canada)

Fax number: 314-447-8029

Elsevier Health Sciences Division
Subscription Customer Service
3251 Riverport Lane
Maryland Heights, MO 63043

*To ensure uninterrupted delivery of your subscription, please notify us at least 4 weeks in advance of move.

Printed and bound by CPI Group (UK) Ltd, Croydon, CR0 4YY

03/10/2024

01040409-0005